Published

Jowsey: Metabolic Diseases of Bone

Forthcoming Monographs in the Series

Burgess: Amputations: Surgical Technique and Postoperative
                   Management

Hughston, Walsh and Puddu: Patellar Subluxation and Dislocation

Mubarak, Hargens and Akeson: Compartment Syndromes

Pappas and Akins: The Child's Hip

Sarmiento and Latta: Functional Bracing of Fractures

Southwick and Johnson: Surgical Approaches to the Spine

ORTHOPAEDIC MANAGEMENT OF CEREBRAL PALSY

by

EUGENE E. BLECK, M.D.

Chief, Orthopaedic Rehabilitation Service,
Children's Hospital at Stanford;
Associate Professor of Clinical Surgery (Orthopaedics),
Stanford University School of Medicine

Volume II in the Series

SAUNDERS MONOGRAPHS IN CLINICAL ORTHOPAEDICS

Consulting Editor
CLEMENT B. SLEDGE, M.D.

1979   W. B. SAUNDERS COMPANY
Philadelphia • London • Toronto

W. B. Saunders Company: West Washington Square
Philadelphia, PA   19105

1 St. Anne's Road
Eastbourne, East Sussex BN21, 3UN, England

1 Goldthorne Avenue
Toronto, Ontario M8Z 5T9, Canada

Orthopaedic Management of Cerebral Palsy   ISBN   0-7216-1730-1

Last digit is the print number: 9   8   7   6   5   4   3   2   1

Foreword

Most conditions which face the orthopedic surgeon arise either from trauma, congenital anomalies, or wear and tear to the human frame. It is appropriate, therefore, to discuss their treatment as isolated anatomical events—hence books on surgery of the elbow, the treatment of congenital dislocation of the hip, etc. Dr. Bleck points out, however, that cerebral palsy is a disease which permeates the entire fabric of the child's life—and that of the parents and siblings.

Since the conquest of polio, cerebral palsy represents the greatest challenge to the orthopedist to be a physician as well as a surgeon, to be a family counselor as well as a therapist. Like polio, it can also be a great "teacher" with the help of an experienced "guide."

It is true that most patients with cerebral palsy are treated in multi-disciplinary clinics with numerous medical and para-medical specialists. Yet the nature of the disease demands that care—in its broadest sense—not be fragmented and that each physician caring for these children—and adults—be knowledgeable with respect to the pervasive nature of the process.

In this book, Dr. Bleck not only has provided a comprehensive discussion of the management of the manifestations of cerebral palsy but has also provided us with an excellent textbook on pediatric orthopedics. He has succeeded in his "synthetic approach" to the point that we will all gain fresh insights into the care of the sick child.

CLEMENT B. SLEDGE, M.D.

Preface

In the past, all the well-springs of orthopaedic knowledge seem to have been organized according to parts of the body, e.g., the hip, knee, ankle, or foot. In the early 1970's, however, Mark M. Hoffer, M.D. suggested a more synthetic approach to the patient with cerebral palsy in the instructional courses given at the annual meeting of the American Academy of Orthopaedic Surgeons. Thus it was decided to organize the course in orthopaedic surgery by three clinical types of cerebral palsy: hemiplegia, diplegia, and total body involvement (the latter term coined by Dr. Hoffer).

My experiences in delivering lectures and attending patient problem conferences at numerous centers in the United States in the past six years have convinced me that a book that reflects this synthetic approach is necessary because the same questions and problems in patient care seem to arise everywhere.

Because the diagnosis of motor disorders and associated central nervous system defects has been discussed in detail in many other publications, in this book I have supplied only enough information to avoid confusion in the terminology used in the text.

In the chapter on orthopaedic assessment, in addition to discussing the clinical examination, I have tried to summarize the data on gait and have suggested ways in which one might record motor dysfunction and the results of treatment. I have relied upon Dr. Wise Young's detailed lecture notes on contemporary neurobiology to bring me and, I hope, other orthopaedic surgeons up to date on known research and data on the neuroplasticity of the central nervous system. This information seems particularly applicable because of the great interest of therapists and other practitioners in the use of nonsurgical treatment methods in their efforts to alter the damaged motor system of the brain. I am grateful to Dr. Young for his scholarship and his clear exposition of this complicated subject.

It was necessary to include a review of the structural changes in the skeletal system that result from spastic paralysis because one must be realistic in facing the future of children: they become adults whose life span is at least three times longer than the duration of childhood.

If one reads this book from cover to cover, some repetition will be discovered. The rationale for this repetition is that texts are not usually read in this fashion, and therefore each of the chapters on hemiplegia, diplegia, and the patient with total body involvement must be able to stand alone. Also, there is a reliable motto: *Repetitio est mater studiorum.*

At times I have engaged in philosophy and, perhaps, polemics; no apology is made for including opinions in the text. Those who treat children with cerebral palsy need a goal or end-point toward which their efforts can be directed. At this time, our goal should be to "demedicalize" the child and his family, to integrate the child with society, not segregate him as a permanent patient, and to do everything we can to allow the individual to enter the community as a responsible citizen.

In discussing surgical treatments I have tried to describe what seems to be effective and what is not effective and to supply the reasons for failures.

I am particularly indebted to those orthopaedic surgeons who have helped to improve the quality of patient care both in practice and by their publications. Their names tend to reappear in the literature: Doctors Phelps, Cooper, Green, Baker, Goldner, Keats, Sharrard, Samilson, Evans, Banks, Frost, Duncan, Hoffer, Perry, and MacEwen.

The three journals in which most of the papers have been published deserve recognition: *The Journal of Bone and Joint Surgery, Developmental Medicine and Child Neurology,* and *Clinical Orthopaedics and Related Research.* The instructional courses of the American Academy of Orthopaedic Surgeons and the American Academy for Cerebral Palsy and Developmental Medicine have contributed much to my continuing education, and this is reflected throughout the text. The United Cerebral Palsy Research and Education Foundation in the United States and the Spastics Society in the United Kingdom have contributed, both by research support and by improved care of persons with cerebral palsy, to creating a milieu that is conducive to such efforts as this book.

Very special credits must be accorded to Charlene Levering, the Director of the Division of Instructional Media, Stanford University School of Medicine, and her staff of artists, especially Halcyon Cowles and S. N. Kelly.

My wife has my deep appreciation for her unending patience and support throughout the writing of this book.

My thanks are also due to Stanford University and the Children's Hospital at Stanford for the sabbatical leave that permitted me to complete this book. And finally, the gracious people of the lovely city of Lyon, France, have our gratitude for housing and feeding us so well during most of the writing—*Je suis enchanté d'avoir fait votre connaissance.*

EUGENE E. BLECK

Palo Alto, California, 1979

Contents

Chapter One

DEFINITIONS

"Cerebral palsy" is a name popularized in 1937 by Dr. Winthrop Phelps to describe a syndrome of motor disorders and associated defects that result from a static encephalopathy. This diagnosis implies the presence of a non-progressive brain condition arising from prenatal, perinatal, or postnatal causes.

This monograph is concerned mainly with the orthopaedic management of the spastic type of cerebral palsy. If orthopaedic surgery is planned, differentiation of the type of motor disorder is important (for example, pure non-tension athetosis rarely results in a deformity). Occasionally, a patient who has athetosis may develop a painful subluxation of the hip, a dislocation of the shoulder, scoliosis, or degenerative joint disease of the wrist, hip, or cervical spine. Management of these problems is similar to that of the same conditions in "normal" persons, although treatment is more difficult because of the superimposed movement disorder.

The types of movement disorders were classified by the American Academy for Cerebral Palsy (Minear, 1956). A few minor modifications of the original classification have occurred through common usage, e.g., the term "spastic diplegia."

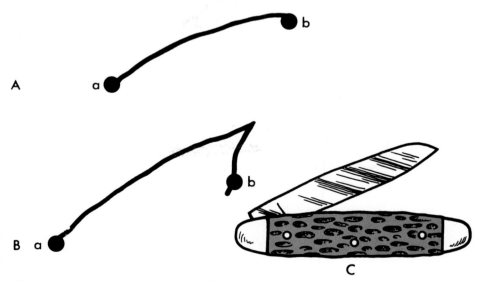

Figure 1–1   A. Graphic representation of normal motor control from points *a* to *b*. B. Graphic representation of spastic motor control—the patient overshoots the mark. C. Symbol of hypertonicity. (Redrawn from Gesell, A., and Amatruda, C. S.: *Developmental Diagnosis,* 2nd ed., Hoeber Division of Harper and Row, New York, 1947.)

CLASSIFICATION OF MOVEMENT DISORDERS

Type	Major Clinical Findings	Common Etiology
Physiological (according to the movement disorder)		
Spasticity (pyramidal)	Increased stretch reflex in muscles, i.e., hypertonicity of "clasp-knife type" (Fig. 1–1 A,B,C)	Prematurity Perinatal hypoxia Cerebral trauma Rubella (maternal)
	Hyperreflexia (deep tendon reflexes) Clonus Positive Babinski sign Esotropia or exotropia	Familial
Athetosis Tension type	Tension can be "shaken out" of limb by examiner (Fig. 1–2) Extensor pattern (usually) Normal or depressed reflexes Paralysis of upward gaze Deafness (often)	Kernicterus due to Rh incompatibility

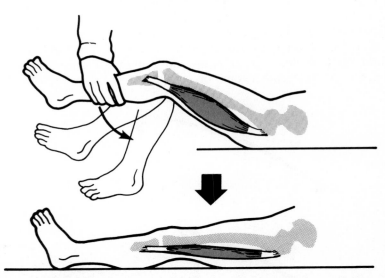

Figure 1–2   A tense spastic hamstring muscle loosens with repetitive movements of the knee — characteristic of tension athetosis.

CLASSIFICATION OF MOVEMENT DISORDERS (*Continued*)

Type	Major Clinical Findings	Common Etiology
Dystonia	Intermittent distorted posturing of limbs, neck, trunk (Fig. 1–3) No contractures Full range of joint motion when relaxed	
Chorea	Spontaneous jerking of distal joints (fingers and toes) (Fig. 1–4)	Neonatal jaundice Hyperbilirubinemia Cerebral anoxia Encephalitis, meningitis, or both

Table continued on the following page

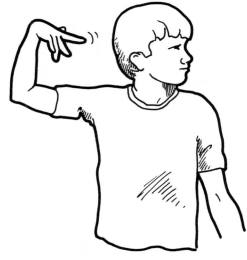

Figure 1–3 Dystonic posturing. (Redrawn from Bleck, E. E., and Nagel, D. A.: *Physically Handicapped Children: A Medical Atlas for Teachers*, Grune & Stratton, New York, 1975.)

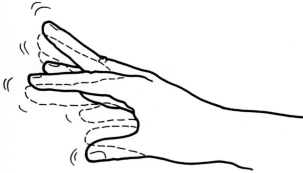

Figure 1–4 Chorea—involuntary movements of distal joints. (Redrawn from Bleck, E. E., and Nagel, D. A.: *Physically Handicapped Children: A Medical Atlas for Teachers*, Grune & Stratton, New York, 1975.)

CLASSIFICATION OF MOVEMENT DISORDERS (*Continued*)

Type	Major Clinical Findings	Common Etiology
Ballismus (rotary, flailing)	Uncontrolled involuntary motions of proximal joints (shoulders, elbows, hips, knees) (Fig. 1–5)	
Rigidity	Rigid limbs Lead pipe type—continuous resistance to passive motion (Fig. 1–6A) Cog wheel type—discontinuous resistance to passive motion (Fig. 1–6B)	

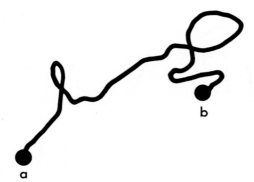

a

b

Figure 1–5 Graphic depiction of motor control in athetosis. (Redrawn from Gesell, A., and Amatruda, C. S.: *Developmental Diagnosis,* 2nd ed., Hoeber Division of Harper and Row, New York, 1947.)

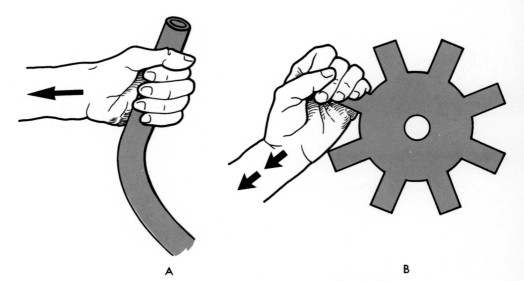

A

B

Figure 1–6 Rigidity. *A.* Lead pipe type. B. Cog wheel type.

CLASSIFICATION OF MOVEMENT DISORDERS (*Continued*)

Type	Major Clinical Findings	Common Etiology
Ataxia	Lack of balance Uncoordinated movement Dysmetria (Fig. 1–7A) Dysarthria Wide-based gait (patient sways as he walks) (Fig. 1–7B) Pes valgus (flexible) common	Head injury Cerebral maldevelopment

Table continued on the following page

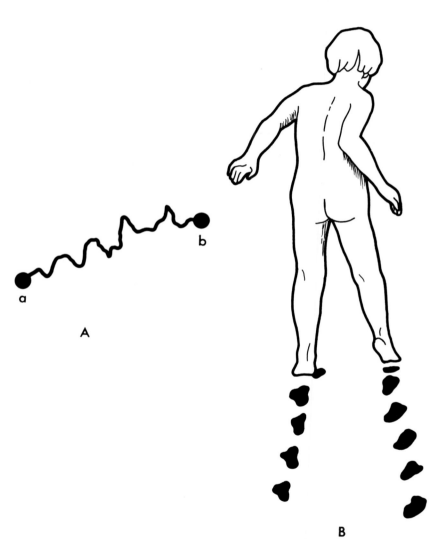

Figure 1–7 A. Graphic representation of ataxic motor performance. B. Typical ataxic wide-based gait. (Redrawn from Gesell. A., and Amatruda, C. S.: *Developmental Diagnosis,* 2nd ed., Hoeber Division of Harper and Row, New York, 1947, and Ducroquet, P.: *Walking and Limping,* Lippincott, Philadelphia, 1968.)

CLASSIFICATION OF MOVEMENT DISORDERS (*Continued*)

Type	Major Clinical Findings	Common Etiology
Tremor	Rare Intentional or non-intentional (Fig. 1–8) Rhythmic or non-rhythmic	
Atonia	Rare Hypotonia of limbs and trunk (Fig. 1–9) Often evolves into athetosis as child matures	Cerebral anoxia

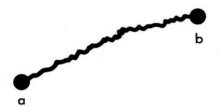

b

Figure 1–8   Graphic representation of tremor. (Redrawn from Gessell, A., and Amatruda, C. S.: *Developmental Diagnosis,* 2nd ed., Hoeber Division of Harper and Row, New York, 1947.)

Figure 1–9   Graphic representation of hypotonicity. Motor control permits going from one point to another, but weakness causes the limb to "fall off" the terminal point. (Redrawn from Gesell, A., and Amatruda, C. S.: *Developmental Diagnosis,* 2nd ed., Hoeber Division of Harper and Row, New York, 1947.)

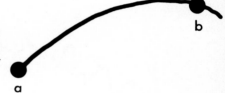

a

CLASSIFICATION OF MOVEMENT DISORDERS (*Continued*)

Type	Major Clinical Findings	Common Etiology
Mixed types	Spasticity and athetosis usual Total body involvement usual	Encephalitis Cerebral anoxia Birth trauma
Topographical Monoplegia	One limb involved Spasticity (usually) Patient should run to exclude hemiplegic pattern	
Hemiplegia	Spastic upper and lower limb on same side (Fig. 1–10)	
Paraplegia	Lower limb involvement only Rare in spastic type of cerebral palsy Common in familial type Spasticity	

Table continued on the following page

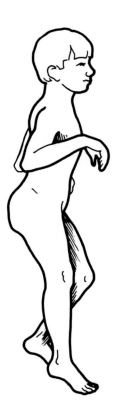

Figure 1–10 Hemiplegic posture—flexed elbow, wrist, and fingers: foot and ankle equinus position.

CLASSIFICATION OF MOVEMENT DISORDERS (*Continued*)

Type	Major Clinical Findings	Common Etiology
Diplegia	Minor involvement of upper limbs (slight incoordination of finger movement) Major involvement of lower limbs (Fig. 1–11) Spasticity	
Triplegia	Three limbs involved Spasticity	
Quadriplegia	Total body involvement (all four limbs, head, neck, and trunk) (Fig. 1–12) Spastic, athetoid, and mixed types	

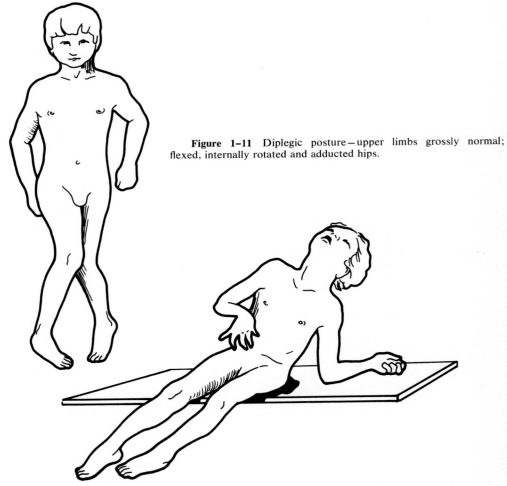

Figure 1–11 Diplegic posture—upper limbs grossly normal; flexed, internally rotated and adducted hips.

Figure 1–12 Total body involvement—spastic or athetoid or mixed quadriplegia—usually a predominant extensor postural pattern.

Today in the United States and, I suspect, throughout the Western world, the majority of patients who have cerebral palsy seem to manifest either spastic hemiplegia, spastic diplegia, or total body quadriplegia. Hence, this text is addressed to the orthopaedic management of these three main forms of the disease.

REFERENCES

Denhoff, E., and Robinault, I. (1960) *Cerebral Palsy and Related Disorders,* New York, McGraw-Hill.

Jones, M. (1975) Differential diagnosis and natural history of the cerebral palsied child. *Orthopaedic Aspects of Cerebral Palsy* (Ed. Samilson, R. L.), Philadelphia, J. B. Lippincott.

Minear, W. L. (1956) A classification of cerebral palsy. *Pediatrics* 18:841–852.

Phelps, W. M. (1932) *Cerebral Birth Injuries, Their Orthopaedic Classification and Subsequent Treatment,* New York Academy of Medicine, January 15.

Chapter Two

ORTHOPAEDIC ASSESSMENT

Discussion of the defects associated with speech, hearing, vision, and intellect is beyond the scope of this monograph. Several texts dedicated to these important defects are listed in the references. Problems concerning the whole child are important to orthopaedic surgeons, and it is presumed that the competent orthopaedist who deals with patients with cerebral palsy will consult the numerous publications, as well as attend postgraduate education courses, on the subject.

ORTHOPAEDIC EXAMINATION

The sequence and content of the orthopaedic examination depends upon the extent of motor development of the particular patient. The following description of the orthopaedic examination presents an orderly method that may enhance observation, encourage an accurate recording of details, and lead to the best possible analysis of the problem so that the treatment that follows can be effective and can be subsequently evaluated.

Posture

If we take our cue from Sherrington, who said that posture accompanies movement like a shadow and that every movement begins in posture and ends in posture, then this is where we should begin (Rushworth, 1964).

The *supine posture* of the infant who has a lesion of the central nervous system is most often characterized by shoulder retraction and abduction, elbow flexion, and trunk and lower limb extension. When such infants are placed prone, the upper and lower limbs assume the flexed position. These postural abnormalities, described by Magnus, are thought to be manifestations of the tonic labyrinthine reflexes, which originate in the brain stem and are mediated through the upper cervical nerve roots (Bobath, 1954) (Fig. 2-1).

The *sitting posture* is either supportive (propped) or unsupportive. Children who are hypotonic, or who have cerebral damage, or both, usually do not have the normal lumbar lordotic curve and, as a result, the spine is rounded. When the child is brought from the lying to the sitting position, the presence of head lag indicates

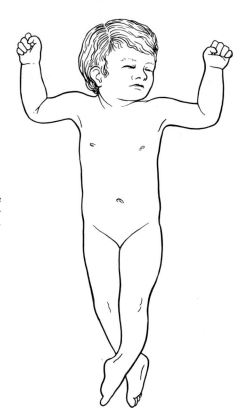

Figure 2–1 Tonic labyrinthine reflex. When the baby is supine, the shoulders are flexed, the spine is extended, and the lower limbs are extended and adducted.

delayed development. When the child is sitting, note whether or not the upper and lower limbs are extended, as is often the case in the severe spastic quadriplegic. Automatic protective placement of the extended arm denotes good function.

Observation of the *standing posture* is important. It is first observed from the side to assess head position, thoracic kyphosis, lumbar lordosis, and pelvic inclination as well as the position of the hip, knee, ankle, and foot. The degree of kyphosis and lordosis can be estimated by placing a straight edge ruler against the thoracic spine and sacrum; with thoracic kyphosis the straight edge will deviate posteriorly from the perpendicular, and the distance between the edge of the ruler and the midlumbar spine is a clinical measurement of the lordosis. In normal children this distance is usually no more than 4 cm (Fig. 2–2).

Because scoliosis occurs more frequently in children who have cerebral palsy, the posture should also be observed from the back (Robson, 1968; Samilson, 1973; Balmer and MacEwen, 1970). The level of the shoulders and pelvis, and any shift of the trunk that creates loin fullness, is noted. The child is asked to bend forward 90 degrees at the hips with the arms extended and the hands together so that any asymmetry of the posterior rib cage can be seen (Fig. 2–3). A rib hump may indicate rotation of thoracic vertebrae; this is an indication for a radiologic examination of the spine. The position of the heel, whether neutral, valgus, or varus, is also noted.

From in front the examiner can observe: (1) asymmetry of the limbs; (2) the

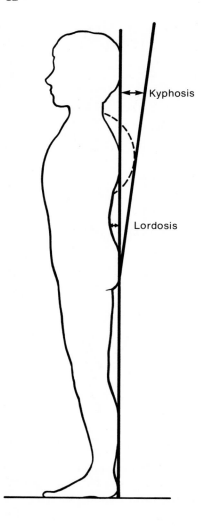

Figure 2-2 Standing posture with straight edge placed against sacrum and apex of thoracic kyphotic curve. With kyphosis, the straight edge deviates posteriorly from the perpendicular and the distance from the straight edge to the mid-lumbar spine is a gross estimate of the lordosis (normal 3 to 4 cm).

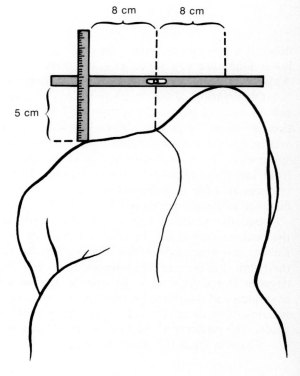

Figure 2-3 Scoliosis. With 90 degree flexion from the hip, a rib hump can be seen and measured.

femur: internal, external, or neutral rotation and adduction; (3) the position of the patella, above or below the femoral condyles; (4) the foot: external or internal rotation; (5) the mid- and forefoot: varus or valgus inclination, or adduction; (6) the toes: flexion, clawing, hallux valgus, or normal position. Because the trunk, head, and arms represent 70 per cent of the body weight, this mass, often referred to as HAT, has to be balanced and supported by the legs. With anatomical shifts of the trunk, such as those occurring in scoliosis, balance is shifted off-center. The lower limbs accommodate to these changes, usually by bringing the feet wider apart (Perry, 1975).

Gait

Gait has been defined by Inman as "bipedal plantigrade progression. It is distinctly human; it permits us to view the world in an upright manner though not always acting in an upright way." The walking pattern of a child is best observed in a wide corridor (preferably carpeted), at least 20 feet long. The examiner should first look at the positions of the head, arms, trunk, pelvis, hips, knees, ankles and feet during both the stance and swing phases of gait. Stance phase begins with heel contact and ends with toe-off. Stance is 60 percent and swing is 40 percent of the gait cycle.

The *gait cycle* has been broken down into several phases for the purpose of describing joint and muscle function (Perry, 1967, 1975) (Figs. 2–4 and 2–5). Stride length can be estimated. Perry (1975) has pointed out that the stride length is dependent upon the stance limb rather than the swing limb during walking. In cere-

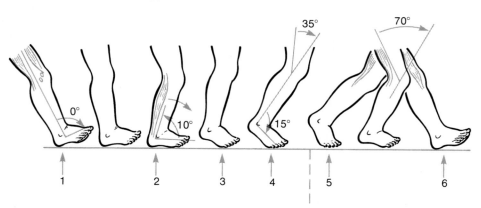

Figure 2–4 Terminology of events of the gait cycle 1. Heel strike: the ankle is flexed zero degrees, knee extended, and the hip flexed 30 degrees; synchronous activity of the hamstrings and quadriceps. 2. Mid-stance: foot flat on the floor, ankle dorsiflexed 10 degrees; gastrocnemius-soleus contracts to prevent forward acceleration of tibia. 3. Terminal stance ("roll-off"): this is not a push but rather a rocker action of the foot to advance the trunk. 4. Pre-swing: 35 to 40 degrees of knee flexion. 5. Initial swing ("pick-up"): knee flexes additional 35 degrees to prevent toe drag: hip flexion need be only 30 to 35 degrees. After pick-up, the knee flexors (biceps and gracilis) relax. Ankle progressively dorsiflexes; when the limb passes the supporting limb, the ankle plantar flexes once again (15 to 20 degrees). Toe clearance is not great and may be as little as 1 cm. 6. Terminal swing ("reach"): the knee extends for maximum stride length, hip flexes about 30 degrees, and the ankle remains in flexed position. Knee is extended primarily by swinging passively. (Adapted from Perry, 1967.)

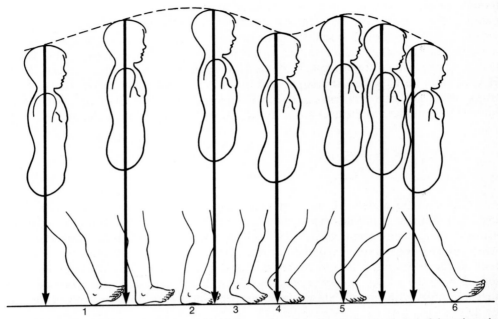

Figure 2–5 Progression of the trunk in relation to that of the foot in the six phases of the gait cycle. The trunk is posterior to the foot at the point of heel contact (1) and gradually progresses forward to mid-stance (2). At terminal stance ("roll-off") (3) the trunk is posterior to the foot once again. Pre-swing (4) is followed by initial swing ("pick-up") (5) and then terminal swing ("rock") (6). Dotted line over the head is a sinusoidal curve that represents normal vertical displacement of the body during walking on the level.

bral palsy, the stride length is limited by the respective ranges of motion of the hip, knee, and ankle, which account for the short swing by the opposite limb in mid-stance. Our studies have demonstrated that the majority of spastic diplegic patients have shorter stance phases and faster cadence than normal (Bleck et al., 1975) (Figs. 2–6 and 2–7). Patterned gait with either predominantly flexor or extensor

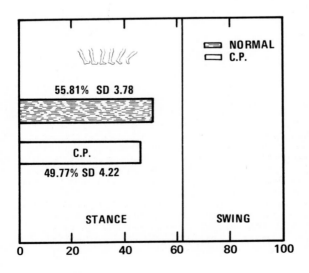

Figure 2–6 Comparison of percent of gait cycle occupied by stance in normal gait, and in cerebral palsy, spastic type. Note that the stance phase is shorter in spastic gait patterns.

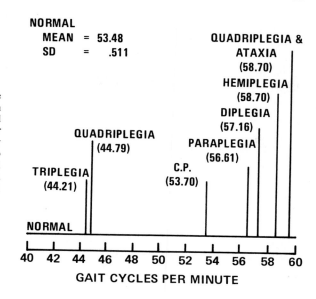

Figure 2–7 Graph showing the cadence of normal gait compared with that of spastic gait. The normal child had a mean of 53.48 gait cycles per minute. With the exception of a few spastic quadriplegics and triplegics, who are slower than normal, the typical diplegic gait is faster—a confirmation of clinical observations; these children cannot slow down (Bleck et al., 1975).

muscle action is characteristic of spastic paralysis. However, many patients who have cerebral palsy have some voluntary and selective control, and so can modify their gait patterns, an ability that probably accounts for the "clinic walk." A more detailed account of the events during gait can be found in Perry's descriptions (1967,

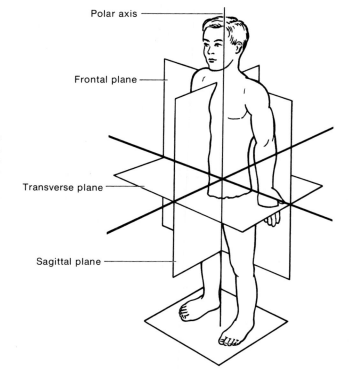

Figure 2–8 The point where all the body planes, coronal, sagittal, and transverse, converge is the center of gravity of the human body (anterior to the second sacral segment). (Redrawn from Kelley, D. L., *Kinesiology,* Prentice Hall, Englewood Cliffs, N.J., 1971.)

1975). Muscle function and timing during normal gait are summarized in the description of electromyographic examinations in this chapter.

The vertical displacement of the center of gravity and its progression in a low sinusoidal curve during walking in order to conserve energy are dependent upon the major determinants of the gait pattern described by Saunders et al. (1953). The center of gravity is defined as a fixed point in a body through which the force of gravitational attraction acts (Kelley, 1971) (Fig. 2–8). In the human body the center of gravity is located just anterior to the first or second sacral segments (Akerblom, 1948; Braune and Fischer, 1898, cited by Brunnstrom, 1962). The center of gravity of the trunk alone is at the eleventh thoracic vertebra (Hellebrandt, 1938, cited by Brunnstrom, 1962). According to Hellebrandt, the mean height of the center of gravity of the body when standing is 55 percent of the height measured from the soles of the feet.

The most efficient example of the principle of the center of gravity is the wheel — its axis stays level throughout its progression. If the legs in humans were non-articulated sticks, a "compass gait" with great energy expenditure would occur as the center of gravity rose and fell (Fig. 2–9). The five determinants of the gait pattern that should be observed are:

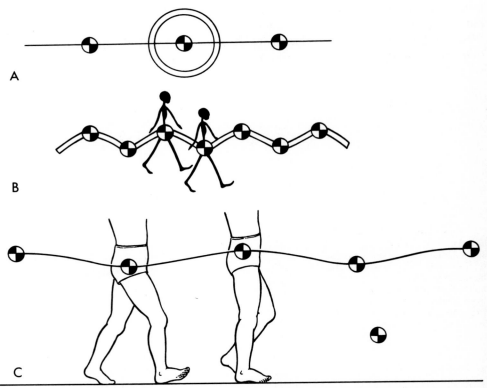

Figure 2–9 Paths of center of gravity. A. The wheel—the most efficient instrument of motion because center of gravity remains horizontal. B. Human gait if knee joint is eliminated—a compass gait results with the center of gravity rising and falling precipitously, causing increased energy expenditure. C. Low sinusoidal curve of the center of gravity in normal gait—the major determinants of gait in the lower limb (pelvis, hip, knee, foot, and ankle) serve to bring the center of gravity as close to the wheel as possible and thus conserve energy.

1. *Pelvic rotation.* Four degrees to either side.
2. *Pelvic tilt.* Angular displacement of 5 or more degrees.
3. *Knee flexion* in the stance phase.
4. *Foot and knee mechanisms.* At heel strike the ankle plantar flexes and the knee flexes to shorten the limb. As the trunk passes over the leg, the knee extends and the heel rises to lengthen the limb.
5. *Lateral displacement of the pelvis.* The shift of the trunk is normally no more than 4 to 5 cm. Excessive displacement (that would occur if the lower limbs were parallel to each other) is prevented by adduction of the femora and by the valgus angle assumed by the tibia and femur.

This quantitative information finds its parallel in data on normal ranges of joint motion during gait (Fig. 2–10). In general, the pelvis and lower limb segments rotate internally throughout the swing phase to mid-stance, when abrupt external rotation occurs. The subtalar joint of the foot absorbs the torque generated by the foot-to-floor reaction. If hip joint rotation is limited, pelvic rotation is also restricted (the angle of hip internal rotation equals the angle of pelvic external rotation), and the arc of the center of gravity is heightened and the gait made less efficient. If knee flexion is limited (e.g., by spastic quadriceps), then the gait becomes compass-like, raises the arc of the center of gravity, and increases the energy expenditure. When ankle motion is restricted, the knee and hip compensate by exaggerated movement. In spastic paralysis, however, neural integration is often deficient, so deformity and limitation of motion at one joint are not as easily compensated for as they are when the central nervous system is intact.

The lack of normal equilibrium reactions in patients who have cerebral palsy creates pathological patterns because muscle function and concomitant joint action attempt to overcome the lack of postural control. Many of the gait abnormalities observed in such patients are actually compensatory attempts to keep from falling. To test the effects of dysequilibrium on the abnormal gait in patients who walk without support, the examiner can stabilize the posture by holding the head of the patient and walking with him. Crutches, walkers, and parallel bars accomplish the same thing.

Upper Limb Assessment

Assessment of the upper limbs is begun by giving the child an object that forces him to use both hands. A toy, such as eggs within larger eggs or plastic barrels within larger barrels, is ideal. When the child grasps this toy, the lateralization of hand function, the degree of grasp and release, and the ability of the hands to cross the midline can be observed. Gross grasp and release can be tested by handing the child a cylindrical stick or similar object (Fig. 2–11). To test fine motion of the fingers and pinch, small wooden beads or candies serve the purpose well (Fig. 2–12). A child who can talk (or communicate with symbols if non-verbal) is tested for stereognosis by asking him to identify objects (pieces of wood cut into a triangle, square, and circle) while he is blindfolded or his vision is occluded with the examiner's hands, first with the abnormal hand, as in a hemiplegic, and then with the normal hand. Two

Text continued on page 25

PELVIC ROTATION

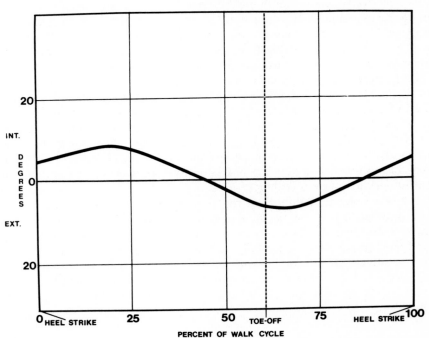

Figure 2–10 Graphic representations of normal range of motion during level gait. Note that, during swing (75 to 100 percent—heel strike on the graph) and early stance (0 to about 40 percent mid-stance), the pelvis, femur, and tibia all internally rotate. At mid-stance, external rotation occurs fairly abruptly. The foot, however, does not rotate internally, but remains in external rotation throughout the cycle. In early stance when other segments are internally rotating, the foot remains externally rotated owing to the torque-absorbing mechanism of the subtalar joint. (Courtesy of Mann, R., and Hagy, J., Shriner's Hospital for Crippled Children, San Francisco.)

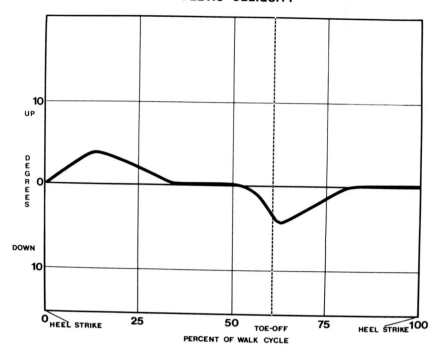

PELVIC OBLIQUITY

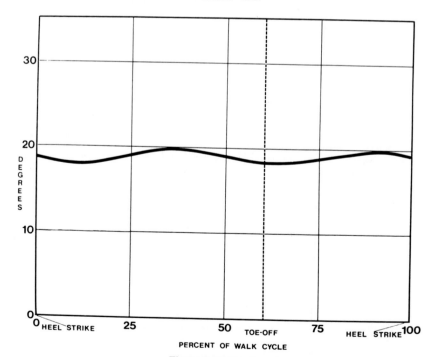

PELVIC TILT

Figure 2–10 *Continued*

Illustration continued on the following page.

FEMORAL ROTATION

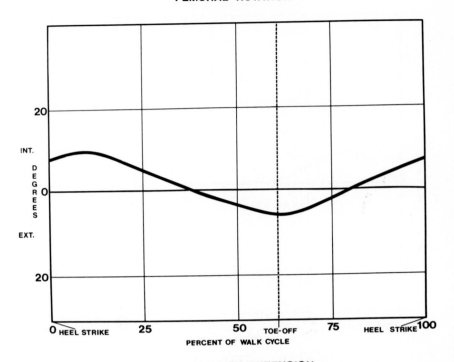

HIP FLEXION-EXTENSION

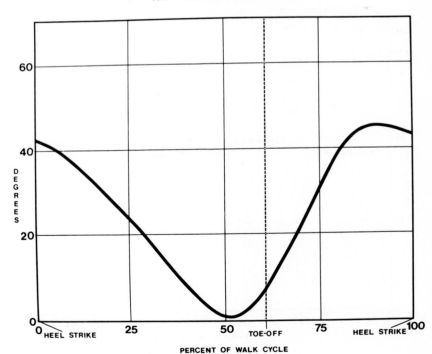

Figure 2–10 *Continued*

HIP JOINT ROTATION

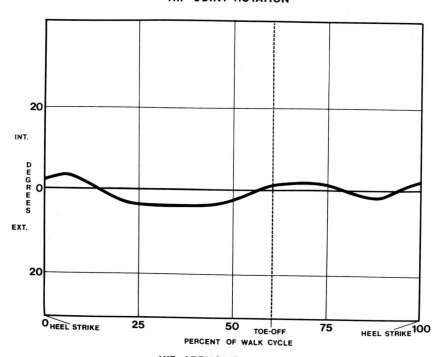

HIP ABDUCTION - ADDUCTION

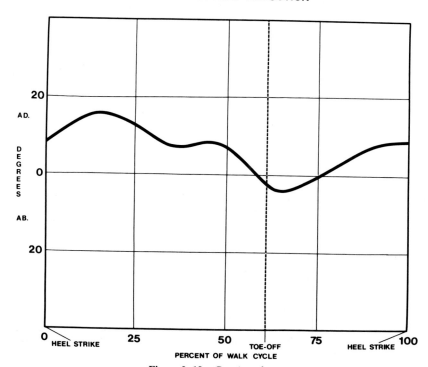

Figure 2–10   *Continued*

Illustration continued on the following page.

KNEE FLEXION-EXTENSION

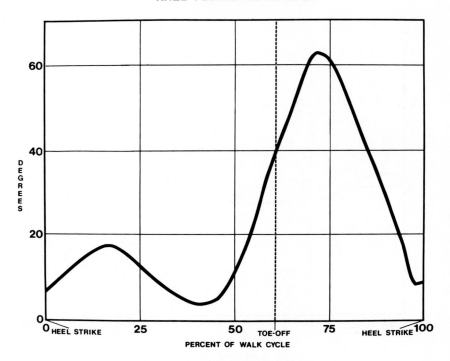

KNEE JOINT ROTATION

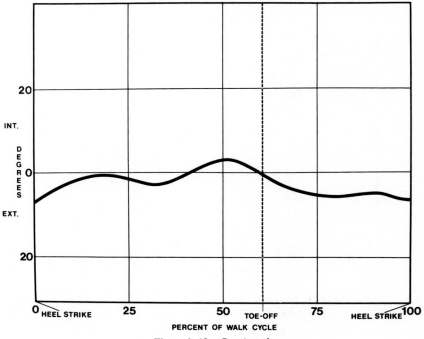

Figure 2–10 *Continued*

TIBIAL ROTATION

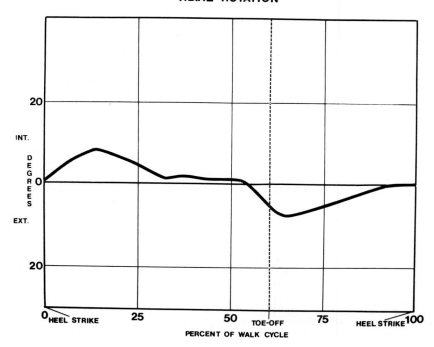

PLANTAR FLEXION-DORSIFLEXION

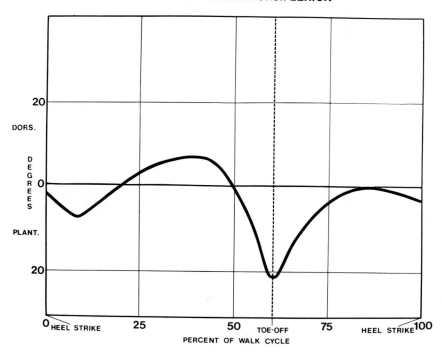

Figure 2–10 *Continued*

Illustration continued on the following page.

FOOT ROTATION

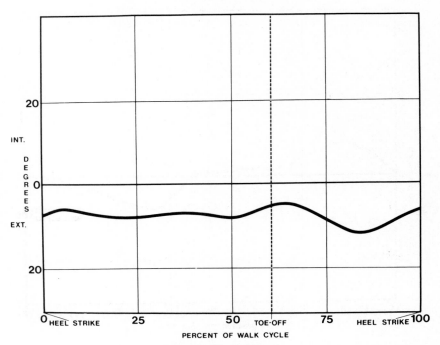

Figure 2–10   *Continued*

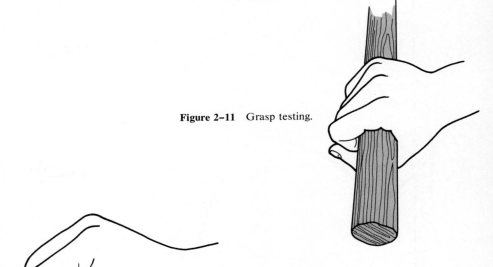

Figure 2–11   Grasp testing.

Figure 2–12   Pinch testing.

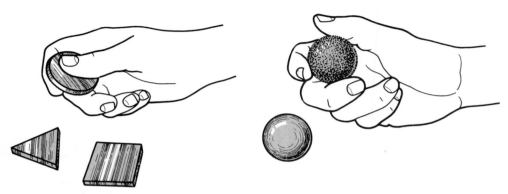

Figure 2–13   Stereognosis test equipment: ¼ inch plywood triangle, square, disc for shape recognition; smooth and fuzzy ping-pong balls for texture recognition.

ping-pong balls, one smooth and one fuzzy-coated, can be used to test tactile sensations (Goldner, 1974) (Fig. 2–13).

The examination proceeds with measurement of the ranges of motion of the shoulder, elbow, wrist, and fingers (Fig. 2–14). Estimates of muscle strength and of voluntary control, while not accurate in patients with spastic paralysis, do at least give some very useful information to the orthopaedic surgeon. A time-oriented flow sheet for muscle testing is a help (Fig. 2–15).

Palpation of the spastic wrist flexors as the wrist is extended can identify which of these tendons is spastic and contracted (Fig. 2–16). If the thumb is indwelling, measuring the web space while pulling the thumb into abduction will define the spastic adductor pollicis. Limited extension of the interphalangeal joint of the thumb when the wrist is held in neutral position, and the metacarpal-phalangeal joint is held in extension, will indicate a spastic flexor pollicis longus. If the fingers are flexed, bring the wrist into neutral position and then extend the metacarpal-phalangeal joints; the absence of the ability to extend the middle joints with the distal joints extended determines the extent of spasticity and contracture of the flexor digitorum superficialis (Fig. 2–17A). If the distal joints are flexed and resist extension with the proximal interphalangeal and metacarpal-phalangeal joints held in extension and the wrist in neutral position, the flexor digitorum profundus is spastic as well (Fig. 2–17B).

The ability to extend the fingers actively can be tested in patients who have wrist and finger flexion spasticity by putting the wrist in flexion and asking the patient to extend the fingers. If the fingers extend at the metacarpal-phalangeal joints, then the extensors of the fingers have a chance of functioning when the finger and wrist flexion deformities are relieved surgically. If, in the presence of massive flexion spasticity, the examiner is in doubt about the function of the wrist and finger extensors, the median nerve can be blocked at the elbow with a local anesthetic to eliminate most of the flexor muscle function; after an effective median nerve block at the elbow, the extent of active wrist and finger extension can be measured.

Finally, if the child cannot walk, observe whether or not he can move the wheelchair functionally and, if so, whether with both hands or only one, and in what positions he places his wrist and fingers to move the chair.

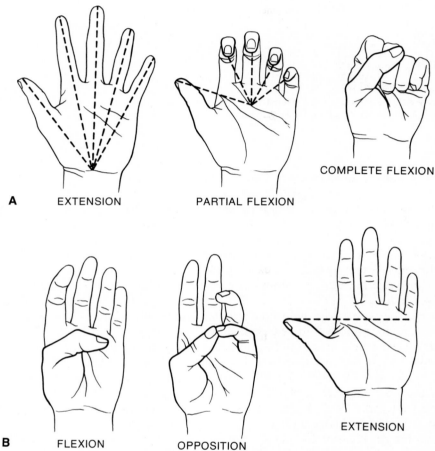

A   EXTENSION   PARTIAL FLEXION   COMPLETE FLEXION

B   FLEXION   OPPOSITION   EXTENSION

Figure 2-14   Linear measurements used to describe opening and closing capacities (range of motion) of the hand. A. Fingers. To describe the opening capacity of each finger, measure the distance in centimeters from the tip of the extended finger to the distal flexion crease of the wrist. To describe the closing capacity of each finger, measure the distance in centimeters from the tip of the finger to the mid-palmar crease, over the third metacarpal. The resulting intervals between full opening and full closing for each finger give a diagrammatic picture of finger excursion. B. Thumb. To measure the opposing capacity of the thumb and fingers, measure the distance in centimeters between the tip of the thumb and the tip of each finger. To measure the opening and closing of the thumb in extension/abduction-flexion/adduction, measure in centimeters the distance from the tip of the thumb to the head of the fifth metacarpal in full extension/abduction and in full flexion/adduction.

TIME-ORIENTED RECORD
MUSCLE TESTING

KEY:	Combinations of Numbers may be placed in each visit square to evaluate the muscles tested.

0 = Blank	9 = Could not position
1 = Zero	properly
2 = Trace	10 = Limited Range
3 = Poor	11 = Patient Uncooperative
4 = Fair	12 = No isolated Movement
5 = Good	Record Left & Right [L \ R]
6 = Normal	
7 = Unable to Grade – Pain Present	GRADING: The grading is based on the procedures described by Daniels and Worthingham (3rd edition, 1972) with some modifications made.
8 = Spastic Antagonist	

VISIT NUMBER	Past	1	2	3
MUSCLE TEST – Upper Limb				
Wrist:				
Flexors–				
Flexor Carpi Radialis				
Flexor Carpi Ulnarius				
Palmaris Longus				
Extensors–				
Extensor Carpi Radialis Longus				
Extensor Carpi Radialis Brevis				
Extensor Carpi Ulnaris				
Fingers:				
Flexor Digitorum Profundus				
Flexor Digitorum Superficials				
Extensor Digitorum Communis				
Extensor Indices Proprius				
Lumbricales and Interossei				
Thumb:				
Opponens				
Flexor Pollicis Longus				
Flexor Pollicis Brevis				
Extensor Pollicis Longus				
Extensor Pollicis Brevis				
Abductor Pollicis				

Figure 2–15 Sample portion of a time-oriented flow sheet for muscle testing, upper limb. Up to 14 serial tests can be put on one page; boxes are divided for grading right and left sides. If computer program is desired, use: 1–no muscle activity, 2–trace, 3–poor, 4–fair, 5–good, 6–normal, 7–unable to grade, 8–spastic antagonist, 9–could not position properly, 10–limited range, 11–patient uncooperative, 12–no isolated movement.

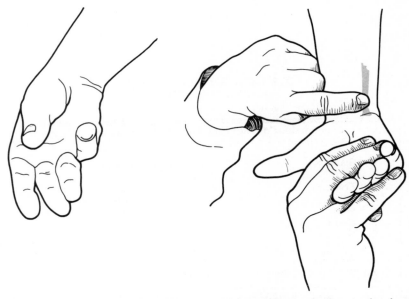

Figure 2–16 To test for a spastic wrist flexor: flex wrist and then gradually extend; palpate the contracted and spastic tendon (flexor carpi ulnaris or radialis).

It is presumed that the examiner will be able to differentiate athetosis from spasticity in the upper limb. Dystonic athetosis can mimic spasticity, but with careful examination and gradual relaxation of the patient, dystonic posturing of the wrist and fingers will become evident.

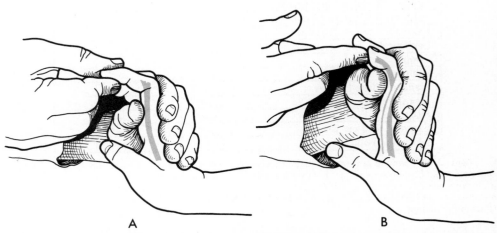

A   B

Figure 2–17 A. Test for spastic and contracted flexor digitorum superficialis: wrist extended, metacarpophalangeal joint extended. Then attempt to extend the proximal interphalangeal joint. B. Test for spastic and contracted flexor digitorum profundus: wrist extended, metacarpophalangeal and proximal interphalangeal joints extended. Then attempt to extend the proximal interphalangeal joint.

Lower Limb Assessment

Hip. The passive range of motion and muscle power of the hip can be measured in the standard way and recorded on the time-oriented flow sheet (Figs. 2–18 and 2–19). The degree of adduction contracture should be measured with the hips flexed 90 degrees and also extended. Hip flexion contracture is measured in two ways. In the Thomas test, the hip is flexed on the abdomen to flatten the lumbar spine, and the opposite hip is gently pushed into its maximum extension. The angle that the femur subtends with the table top is a measure of the degree of hip flexion deformity (Fig. 2–20A). Unfortunately, a variety of hip flexion deformities can be produced in the same patient, depending upon how far the hip is pushed on the abdomen and how much pelvic femoral fixation has occurred because of spastic and contracted hamstrings and a contracted hip joint capsule (Fig. 2–20B and C). I have found that the Thomas test can delineate spasticity and contracture of the iliopsoas in the following manner. Grasp the femoral condyles of the side to be measured and attempt to rotate the femur externally; external rotation is blocked when the iliopsoas is spastic. In contrast, the hip can be externally rotated easily in patients who have a hip flexion contracture due to shortening of the iliotibial band. This condition is seen most often in flaccid paralysis resulting from poliomyelitis or muscular dystrophy.

A second method of measuring hip flexion contracture has been found to be more accurate (Staheli, 1977). The patient lies prone with the pelvis over the edge of the table and the lower limbs hanging free in flexion. The examiner places one hand on the posterior superior iliac spines, while the other hand brings the lower limb gradually into extension. The point at which the pelvis begins to move anteriorly is the point of hip flexion deformity; the angle subtended by the femoral shaft and the horizontal plane is measured (Fig. 2–21). When hip internal and external rotation are measured, the patient should be prone and the pelvis stabilized with the examiner's hand to avoid overestimation of hip internal rotation due to lateral rolling of the pelvis (Fig. 2–22A and B).

With the patient still prone, quadriceps spasticity can be estimated by the prone-lying rectus femoris test, in which the knee is rapidly flexed and its resistance to flexion is felt. Buttock elevation is indicative of a positive test (Fig. 2–23). Stretch electromyograms have demonstrated that in this test the iliopsoas muscle fires almost the same number of action potentials as the rectus femoris (Perry, 1976).

Stretch tests about the hips are limited in specificity (Perry, 1976). On the basis of this evidence, the gracilis test* can be eliminated (I have not used it for 20 years). Electromyographic data show that both the straight leg raising and gracilis tests induce the same amount of electrical activity of the medial hamstrings. The Thomas test and the prone-lying rectus femoris test also produce about the same amount of electrical activity in the iliopsoas and the rectus femoris. The adductors are sensitive to the hip adductor stretch with the hips and knees flexed, to the gracilis test, and to the Thomas test.

Knee. Spasticity and contracture of the hamstrings are reliably measured with the straight leg raising test. The hamstrings almost exclusively are active on the electromyogram with straight leg raising. To palpate the hamstrings and obtain a

Text continued on page 33

---

*Gracilis test of Phelps: With patient prone, knees flexed, and hips abducted, extend knees. Adduction of thighs indicates gracilis spasm and contracture (Keats, 1965).

TIME-ORIENTED RECORD
RANGE OF MOTION

Use passive range. Record in 5° increments. Anatomical position is 0°. Contracture = degrees from normal.	N = normal range S = sitting U = unable to perform motion P = motion limited by pain √ = flexed / = extended			
VISIT NUMBER	**Past**	**1**	**2**	**3**
LOWER LIMB				
Hip:				
Rt. Flexion – 0–110° or 120°				
Lt. Flexion – 0–110° or 120°				
Rt. Flexion Contracture (knee √)				
Lt. Flexion Contracture (knee √)				
Rt. Flexion Contracture (knee /)				
Lt. Flexion Contracture (knee /)				
Rt. Internal Rot. (hip √) 0–45°				
Lt. Internal Rot. (hip √) 0–45°				
Rt. Internal Rot (hip /) 0–45°				
Lt. Internal Rot. (hip /) 0–45°				
Rt. Ext. Rot. (hip √) 0–45°				
Lt. Ext. Rot. (hip √) 0–45°				
Rt. Ext. Rot. (hip /) 0–45°				
Lt. Ext. Rot. (hip /) 0–45°				
Rt. Abduction (hip √) 0–45° or 60°				
Lt. Abductn (hip √) 0–45° or 60°				
Rt. Abductn (hip /) 0–45°				
Lt. Abductn (hip /) 0–45°				
Rt. Adductn (hip /) 0–30°				
Lt. Adductn (hip /) 0–30°				
Straight Leg Raise – in Degrees				
Knee:				
Rt. Flexion Contracture (supine)				
Lt. Flexion Contracture (supine)				
Rt. Flexion Contracture (prone)				
Lt. Flexion Contracture (prone)				
Rt. Extension Contracture (prone)				
Lt. Extension Contracture (prone)				
Rt. Hyper-extension				
Lt. Hyper-extension				
Ankle:				
Rt. Dorsi-flexion (knee √) 0–20°				
Lt. Dorsi-flexion (knee √) 0–20°				
Rt. Dorsi-flexion (knee /) 0–20°				
Lt. Dorsi-flexion (knee /) 0–20°				
Rt. Plantar Flexion (knee √) 0–50°				
Lt. Plantar Flexion (knee √) 0–50°				
Foot: (forepart)				
Right Inversion 0–35°				
Left Inversion 0–35°				
Right Eversion 0–15°				
Left Eversion 0–15°				

Figure 2–18   Sample portion of a time-oriented flow sheet for recording lower limb range of motion. Anatomical position is 0. All ranges passive. Record in 5 degree increments.

TIME-ORIENTED RECORD
MUSCLE TESTING

KEY: Combinations of Numbers may be placed in each visit square to evaluate the muscles tested.

0 = Blank
1 = Zero
2 = Trace
3 = Poor
4 = Fair
5 = Good
6 = Normal
7 = Unable to Grade — Pain Present
8 = Spastic Antagonist

9 = Could not position properly
10 = Limited Range
11 = Patient Uncooperative
12 = No isolated Movement
Record Left & Right   [L / R]

GRADING: The grading is based on the procedures described by Daniels and Worthingham (3rd edition, 1972) with some modifications made.

VISIT NUMBER	Past	1	2	3
MUSCLE TEST — Lower Limb				
Hip:				
Flexors— (Psoas Major & Iliacus)				
Extensors— (Gluteus Maximum)				
Abductors— (Gluteus Medius)				
Adductors— (Adductor Magnus, Brevis, Longus)				
Longus				
Lateral Rotators				
Medial Rotators— (Gluteus Minimus)				
Knee:				
Flexors —				
Biceps Femoris				
Semitendinosus				
Semimembranosus				
Extensors — (Quadriceps Femoris)				
Ankle:				
Plantar Flexion — (Gastrocnemius Soleus)				
Dorsi— Flexors— (Tibialis Anterior)				
Invertors — (Tibialis Posterior and Anterior)				
Evertors — (Peroneus Longus & Brevis)				
Foot:				
Toe Flexors				
Toe Extensors				

Figure 2–19 Sample portion of a time-oriented flow sheet for testing lower limb muscle. See Figure 2–15 for grading system.

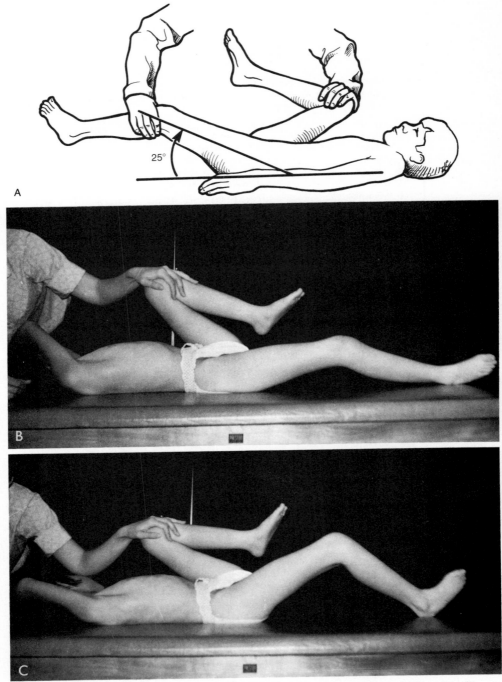

Figure 2–20   A. The Thomas test for hip flexion contracture. B and C. The variability of the Thomas test in measuring hip flexion contracture in the same patient.

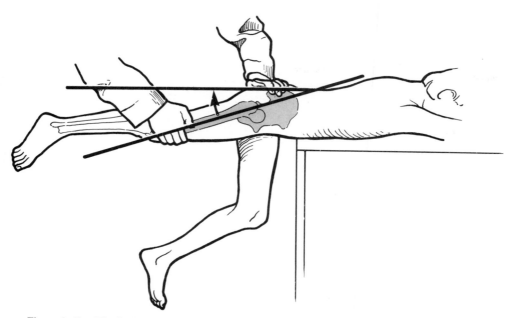

Figure 2-21 Hip flexion contracture test in prone position (Staheli, 1977). Patient lying prone with pelvis off examining table. Put one hand on posterior superior iliac spine region. As one hip is brought up into extension, the point of contracture is reached when the pelvis begins to roll anteriorly.

closer estimate of contracture, I have found it preferable to flex the hip 90 degrees and then extend the knee to its limit. The degree of contracture is measured as the angle that the tibia subtends with the knee joint at the extended (zero) position (the popliteal angle) (Fig. 2-24). The position of the patella is noted, whether it is high (riding above the patellar femoral articulation) or is in a normal position. The degree of flexion contracture of the knee joint owing to capsular contracture is measured when the limb is laid flat. If firm pressure on the anterior aspect of the knee joint fails to extend the knee to the zero position, a flexion contracture of the knee joint is likely. Quadriceps strength within the range allowed by knee flexion contracture can be estimated with the patient lying on his back with his legs flexed over the edge of a table (Evans, 1975). Simultaneous extension of both knees is easier for most patients, although those who have unilateral voluntary control of knee extension have better walking patterns. This same position can be used to elicit quadriceps spasticity by gently pushing the knees into flexion. Those patients who have severe quadriceps spasticity will not be able to flex their knees 90 degrees, and the increased stretch reflex can be easily appreciated.

Leg, Foot, and Ankle. The degree of tibial-fibular torsion can be measured with the patient sitting with his knees flexed 90 degrees over the table edge. If the hip is placed in neutral rotation, an imaginary line can be drawn through the femoral condyles that is almost parallel to the transcondylar line through the proximal tibia. This line then intersects with a line drawn through the tips of the malleoli. The table edge becomes the transcondylar line. One arm of a goniometer is placed parallel to the table edge while the other arm is placed in line with the oblique line through the tips of the malleoli (Fig. 2-25A and B). With this method of measurement, the normal

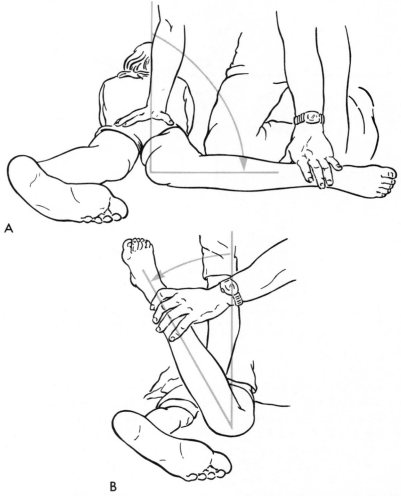

A

B

Figure 2-22   A. Measurement of internal rotation of hip with hip in extension. One hand should always be placed on the pelvis to stabilize it so that pelvic rotation is minimized. B. Measurement of external rotation of hip with hip in extension. Note hand on pelvis.

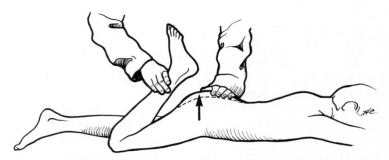

Figure 2-23   Rectus femoris test (Ely test) with patient lying prone. Rapid flexion of the buttocks causes them to rise if there is spasticity of the rectus femoris (quadriceps spasm). This test also causes contraction of the iliopsoas.

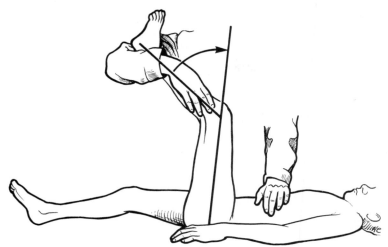

Figure 2–24 Test for hamstring spasm and contracture. Patient is lying supine with hip flexed 90 degrees and knee extended to point of contracture. The angle is termed "popliteal angle."

means for external tibial-fibular torsion according to age are: 0 to 12 months, 7.6 degrees (S.D., 4.1 degrees); 13 to 24 months, 10.6 degrees (S.D., 2.3 degrees); and 25 months to 13 years, 13.1 degrees (S.D., 2.7 degrees). In the skeletally mature patient, this angle is 22 degrees. An alternative, and probably more accurate, method of measuring tibial-fibular torsion is that of Staheli and Engel (1972). The normal values obtained by their method are slightly lower than those just described.

The range of dorsiflexion of the hindfoot is measured with the heel held in varus position to lock the mid-tarsal joint. If dorsiflexion of the foot with the knee flexed is much greater than that with the knee extended, then the gastrocnemius is likely to be the site of the main contracture (Fig. 2–26). If there is no change in the dorsiflexion with this maneuver, there is contracture of both the gastrocnemius and the soleus muscles (Silfverskiöld, 1924). Electromyographic studies of the gastrocnemius and soleus muscles in performance of the Silfverskiöld test have cast doubt on its validity in differentiating spasm and contracture of these two muscles (Perry et al., 1974). Although the test may be positive, the underlying neural mechanism causes a total extensor response so that both muscles are spastic. In three of Perry's eight cases no demonstrable differences in gastrocnemius and soleus spasticity were found on electromyographic examination in spite of positive Silfverskiöld tests in all.

If the hindfoot is in varus position and quickly everted, palpation of the posterior tibial tendon reveals its spasticity. Conversely, if the foot is in valgus position and rapidly inverted, the peroneal tendons may be palpated and spasticity confirmed.

Voluntary dorsiflexion of the foot with the knee extended, even in the presence of equinus deformity, is worth noting. Frequently the foot can be actively dorsiflexed only with the flexor withdrawal reflex ("confusion reflex"), which is elicited by flexing the knee 90 degrees over the edge of the table and asking the patient to flex his hip actively while hip flexion is resisted by manual pressure on the anterior distal thigh. With this maneuver, automatic dorsiflexion of the foot constitutes a positive response (Fig. 2–27).

The foot is inspected for forefoot adduction. The examiner holds the heel in one

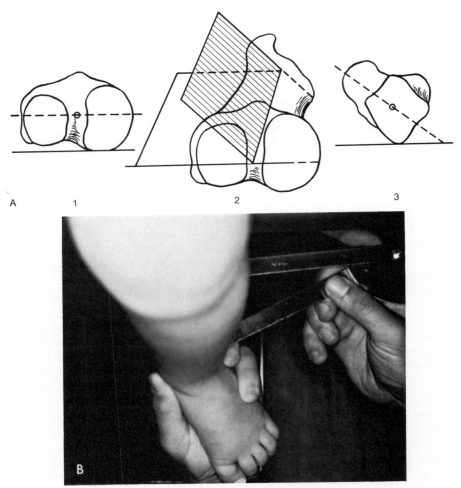

Figure 2–25 A. Tibial torsion: 1. Proximal articular surface of tibia with line through polar axis to represent coronal plane. 2. Intersection of the two planes represented results in dihedral angle that measures the twist between the proximal and distal ends of the tibia. 3. Distal articular surface of tibia with line bisecting the medial malleolus and articular facet for fibula. B. Clinical measurement of tibial-fibular torsion; knee flexed 90 degrees over the table; hip in neutral rotation. One limb of goniometer is parallel to table edge and the other limb is parallel to the line through the tip of the fibular and medial malleoli. This is a gross measurement but reasonably accurate for a clinical estimate of the amount of tibial-fibular torsion.

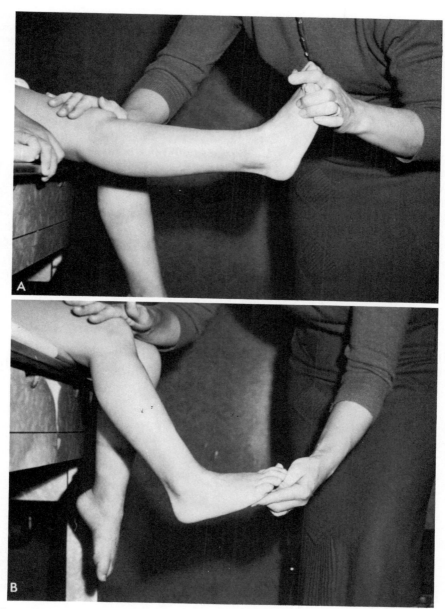

Figure 2-26 A. and B. Silfverskiöld test for gastrocnemius vs. soleus contracture. With the knee extended, the foot is held in varus position and dorsiflexion of the ankle is attempted; then the knee is flexed 90 degrees and dorsiflexion of the ankle is again attempted. If the foot remains in equinus position with the knee flexed, the gastrocnemius and soleus are both contracted. If the foot dorsiflexes above neutral at the ankle with the knee flexed, then only the gastrocnemius is contracted. For explanation of the pitfalls and a critique of this traditional test, see text.

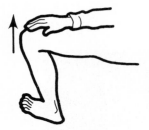

Figure 2-27 Flexor withdrawal reflex ("confusion reflex"). Patient is seated, with hip and knee flexed 90 degrees. Examiner's hand is on the anterior surface of the distal thigh. The patient is instructed to flex hip against resistance of examiner's hand. Automatic dorsiflexion of the foot occurs in a positive response.

hand and the palm of the other hand against the head of the first metatarsal; limited passive abduction of the forefoot will indicate a fixed forefoot adduction deformity. One way to record the metatarsal adduction deformity is to visualize the plantar weight-bearing surface of the heel as an ellipse (Bleck, 1971). The major axis of this ellipse is the central axis of the foot. In the normal foot, this axis passes between the second and third toes; in moderate metatarsus adductus it passes between the third and fourth toes; and in more severe adductus, between the fourth and fifth toes (Fig. 2-28). With passive abduction of the forefoot, the tendon of the abductor hallucis muscle on the medial aspect of the neck of the first metatarsal can be palpated in patients with dynamic spastic forefoot adduction.

NEUROLOGICAL EXAMINATION

Type of Movement Disorder

Because the diagnosis of spasticity is based upon the increased stretch reflex, the presence or absence of spasticity in the limbs can be determined by repetitive

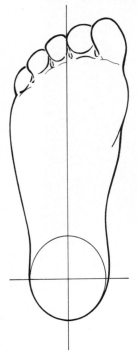

Figure 2-28 Configuration of the plantar aspect of the normal foot. The weightbearing surface of the heel can be visualized as an ellipse: thus, its major axis can be visualized. When this axis is extended, it becomes the center line of the foot. Normally, the center line passes between the second and third toes. In moderate metatarsus adductus, it bisects the foot between the third and fourth toes; in more severe cases, the fourth and fifth toes.

quick motions of the major joints. In tension athetosis, rapid motions of the lower limb result in decreased tension of the muscles. Athetosis, dystonic posturing, and chorea can be observed when the patient is at rest or when he attempts purposeful movement.

Deep Tendon and Plantar Reflexes

The biceps, triceps, and periosteal-radial reflexes in the upper limb, and the quadriceps and Achilles reflexes in the lower limb, are hyperactive in spasticity and normal or absent in athetosis and ataxia. Rigidity may be so severe that deep tendon reflexes are obliterated. The Babinski sign is best elicited by gently stroking the lateral plantar aspect of the foot with a blunt instrument such as a key or the handle of a reflex hammer. Another useful sign of upper motor neuron paralysis, especially in mild cases of spastic hemiplegia, is Chaddock's sign. The lateral aspect of the dorsum of the foot is gently stroked from the heel to the forefoot, and fanning of the toes and hyperextension of the great toe is a positive sign and comparable to the positive Babinski sign.

The Head

The *head* circumference should always be measured and compared with normal measurements (Fig. 2–29). The fontanelles should be palpated for closure. I always auscultate the skull for a bruit. Rarely, one may find a vascular anomaly of the brain to explain the etiology of spastic hemiplegia.

CRANIAL NERVES

III, IV, and VI. Eye mobility is frequently affected in cerebral palsy. The presence of esotropia or exotropia should be noted. According to Perlstein, esotropia is six times as common as exotropia. Pupil inequality is uncommon and is most often seen in patients with hemiplegia of cerebrovascular or brain tumor origin. Paralysis of upward gaze is common in patients who have tension athetosis due to kernicterus (Rh incompatibility hyperbilirubinemia).

VII and XII. On inspection of the mouth and face, inequality of muscle function is sometimes noted in cases of hemiplegia in which there is residual seventh cranial nerve paralysis. Athetoid movements of the tongue and lips often accompany these movement disorders.

IX. If the patient can open his mouth, paralysis of the pharyngeal musculature may be seen. Paralysis of the ninth cranial nerve musculature may be suspected if the palate fails to rise when the child says "aaah." If swallowing is more difficult with fluids, spasm of the pharyngeal musculature should be suspected; if difficulty is greater with solids, paralysis of the pharyngeal muscles may be present (Perlstein).

VIII. Gross hearing defects can be ascertained by asking the parents whether they think the child hears and by watching the child's reactions to shaking a few grains of sand in a cardboard cylinder or to the sound from a cat meow or moo box. In suspicious cases, audiometric examinations should be done.

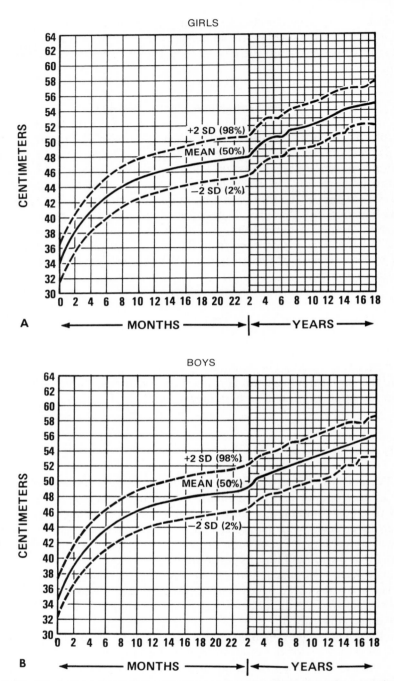

Figure 2–29 Head circumferences for girls (A) and boys (B). Head circumference below minus 2 standard deviations almost always indicates mental retardation. If head circumference approaches minus 4 standard deviations, more serious mental retardation would be likely. Children with growth failure, but with normal intelligence, have normal head circumference. (Redrawn from O'Connell, E. J., Feldt, R. H., and Stickler, G. B., Head circumference, mental retardation, and growth failure. *Pediatrics* 36:62–66, 1965.)

Infantile Automatism and Postural Reflexes

To determine locomotor prognosis the child should be tested for seven infantile reflexes, but the tests are to be considered valid for prognostic purposes only after the age of 12 months (Bleck, 1975). The testing proceeds in the following sequence:

1. *Asymmetrical tonic neck reflex.* With the child lying supine, the head is turned to one side and then the other. A positive response is flexion of the upper and lower limbs on the skull side and extension on the face side. The reflex may be present to a minor degree in normal infants, but it is never normal if it can always be imposed and the child cannot move his limbs out of position while the head is held turned to the side (Fig. 2–30). In some children who have cerebral palsy, only the upper limb may manifest the obvious reflex concomitant with lesser degrees of postural change in the lower limb. The reflex may be positive with the head turning to one side only.
2. *Neck righting reflex.* This sign is positive if, when the head is turned, the shoulders and trunk immediately turn also. The occurrence of this reflex is never normal if the child can be rolled over and over as if he were a log (Fig. 2–31).
3. *Moro reflex.* With the child supine, the reflex is elicited by suddenly dropping the head into 20 to 30 degrees of extension. Other traditional methods are a loud noise made by jarring the table on which the child is lying, or pinching of the abdominal skin. The positive response is shoulder abduction and spreading of the fingers, followed by an embrace. The complete Moro reflex may be present up to 6 months of age (Fig. 2–32).
4. *Symmetrical tonic neck reflex.* The child is placed in the quadriped or crawl position. When the head is flexed ventrally, flexion of the arms and extension of the legs result; dorsiflexion of the head causes extension of the arms and flexion of the legs. A positive reflex is normal up to the age of 6 months (Fig. 2–33).
5. *Parachute reaction.* The child, held prone by the trunk, is lifted from the table and then tipped quickly to the table top. With this movement, protective exten-

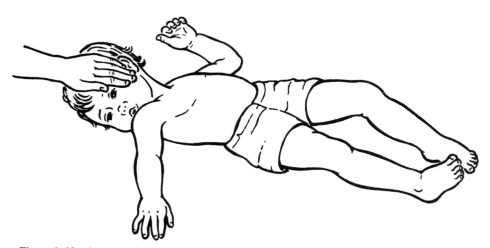

Figure 2–30 Asymmetrical tonic neck reflex. With head turning, the limbs on the skull (occipital) side flex and those on the face side extend.

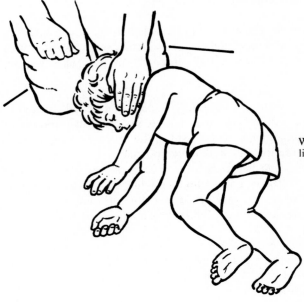

Figure 2–31 Neck righting reflex. With head turning, the entire trunk and all limbs turn to the same side.

Figure 2–32 Moro reflex elicited by a loud noise, by a jar of the examining table, by 20 to 30 degrees extension of the head, or sometimes by pinching the upper abdominal skin. The complete response is abduction of the upper limbs followed by the embrace.

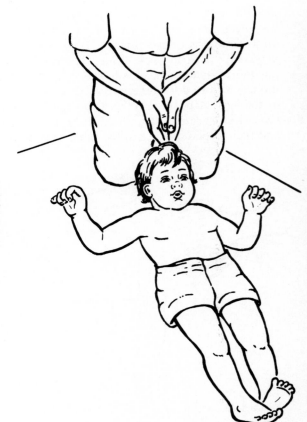

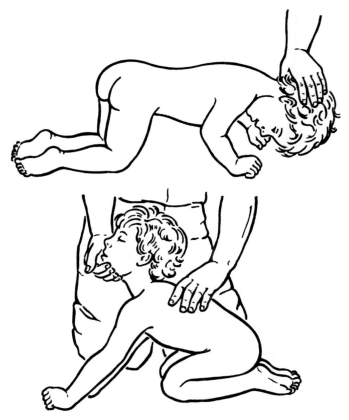

Figure 2–33 Symmetrical tonic neck reflex. With flexion of the head, the upper limbs flex and the lower limbs extend. With extension of the head, the upper limbs extend and the lower limbs flex.

sion of the hands and arms occurs (Fig. 2–34). It is abnormal for this reflex to be absent after 11 months of age.

6. *Foot placement reaction.* The child is held by the chest and axillae and, with the lower limbs extended, the dorsa of the feet are brought upward against the edge of a table top or chair. (Usually a plain wooden edge on a table top or chair is best.) Automatic foot placement occurs either symmetrically or asymmetrically. This response is normal in babies and becomes voluntarily inhibited by the age of 3 to 4 years (Fig. 2–35). The absence of this response is abnormal. The absence of the foot placement reaction often coexists with persistent extensor thrust, the test described next.

7. *Extensor thrust.* The child is lifted by the axillae and his feet are gently touched to the floor. A response of definite and progressive extension of the legs, beginning with the feet and extending upward through the legs and into the trunk, is always abnormal (Gesell and Amatruda, 1947) (Fig. 2–36). Normal infants will flex their legs with this maneuver.

The Landau reflex seems to be useful in determining the presence of hypotonia. This reflex is elicited by holding the child prone while supporting the trunk. The normal child will extend the trunk and head. Flexing the head normally causes the

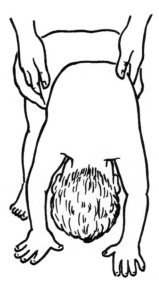

Figure 2–34 Parachute reaction. The prone child is lifted by the trunk and suddenly lowered or tipped to the table top. The normal response is automatic extension of the upper limbs and placement of the hands on the surface of the table.

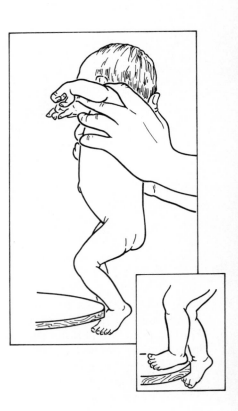

Figure 2–35 Foot placement reaction. The child is lifted by the axillae so that the dorsa of the feet come up against the underside of a table top or chair. Symmetrical or asymmetrical placement of the feet on the surface is the normal response.

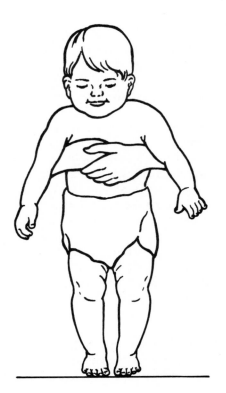

Figure 2–36 Extensor thrust. The child is held erect and the feet are lowered to the floor or table top. Progressive extension of the lower limbs upward toward the trunk is an abnormal response.

hips to flex, while the hypotonic child will collapse into an inverted letter U (Paine, 1966). This reflex has also been used to assess the motor development of infants (Cupps et al., 1976).

Equilibrium Reactions

The sitting equilibrium reactions are tested by gently pushing the child from side to side, forward, and backward. The plane in which the child cannot maintain balance is recorded. If the child can stand, the standing equilibrium reactions are tested by gently pushing the child from side to side, forward, and backward (Fig. 2–37). Normal children will maintain their balance with ease, but children who have deficient equilibrium reactions will topple over like "felled pine trees" (Hagberg et al., 1972) (Fig. 2–37A).

Equilibrium reactions of the feet can be observed in standing children by pushing them backward and laterally (Gunsolus et al., 1975). The normal foot response to posterior displacement is toe dorsiflexion and no clawing of the toes (spastic children have significantly more clawing). With lateral displacement, normal children consistently invert the mid-foot (called "medical arch reaction") and step. Children who have cerebral palsy invert the foot and step to a lesser extent. Tests for equilibrium reactions are not complicated, are easy to interpret, and provide very important and useful information. Responses to equilibrium testing help determine whether mobility and walking aids are needed.

PHYSICAL THERAPIST'S ASSESSMENT

The physical therapist is a valuable assistant to the physician in the complete motor assessment of the child with cerebral palsy. The following examinations are recorded on special forms so that progress can be followed as the child matures: (1) range of motion tests of the major upper and lower limb joints; (2) manual muscle tests (the observation of selective motor control is important); and (3) motor maturity evaluation. The motor age of the child is determined from the results of a series of postural and neurological tests performed in an organized and serial fashion (Fig. 2–38). The therapist should be able to describe the gait pattern, the predominant synergies of muscle groups, and the type of motor disorder. The therapist can point out problem areas that may not have been noticed by the physician, can assess the child's overall behavior, and can often bring out parental concerns or misunderstandings. Other areas in which the physical therapist can help are use of measuring devices and equipment for gait analysis, testing of postural reactions, and evaluation of treatment methods.

OCCUPATIONAL THERAPIST'S ASSESSMENT

The occupational therapist, along with the physical therapist, is the orthopaedic physician's assistant and can define the child's functional level, his ability to cope with everyday living, and his perceptual and visual-motor abilities. We recommend and use: (1) A functional test. Numerical scores enable us to review the functional

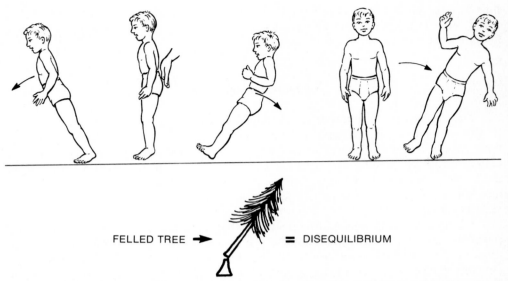

FELLED TREE ➡   = DISEQUILIBRIUM

Figure 2–37 Standing equilibrium reactions. The child is gently pushed forward, backward, and from side to side. Lack of normal equilibrium reactions is easily demonstrated—the child topples over, without the usual stepping response, as a "felled pine tree."

level of the patient quickly and allow for serial review on follow-up. (2) Activities of daily living test (Fig. 2–39). As the child gets older (7 to 8 years) and "more therapy" is requested, this test will highlight the realities of treatment planning. As in the functional test, numerical scores facilitate assessment. A review of deficiencies determines whether or not remedial therapy will be of use or whether adaptive equipment to compensate for the loss of function will be necessary. (3) Perceptual and visual motor tests. Such tests, currently in fashion, were originally designed for children with learning disabilities (Frostig, 1963, 1964; Ayeres, 1972). These and other tests have been extensively applied to children with cerebral palsy (Abercrombie, 1964). Educators in particular have requested such tests in the hope that remedial occupational therapy would assist the child's learning processes. These tests, to be of value, should be used both prior to and after a course of treatment. If no progress has been made, then either the treatment should be modified or discontinued, or remedial therapy should be given up and adaptive compensatory methods substituted.

The hand and its function are the special province of the occupational therapist. Detailed hand function evaluations are essential when surgery is contemplated. These include range of motion testing of all joints, measurement of contractures, testing of muscle strength, observation of non-functioning muscles, testing of the functional ability of the hand in pinch, grasp, and release, and testing of manual dexterity and, most importantly, of tactile sensation.

Like the physical therapist, the occupational therapist can inform the physician of the patient's emotional and behavioral problems and parental concerns and expectations. Advice on coping with the handicap most often becomes the role of the occupational therapist.

Text continued on page 55

Motor Development:	3 = Passes motor item unassisted and in a normal manner
	2 = Passes motor item unassisted but has abnormal pattern
	1 = Can complete motor item with assistance (holds posture at least 30 seconds after placed in position)
	0 = Fails motor item
Abnormalities of Postural/Movement Control:	+ = Present

VISIT NUMBER				
DATE				
MOTOR DEVELOPMENT: PRONE				

mo.

3	Holds chin and shoulders off table, weight on forearms				
3	Pelvis is flat when plane of face is 45° to 90° to table				
4	Head in mid-line				
4	Prone swimming, jerky movements				
5	Arms forward, fully extended for support				
5	Arms retracted and flexed (hands off support)				
5	Support on one forearm and reaches for toys				
5	Free kicking of legs				
6	Rolls prone to supine (purposeful)				
7	Commando-crawls				
7	Assumes quadruped position				
8	Pivots				
9	Goes from prone to sitting				
10	Creeps on hands and knees				

MOTOR DEVELOPMENT: SUPINE

mo.

3	Limb posture is flexion				
3	Limb and trunk postures becoming symmetrical				
4	Bilateral activities at mid-line				
4	(Resting) legs are in flexion, abduction, and outward rotation				
4	(Active) able to flex hips and extend legs, lifting them an inch				
5	Back arches and child raises hips (bridges, no progression)				
6	Rolls supine to prone				
6	Reaches forward with extended arms to be picked up				
6	Lifts legs and plays with feet				
7	Lifts head off table				
8	Does not like supine position				

Figure 2-38 Basic motor maturity tests.

Illustration continued on the following page.

Motor Development:	3 = Passes motor item unassisted and in a normal manner			
	2 = Passes motor item unassisted but has abnormal pattern			
	1 = Can complete motor item with assistance (holds posture at least 30 seconds after placed in position)			
	0 = Fails motor item			
Abnormalities of Postural/Movement Control:	+ = Present			

VISIT NUMBER				
DATE				
MOTOR DEVELOPMENT: PULL TO SIT				
mo.				
3 Head lag in beginning of movement, then keeps head in line with trunk				
3 Head will bob forward when sit is completed				
3 Lower limbs are flexed				
4 Slight head lag in beginning of movement, then keeps head in line with trunk (lower limbs flexed)				
5 Assists and brings head forward, no head lag (lower limbs flexed)				
6 Spontaneous lifting of head				
6 Pulls himself to sitting				
6 Raises extended legs (hips are flexed, knees are extended)				
MOTOR DEVELOPMENT: SITTING				
mo.				
3 Back somewhat rounded				
3 Head mostly held up				
4 Holds head steady, but set forward				
4 Head wobbles when child is swayed				
4 Back shows only a lumbar curvature (slight rounding)				
5 No arm support, arms retracted at shoulders with elbows flexed				
5 Child tends to fall backwards (does not push back)				
5 Head stable when body is mildly rocked by examiner				
6 May sit alone unsupported briefly when placed				
6 Arm support forward				
6 Sits well when propped				
8 Sits unsupported, without hand support for 1 minute				
8 Sits erect				
8 Has arm support sideways				
9 Adjusts posture to reach				
9 Good sitting balance, sits 10 min.				
10 Pivots to pick up objects				
10 Arm support backwards				
10 Leans forward and recovers				
10 Can lean over sideways and recover				
10 Goes forward from sitting to prone				

Figure 2–38 *Continued*

Motor Development:	3 = Passes motor item unassisted and in a normal manner
	2 = Passes motor item unassisted but has abnormal pattern
	1 = Can complete motor item with assistance (holds posture at least 30 seconds after placed in position)
	0 = Fails motor item

**Abnormalities of
  Postural/Movement
  Control:**   + = Present

VISIT NUMBER				
DATE				
MOTOR DEVELOPMENT: STANDING				

mo.

3	Does not accept weight				
4	Accepts some weight				
5	Takes almost full weight				
6	Bounces				
8	Readily bears whole weight when supported (not rigid)				
9	Pulls self to standing				
10	Stands holding on and lifts one foot				
10	Lowers self to floor by holding on				
10	Collapses if not holding on				
11	Walks holding on to furniture				
12	Walks with one hand held				
12	Attempts to stand alone				
13	Stands alone well				
13	Walks alone				
14	Gets to standing unsupported				
15	Stoops and recovers				

Figure 2–38 *Continued*

Key to Scoring: 4 Independent
3 Independent with equipment and/or adaptive technique
2 Completes but cannot accomplish in practical time
1 Attempts but requires assistance or supervision to complete
0 Dependent—cannot attempt activity
– Not applicable

The *Year-Month* vertical column represents the Order of Developmental Sequence or approximate age when the child accomplishes the activity: the horizontal column represents the chronological age of the child being assessed.

VISIT NUMBER			1		2		3	
DATE								
		YR.–MO.						
Bed		*Order Of Dev. Seq.*	*R*	*L*	*R*	*L*	*R*	*L*
1	Supine position	birth						
2	Prone position	birth						
3	Roll to side	1–4 wk.						
4	Roll prone to supine	0.6						
5	Roll supine to prone	0.7						
6	Sit up	0.10						
7	Propped sitting	0.6						
8	Sitting/hands props	0.7						
9	Sitting unsupported	0.10–0.12						
	Reaching:							
10	to midline	0.5						
11	to mouth and face	0.6						
12	above head	–						
13	behind head	–						
14	behind back	–						
15	to toes	1.3						

Figure 2–39 Activities of daily living assessment.

Key to Scoring: 4 Independent
3 Independent with equipment and/or adaptive technique
2 Completes but cannot accomplish in practical time
1 Attempts but requires assistance or supervision to complete
0 Dependent — cannot attempt activity
– Not applicable

The *Year-Month* vertical column represents the Order of Developmental Sequence or approximate age when the child accomplishes the activity: the horizontal column represents the chronological age of the child being assessed.

VISIT NUMBER		1	2	3
DATE				
	YR.–MO.			
Feeding	*Order of Dev. Seq.*	R L	R L	R L
16 Swallow (liquids):	birth			
17 drooling under control	1.0			
18 suck and use straw	2.0			
19 Chew (semisolids, solids)	1.6			
20 Fingerfoods	0.10			
Utensils:				
21 Bottle	0.10			
22 Spoon	3.0			
23 Cup	1.6			
24 Glass	2.0			
25 Fork	3.0			
26 Knife	6.0–7.0			
Toileting				
27 Bowel control	1.6			
28 Bladder control	2.0			
29 Sit on toilet	2.9			
30 Arrange clothing	4.0			
31 Cleanse self	5.0			
32 Flush toilet	3.3–5.0			

Figure 2–39 *Continued*

Illustration continued on the following page.

Key to Scoring: 4 Independent
3 Independent with equipment and/or adaptive technique
2 Completes but cannot accomplish in practical time
1 Attempts but requires assistance or supervision to complete
0 Dependent — cannot attempt activity
– Not applicable

The *Year-Month* vertical column represents the Order of Developmental Sequence or approximate age when the child accomplishes the activity: the horizontal column represents the chronological age of the child being assessed.

Visit Number		1	2	3
Date				
	Yr.–Mo.			
Hygiene	Order of Dev. Seq.	R L	R L	R L
33 Turn faucets on/off	3.0			
34 Wash/dry hands/face	4.9			
35 Wash ears	8.0			
36 Bathing	8.0			
37 Deodorant	12.0			
38 Care for teeth	4.9			
39 Care for nose	6.0			
40 Care for hair	7.6			
41 Care for nails	8.0			
42 Feminine hygiene	puberty			
Undressing				
Lower body:				
43 Untie shoe bow	2.0–3.0			
44 Remove shoes	2.0–3.0			
45 Remove socks	1.6			
46 Remove pulldown garment	2.6			
Upper body:				
47 Remove pullover garment	4.0			

Figure 2–39 *Continued*

Key to Scoring: 4 Independent
3 Independent with equipment and/or adaptive technique
2 Completes but cannot accomplish in practical time
1 Attempts but requires assistance or supervision to complete
0 Dependent—cannot attempt activity
– Not applicable

The *Year-Month* vertical column represents the Order of Developmental Sequence or approximate age when the child accomplishes the activity: the horizontal column represents the chronological age of the child being assessed.

Visit Number		1	2	3
Date				
	Yr.–Mo.			
Dressing	Order of Dev. Seq.	R L	R L	R L
Lower body:				
48 Put on socks	4.0			
49 Put on pulldown garment	4.0			
50 Put on shoe	4.0			
51 Lace shoe	4.0–5.0			
52 Tie bow	6.0			
Upper body:				
53 Put on pullover garment	5.0			
Fasteners				
Unfastening:				
54 Button: front	3.0			
55 side	3.0			
56 back	5.6			
57 Zipper: front	3.3			
58 separating front	3.6			
59 back	4.9			
60 Buckle: belt	3.9			
61 shoe	3.9			
62 Tie: back sash	5.0			

Figure 2–39 *Continued*

Illustration continued on the following page.

Key to Scoring: 4 Independent
3 Independent with equipment and/or adaptive technique
2 Completes but cannot accomplish in practical time
1 Attempts but requires assistance or supervision to complete
0 Dependent—cannot attempt activity
– Not applicable

The *Year-Month* vertical column represents the Order of Developmental Sequence or approximate age when the child accomplishes the activity: the horizontal column represents the chronological age of the child being assessed.

VISIT NUMBER			1	2	3
DATE					
		YR.–MO.			
Fasten:		*Order of Dev. Seq.*	R L	R L	R L
63	Button: large front	2.6			
64	series	3.6			
65	back	6.3			
66	Zipper: front, lock tab	4.0			
67	separating front	4.6			
68	back	5.6			
69	Buckle: belt	4.0			
70	shoe	4.0			
71	insert belt in loops	4.6			
72	Tie: front	6.0			
73	back	8.0			
74	neck tie	10.0			
75	Snaps: front	3.0			
76	back	6.0			

Figure 2–39   *Continued*

PHOTOGRAPHIC RECORDING

Photography is a useful adjunct to recording changes in posture as the child develops (Fig. 2–40). Gait and movement are best recorded by motion pictures, and I have found that the Super-8 movie camera is most efficient and least costly. The surgeon or his assistant can easily take motion pictures. Generally, 100 feet of film per child per year is sufficient for the clinical record. Super-8 film can be optically transferred to 16 mm film if special films are desired for teaching. The major disadvantage of motion picture recording is the need to splice serial films of one patient into sequence. For research, slow-motion pictures can be made with phonosonic cameras.

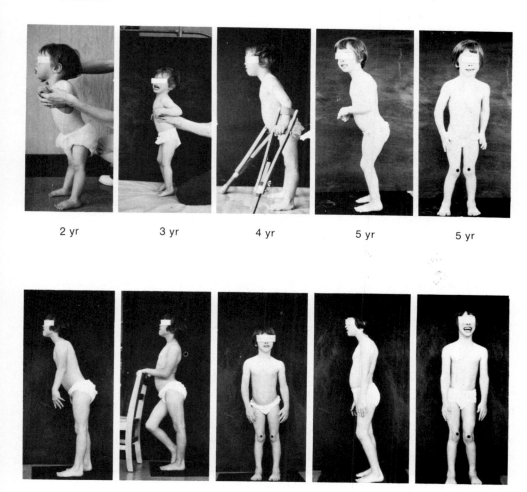

| 2 yr | 3 yr | 4 yr | 5 yr | 5 yr |

| 7 yr | 7 yr | 7 yr | 8 yr | 8 yr |

Figure 2–40 Photographs taken at various ages to show the progressive postural problems of a child who has spastic diplegia. This series of photographs shows the persistence of a hip flexion deformity and of hip internal rotation. After bilateral derotation subtrochanteric femoral osteotomies at age 10.5 years, her hip flexion deformity increased and, to compensate for this and remain erect, knee flexion contractures developed (see Chapter 6, Spastic Diplegia, for an analysis of this problem and its prevention).

Illustration continued on the following page.

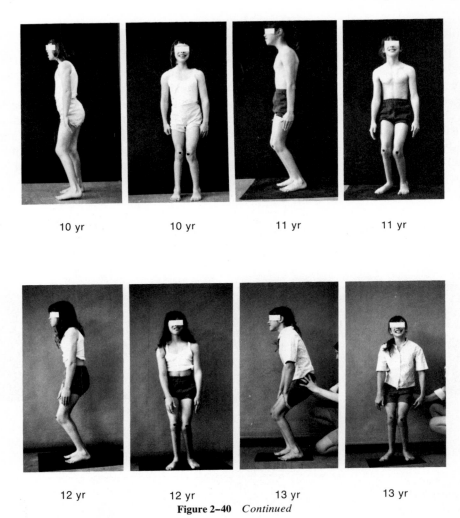

| 10 yr | 10 yr | 11 yr | 11 yr |

| 12 yr | 12 yr | 13 yr | 13 yr |

Figure 2–40 *Continued*

Videotape recordings of gait and motion permit immediate review. Their major disadvantages include the need to splice tapes depicting serial development and the tendency to shoot more footage of tape than is necessary. While display of video-tapes is feasible for teaching large audiences, the technology has not yet been widely accepted by scientific academies. It appears, however, that the use of videotape cassettes is gaining acceptance and may ultimately replace the standard 16 mm film that has enjoyed widespread use in teaching. Television is now being used more extensively in laboratories investigating gait patterns.

We have used photographic recording of the light trajectories formed during gait when small colored lights (BP 2/60 2 AMP/MURA) are placed on the target areas of the body (Fig. 2–41): the head, shoulder (tip of the acromion), wrist (dorsum of the distal radius), pelvis (anterior superior iliac spine), distal lateral thigh, lateral malleo-lus of the ankle, and fifth metatarsal head. The patient walks at a set distance from a camera with a wide-angle (28 mm) lens. A time exposure is made to record the light

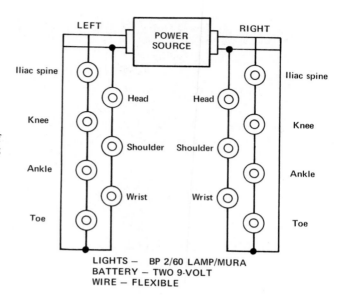

Figure 2-41 Arrangement of lights on target areas for recording light patterns during gait cycle.

trajectories on high-speed film (Ektachrome ASA 160) during gait. Measurements made on the resulting color transparencies can be used to determine the vertical displacement of the body during gait; the normal light pattern is that of the sinusoidal curve made by the center of gravity of the body during walking (Saunders et al., 1953). The highs and lows of this curve can be related to the swing and stance phases of gait (Aptekar et al., 1976) (Fig. 2-42 through 2-44). Because the amount of vertical displacement of the center of gravity is an indication of the efficiency and function of the pelvic and lower limb determinants of walking, this light pattern provides a simple, inexpensive, and easily stored record from which the status of the patient's

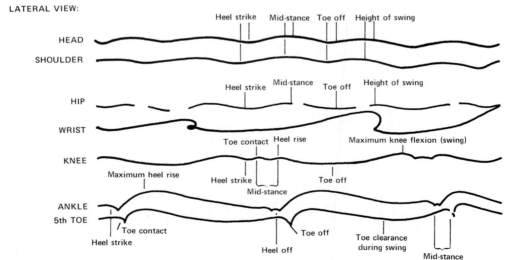

Figure 2-42 A light pattern of a normal child's gait. Note smooth sinusoidal curve of head as gait progresses. The phases of the gait cycle are labeled on the drawing.

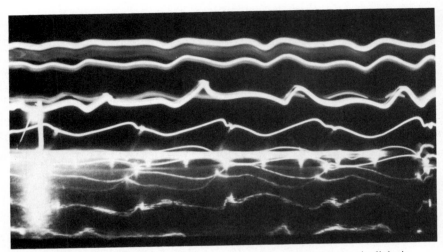

Figure 2–43   Preoperative light pattern of gait of a child with spastic diplegia.

walking pattern can be judged. This method is capable of measuring only one aspect of walking. It can be used to determine the effects of treatment on the gait pattern of the child (Ford et al., 1976) (Fig. 2–45). The patient's progress, lack of progress, or retrogression during treatment and over a period of years can be recorded, and decisions regarding treatment can be made accordingly. A more sophisticated method of measuring light patterns of the limbs and trunk during gait uses light-emitting diodes on target areas that are followed by special cameras linked to an x–y coordinate system and computerization (Selspot, Selcom Electronic Inc., P.O. Box 100, Valdese, N.C.).

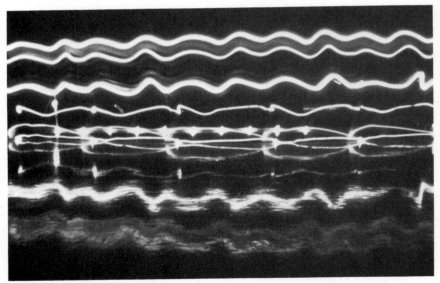

Figure 2–44   Postoperative light pattern of the child shown in Figure 2–43 after iliopsoas recession and hamstring lengthening. Note that, although the pattern of the head trajectory is more regular, the peaks and valleys of the curve are greater, indicating the possibility of more energy expenditure. The exaggerated sinusoidal curve of the head probably indicates more quadriceps activity, after hamstring lengthening. There is a resultant loss of the knee flexion function during early swing, causing a more compass-like, or vaulting, gait.

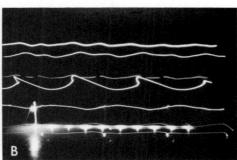

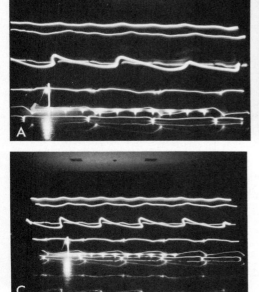

Figure 2-45 A light pattern of gait before, during, and after drug therapy designed to reduce spasticity. A. Pre-Dantrolene. B. On Dantrolene. C. Six weeks off Dantrolene.

PEDOGRAPHS

Another simple and inexpensive way to record and measure some elements of gait is to measure footprints during walking. The method comprises a number of steps. First, dip the patient's feet in a pan of finely ground charcoal powder. He then walks on a strip of white paper 5 meters long and 1 meter wide; a mirror is placed beyond the end of the paper pathway (about 2 meters) so the patient may watch his progress. The patient should continue to walk off the end of the paper and onto the floor so that walking speed and pattern are not distorted. From the resultant foot-prints, the extent of foot contact at mid-stance (consistent toe-walking will be evident) and toed-in or toed-out gait may be observed. Measurements are made according to the technique of Chodera and Levell (1973) that relates measurements to the continually changing direction of walking (for details, see Appendix A). The following information can be obtained: (1) step length—the toe-to-toe distance between two successive footprints of the lower limbs, either right-to-left or left-to-right; (2) stride length — a toe-to-toe distance between two successive footprints of the same foot; (3) distance from heel-to-heel; and (4) angle of foot placement. Footprint analysis can be used to determine the efficacy of treatment programs designed for a specific purpose, e.g., elimination of equinus deformity, correction of in-toeing, narrowing of the base of the gait. We have used pedographs as one of several measurements in drug therapy evaluation (Ford et al., 1976) (Fig. 2–46).

ELECTROMYOGRAPHIC EXAMINATIONS

Electromyographic examinations of muscle function during gait and the accom-panying measurements of gait sequences are proving more and more valuable. In

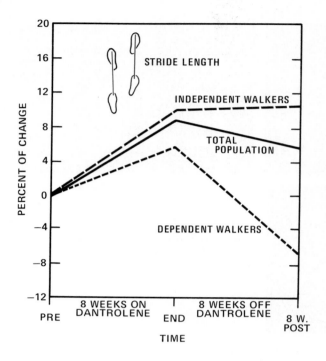

Figure 2–46. Pedographic analysis of stride length (toe to toe) to assess the results of drug therapy.

difficult gait problems, in which surgical decision-making may be compromised because of inadequate information or inability to examine the muscles responsible for the gait problem, electromyographic examination in a motion analysis laboratory can be helpful (Sutherland and Hagy, 1972; Perry et al., 1974, 1976; Simon, 1976). Our own technique consists of an electromyographic FM/FM telemetry system. The child wears a central transmitter and the receiver-recorder unit is placed in a remote location (range 30 meters). Any number of channels may be used (four to eight seem most practical at any one time). To record muscle activity, miniature bipotential skin electrodes or needle electrodes (50 μm nylon-shielded copper wire) are used. Skin electrodes record only mass muscle activity, whereas needle electrodes record activity of the isolated muscle. Each has its use, depending upon the needs of the study. Without question, needle electrodes are the more accurate of the two. Their main disadvantage is that most children (and many adults) are needle-shy. The surface electrode recordings are fed into an isolation amplifier to reduce artifacts.

To record the sequences of the gait cycle, foot switches that respond to contact are placed under the heel and under the plantar aspects of the heads of the first and fifth metatarsals (Fig. 2–47). These switches record different voltages via one channel of the transmitter and are recorded simultaneously with the muscle action potentials on an oscillograph using light-sensitive paper. The resultant record can then be measured, and the data thus obtained can be analyzed. The graphic data generated (analog) can also be fed directly into a computer for which an appropriate program has been written, thus converting the patterns to digital data, which can be reconstituted into graphic form by a similarly programmed computer (Fig. 2–48). These techniques are continuously undergoing refinement.

Another system of sophisticated gait analysis has been developed by Sutherland and Hagy (1972). This method combines high-speed three-dimensional motion pic-

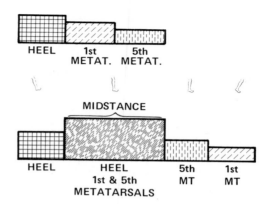

Figure 2–47 Foot switch patterns to record phases of gait electrically. Top drawing shows the individual markings of the heel, first metatarsal and fifth metatarsal. The lower drawing shows how, when the foot switch contacts are combined, the phases of gait during stance can be defined from the graphic record.

tures that are correlated with the electromyographic data with computer measurement of limb and pelvic motions and with additional information from a force plate that measures foot-to-floor reactions. Simon (1976) has designed a similar system with the addition of a graphic stick figure display of the movements of the trunk and lower limbs during gait progression.

As research tools, all of these methods have enhanced our knowledge of muscle function and deformity in cerebral palsy. The art has progressed to the state at which it has become a practical clinical tool for surgical decision-making in selected cases. The validity of a number of clinical examination techniques has been questioned while that of others has been verified. For example, the straight leg raising test does isolate hamstring spasticity (Perry et al., 1976). Consequently it might be hasty to

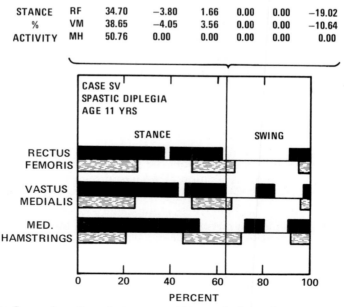

Figure 2–48 Conversion of an electromyographic record of a patient with spastic diplegia into digital form and then into graphic display. The shaded areas represent normal phasic contraction of the muscles recorded; the black areas indicate the spastic muscles.

conclude that *every* patient will need an electromyographic examination before a surgical judgment can be made. The need for such analysis exists only in selected cases.

With the rise and fall of the center of gravity during gait, potential energy is converted into kinetic energy by muscle contraction. Muscle function during normal level gait has been studied in many laboratories. A graphic display of normal muscle function during gait, reproduced in Figure 2–49, can be seen to consist of only short bursts of activity. The hip flexors begin to contract near the end of stance so that the leg can move quickly to the swing phase. During initial swing, knee flexion is necessary for toe clearance. The knee flexors relax at terminal swing. All the hamstrings act to decelerate the hip and then the knee. The soleus muscle is about twice the size of the gastrocnemius; these two muscles prevent forward acceleration of the calf during stance and thus restrain dorsiflexion of the ankle. Of all the plantar flexors, the posterior tibial and peroneals are the least efficient and serve mainly as restrainers. A large part of plantar flexion during terminal stance is due not to muscle action but rather to a rolling action on the plantar surface of the foot (Perry, 1975). These brief comments are pertinent to surgical procedures and orthotics designed to improve muscle function during gait. In the following chapters, specific surgical procedures are described and there is additional discussion on the subject of muscle function.

MEASUREMENT OF BALANCE

We have used strain gauges in foot plates that measure the vertical displacement of the body in various standing and tilted positions. The electrical output from these gauges is then amplified, graphically displayed by an oscilloscope, and converted to digital output that is reconverted to graphic display with the aid of a computer (Fig. 2–50). Piezoelectric force plates have been used for similar purposes (Murray et al., 1975). These data should help determine the degree of dysequilibrium in the patient. In this way an important neurological determinant of postural problems in cerebral palsy can be analyzed in the follow-up of treatment methods and in the development of the child.

MYONEURAL BLOCKS

When the physician is in doubt about the possible effects of surgical treatment or about whether temporary relaxation of a spastic muscle is desired in dynamic deformities (e.g., equinus), a myoneural block of the muscle is useful. The agents most commonly used are local anesthetics (lidocaine), alcohol, and phenol.

Local anesthetics injected directly into muscle bellies reduce the stretch reflex, presumably by altering the sensitivity of the muscle spindle receptors. Generally,

---

Figure 2–49 Normal electromyographic data of the phasic contraction of lower limb muscles during gait. (Redrawn from Mann, R., and Hagy, J., Shriner's Hospital for Crippled Children, San Francisco.)

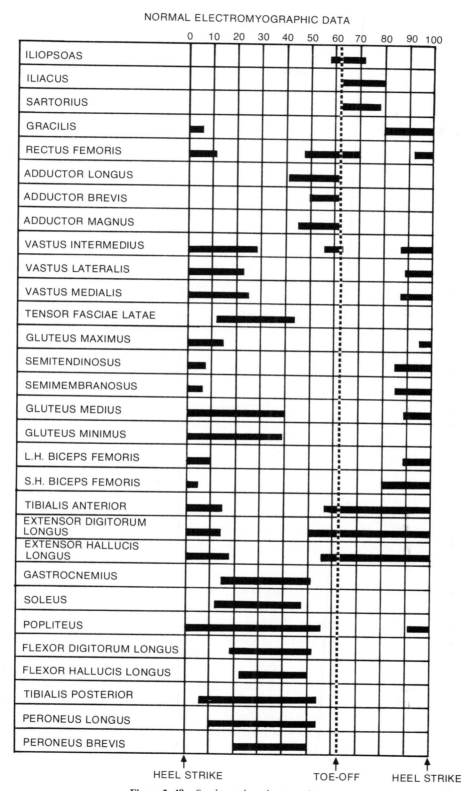

NORMAL ELECTROMYOGRAPHIC DATA

Figure 2–49 *See legend on the opposite page*

POSITION 1

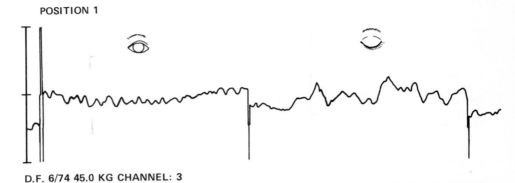

D.F. 6/74 45.0 KG CHANNEL: 3

Figure 2–50 Graphic display of electrical activity recorded with patient standing on strain gauges, with eyes first open and then closed, to measure postural sway and postural adjustment ability.

children do not take well to needles, and local anesthetics often cause dizziness. By the time the procedure is finished the child is frequently too upset to walk and leaves the clinic; since the block wears off in an hour or two, there is insufficient time for an accurate assessment. Adolescents and adults generally respond better than children to local anesthetic myoneural blocks. It is possible that the newer longer-acting local anesthetics such as bupivacaine (Marcaine) will permit a better analysis of the effects of paralyzing a specific muscle in the limb.

In children I prefer to employ a neurolytic agent that has longer effects. We have used 45 percent ethyl alcohol (sterile alcohol for injection is available) (Hariga, 1966; Carpenter, 1972). Under brief general anesthesia the muscle belly is infiltrated with a needle and syringe in two or three locations, with 3 to 4 ml of the alcohol injected in each location. This technique is applicable to muscles close to the surface: the gastrocnemius, hip adductors, medial hamstrings, and biceps brachii (Fig. 2–51). This type of block has been performed on outpatients; hospital admission is not ordinarily required. The effects of the block last from 2 to 6 weeks; thus, the parents, the physical therapist, the patient, and the physician have time to observe them. In children who have a dynamic spastic equinus foot, the relief of the deformity may be permanent. The explanation for this desired result may be that, when the extensor gait pattern is broken, stimulation of the heel pad occurs, and phasic dorsiflexion results because the heel pad is the tonic reflex area for this function (Duncan, 1960).

A myoneural block is contraindicated if contracture of the muscle is present. At times the only way to differentiate a contracture from spasticity is to examine the patient under general anesthesia. We have used these blocks in children who have equinus deformity without contracture but who cannot tolerate an ankle-foot orthosis in the prewalking stage of development. Among approximately 50 patients we have had only one temporary complication. The patient had a post-injection peroneal nerve paralysis from which she completely recovered in 3 months. Carpenter (1972) reported no complications in 35 patients. Biopsies of hip adductor muscles after alcohol blocks have shown no histological changes in the area of injection.

Phenol is another effective blocking agent and has short-term (local anesthetic) and long-term (destructive) effects on nerve tissue. Nerve fibers of all diameters are destroyed. Phenol blocks can effectively relieve spasticity from 6 months to more

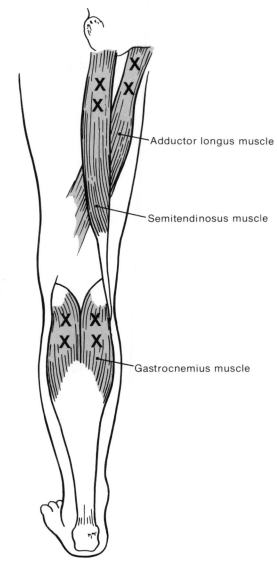

Adductor longus muscle

Semitendinosus muscle

Gastrocnemius muscle

Figure 2–51 Sites of injection for myoneural blocks with 45 percent alcohol. Caution: when injecting into the lateral head of the gastrocnemius, do not go proximal to the mark shown in the drawing. The peroneal nerve crosses the proximal lateral part of the lateral gastrocnemius head and thus may be inadvertently blocked.

than a year. We have not used phenol because, as Herman (1976) pointed out, it is difficult to control the degree of tissue destruction, and direct injection of perineural tissue (open surgical exposure) may cause marked overactivity of the associated muscles. Furthermore, inadvertent subcutaneous injection of phenol may cause skin to slough.

REFERENCES

Abercrombie, M. L. J. (1964) *Perceptual and Visuo-motor Disorders in Cerebral Palsy*, London, William Heinemann Medical Books.
Aptekar, R. G., Ford, F., and Bleck, E. E. (1976) Light patterns as a means of assessing and recording

gait—I: methods and results in normal children. *Developmental Medicine and Child Neurology* 18:31–36.

Aptekar, R. G., Ford, F., and Bleck, E. E. (1976) Light patterns as a means of assessing and recording gait—II: results in children with cerebral palsy. *Developmental Medicine and Child Neurology* 18:37–40.

Ayeres, J. (1972) *Sensory Integration and Learning Disorders,* Los Angeles, Western Psychological Services.

Balmar, G. A., and MacEwen, G. D. (1970) The incidence of scoliosis in cerebral palsy. *Journal of Bone and Joint Surgery* 52B:134–136.

Bleck, E. E. (1971) The shoeing of children: sham or science? *Developmental Medicine and Child Neurology* 13:188–195.

Bleck, E. E. (1975) Locomotor prognosis in cerebral palsy. *Developmental Medicine and Child Neurology* 17:18–25.

Bleck, E. E., Ford, F., Stevik, A. C., and Cosongradi, J. (1975) EMG telemetry study of spastic gait patterns in cerebral palsied children (abstract). *Developmental Medicine and Child Neurology* 17:307.

Bobath, B. (1954) A study of abnormal reflex activity in patients with lesions of the central nervous system. *Physiotherapy,* Sept–Dec:1–30.

Brunnstrom, S. (1962) *Clinical Kinesiology,* Philadelphia, F. A. Davis.

Carpenter, E. B., and Miklail, M. (1972) The use of intramuscular alcohol as a diagnostic and therapeutic aid in cerebral palsy. *Developmental Medicine and Child Neurology* 14:113–114.

Chodera, J. D., and Levell, R. W. (1973) Footprint patterns during walking. *Perspectives in Biomedical Engineering* (Ed. Kennedy, E. M.), Baltimore, University Park Press.

Cupps, C., Plescia, M. G., and Houser, C. (1976) The Landau reaction: a clinical and electromyographic analysis. *Developmental Medicine and Child Neurology* 18:41–53.

Duncan, W. R. (1960) Tonic reflexes of the foot. *Journal of Bone and Joint Surgery* 42A:859–869.

Evans, E. B. (1975) The knee in cerebral palsy. *Orthopedic Aspects of Cerebral Palsy* (Ed. Samilson, R. L.), Philadelphia, J. B. Lippincott.

Ford, F., Bleck, E. E., Aptekar, R. G., Collins, F. J., and Stevick, D. (1976) Efficacy of dantrolene sodium in the treatment of spastic cerebral palsy. *Developmental Medicine and Child Neurology* 18:770–783.

Frostig, M. (1963) Visual perceptual development and school adjustment programs. *American Journal of Orthopsychiatry* 33:367–368.

Frostig, M. (1964) *The Frostig Program for Development of Visual Perception* (Ed. Houne, D.), Chicago, Follett.

Gesell, A., and Amatruda, C. S. (1947) *Developmental Diagnosis,* 2nd Ed., New York, Hoeber Division of Harper and Row.

Goldner, J. L. (1974) Upper extremity tendon transfer in cerebral palsy. *Orthopedic Clinics of North America* 5:389–411.

Gunsolus, P., Welsh, C., and Houser, C. (1975) Equilibrium reactions in the feet of children with spastic cerebral palsy and of normal children. *Developmental Medicine and Child Neurology* 17:580–591.

Hagberg, B., Sanner, G., and Steen, M. (1972) The dysequilibrium syndrome in cerebral palsy. *Acta Paediatrica Scandinavica (Supplement)* 226:1–63.

Hariga, J. (1966) Influences sur la motricité de la suppression des effecteurs gamma par alcoalisation des nerfs périphériques. *Acta Neurologica Belgica* 66:607–711.

Herman, R. (1976) Postural control and therapeutic implications. *The Advance in Orthotics,* London, Edward Arnold.

Keats, S. (1965) *Cerebral Palsy,* Springfield, Illinois, Charles C Thomas.

Kelley, D. L. (1971) *Kinesiology,* Englewood Cliffs, New Jersey, Prentice–Hall.

Murray, M. P., Wood, A. A. S., and Sepic, S. B. (1975) Normal postural stability and steadiness: quantitative assessment. *Journal of Bone and Joint Surgery* 57A:510–516.

Paine, R. (1966) *Neurological Examination of Children,* London, William Heinemann Medical Books.

Perlstein, M. D., and Barnett, H. E. (1952) Natural history and recognition of cerebral palsy in infants. *Journal of the American Medical Association* 148:1389–1397.

Perlstein, M. D. (1960–1966) Lectures in cerebral palsy, American Academy for Cerebral Palsy.

Perry, J. (1967) The mechanics of walking. *Physical Therapy* 117:778–804.

Perry, J., Hoffer, M., Giovan, P., Antonelli, D., and Greenberg, R. (1974) Gait analysis of the triceps surae in cerebral palsy. *Journal of Bone and Joint Surgery* 56A:511–520.

Perry, J. (1975) Lecture notes from Gait Analysis Conference, San Diego.

Perry, J. (1975) Cerebral palsy gait. *Orthopaedic Aspects of Cerebral Palsy* (Ed. Samilson, R. L.), Philadelphia, J. B. Lippincott.

Perry, J., Hoffer, M., Antonelli, D., Plut, J., Lewis, G., and Greenberg, R. (1976) Electromyography before and after surgery for hip deformity in children with cerebral palsy. *Journal of Bone and Joint Surgery* 58A:201–208.

Robson, P. (1968) The prevalence of scoliosis in adolescents and young adults with cerebral palsy. *Developmental Medicine and Child Neurology* 10:447–452.

Rushworth, G. (1964) *The Role of the Gamma System in Movement and Posture,* New York, Association for the Aid of Crippled Children.

Samilson, R. L., and Bechard, R. (1973) Scoliosis in cerebral palsy. *Current Practice in Orthopaedic Surgery,* St. Louis, C. V. Mosby Company.

Saunders, J. B., Dec, M., Inman, V. T., and Eberhart, H. D. (1953) The major determinants in normal and pathological gait. *Journal of Bone and Joint Surgery* 35A:543–558.

Silverskiöld, N. (1924) Reduction of the uncrossed two joint muscles of the one-to-one muscle in spastic conditions. *Acta Chirurgica Scandinavica* 56:313–330.

Simon, S. (1976) Genu recurvatum in spastic cerebral palsy. (Abstract of paper read at the annual meeting of the American Academy for Cerebral Palsy and Developmental Medicine, 1976.) *Developmental Medicine and Child Neurology* 19:119.

Staheli, L. T., and Engel, G. M. (1972) Tibial torsion, a method of assessment and a survey of normal children. *Clinical Orthopaedics* 86:183–186.

Staheli, L. (1977) The prone hip extension test. *Clinical Orthopaedics* 123:1215.

Sutherland, D. H., and Hagy, J. L. (1972) Measurement of gait movements from motion picture films. *Journal of Bone and Joint Surgery* 54A:787–797.

FURTHER READING

Andre-Thomas, Chesni, Y., and Dargassies, S. S. (1960) *The Neurological Examination of the Infant,* London, National Spastics Society.

Beintema, D. J. (1968) *A Neurological Study of Newborn Infants,* London, William Heinemann Medical Books.

Bobarth, K. (1966) *The Motor Deficit in Patients With Cerebral Palsy,* London, William Heinemann Medical Books.

Cahuzac, M. (1977) *L'Enfant Infirme Moteur d'Origine Cérébrale,* Paris, Masson.

Denhoff, E. (1960) *Cerebral Palsy and Related Disorders,* New York, McGraw–Hill.

Denhoff, E. (1967) *Cerebral Palsy – The Preschool Years,* Springfield, Ill., Charles C Thomas.

Holt, K. S. (1965) *Assessment of Cerebral Palsy,* London, Lloyd–Luke.

Keats, S. (1965) *Cerebral Palsy,* Springfield, Ill., Charles C Thomas.

Paine, R. S., and Oppe, T. E. (1966) *Neurological Examination of Children,* London, William Heinemann Medical Books.

Samilson, R. L., Ed. (1975) *Orthopaedic Aspects of Cerebral Palsy.* Philadelphia, J. B. Lippincott.

Chapter Three

NEUROBIOLOGY, PROGNOSIS, AND STRUCTURAL CHANGES

NEUROBIOLOGY

To gain perspective in prognosis and methods of treatment of patients with cerebral palsy (or "static encephalopathy," the term preferred by neurologists), clinicians might review some of the highlights of contemporary neurobiology. Those who wish more in-depth knowledge should consult the references listed at the end of this chapter.

Human Brain Development

The human brain develops in rapid growth spurts. The changes in the brain are so accelerated that they have been compared to driving a car on the highway: the greater the rate of acceleration, the greater the stress on the controlling mechanism, and the greater the chance for disaster when these mechanisms are blocked or sidetracked (Neligan, 1974). Dendritic ramifications commence just after birth. By 6 months of age the rate of growth of dendritic processes is striking. Up to 15 months, the dendrites increase in size and length but not in number. By the age of 2 years neuronal differentiation is essentially complete. After 2 years this growth continues but at a considerably reduced rate (Schade and Von Groenigen, 1961). Experimental retardation of neuronal growth in rats by treatment with corticosteroids clearly demonstrated the mechanism causing the halting of dendritic expansion during the rapid growth phase; this stunting of dendritic growth at a crucial stage of development appears to be incapable of recovery (Oda and Huttenlocker, 1974).

The brain regions do not develop synchronously (Dobbing and Sands, 1973). The most rapid phase of cell multiplication in the forebrain is complete by 18 weeks of gestation. Cell growth and myelination continue rapidly until about the age of 3 years. Cerebellar growth starts about halfway through gestation and is complete by about 18 months of age.

Neuroplasticity*

The ability of the central nervous system to recover from injury is of special interest to clinicians and therapists. The work of Cajal (1928), and later of Windle (1956) and Clement (1964), strongly indicated that the nervous system degenerated *irreversibly* after specific injury.

Despite this experimental evidence that brain degeneration is a *fait accompli,* we do know that some humans do recover from brain injury but only to a limited extent. Even in the nineteenth century, it was recognized that patients often recovered dramatically from strokes (Rosen, 1974). We can conclude from these clinical observations that there is some process that accounts for changes in the central nervous system (sometimes over the course of years) and for the subsequent recovery of lost functions.

MECHANISM OF RECOVERY

In order to reconcile the fact that patients do recover from brain injury despite anatomical data showing lack of regeneration, much experimental work has been done to attempt to explain how uninjured parts of the brain might compensate for lost function (Rosner, 1974). An extreme view was that of Lashley (1938), who proposed the theory of "equipotentiality" or "mass action." He rejected the idea of localization of function in the brain and advocated the idea that it was the mass of brain tissue removed, not its location, that determined the permanence of functional deficits due to injury. Other schools of thought emphasized the ability of the uninjured parts of the nervous system to alter their function (Brodal, 1969), to substitute behavioral tricks to minimize the functional deficit (Sperry, 1947), or to take over lost functions (Kennard, 1938).

Two specific mechanisms of compensation have been proposed and can be supported by experimental data:

1. *Denervation supersensitivity.* The denervated peripheral nervous system structures and muscles are hyper-reactive to the remaining innervation (Sharpless, 1964).
2. *Collateral sprouting of neurons.* Uninjured neuronal axons sprout extra or "collateral" connections with denervated structures (Edds, 1953; Liu and Chambers, 1958).

Circumstantial evidence that both these mechanisms contribute to recovery of function in humans has been reported (McCouch, 1961; Goldberger, 1974; Moore, 1974; Wall and Egger, 1971). However, neither of these mechanisms adequately explains the recovery process.

RECOVERY IN IMMATURE NERVOUS SYSTEMS

It has long been known that lesions in young and immature nervous systems do not provoke symptoms that are as severe as those in adults. Based upon evidence

---

*Abstracted from lecture notes published by Wise Young, M.D., Ph.D.

of the greater regenerative ability of lower vertebrates such as amphibia and reptiles, it has been assumed that the immature nervous system is more "plastic" than that of the adult (Kerr, 1975). This assumption has been refuted by recent research: the immature nervous system is much less "plastic" than was originally thought (Goldman, 1972, 1974; Lawrence and Hopkins, 1972; Berman and Berman, 1973). Recovery apparently occurred not so much by regeneration of lost neural mechanisms as by the early development of behavioral maneuvers that masked the less specific motor functions. Thus, evidence is lacking that infant nervous systems will regenerate central pathways or have greater degrees of collateral axonal sprouting, or develop more denervation supersensitivity than in the adult. The data indicate that damage to the nervous system during its periods of rapid growth may result in more destruction of ultimate function than will injury during the more stable phases of brain development (Teuber, 1971, Goldman, 1972, 1974; Schneider and Jhavery, 1974; Neligan, 1974; Goldberger, 1974; Brunner and Altman, 1974).

MASKING OF NEUROLOGICAL DEFICITS

Spectacular examples of the degree to which specific neurological deficits are masked abound in the clinical and experimental literature (Geschwind, 1974). Cases of near normal behavior attained after hemispherectomies, and of normal speech after repeated ablations of the speech cortex, have been reported; recovery occurred despite demonstrations of a lack of significant healing processes in these brains. Despite these examples of dramatic recovery, there are many patients who do not recover from neural damage. Small lesions have produced large functional deficits. What are the possible reasons for this result? Experiments suggest that function is often recovered but that the recovery process may be inhibited by the remaining intact system. If a single limb in a monkey is deafferentated by cutting the dorsal spinal root nerves, permanent impairment of all spontaneous limb movement results (Mott and Sherrington, 1895; Lassek, 1953; Twitchell, 1954). In addition, reflex activity unrelated to dorsal root sensory nerves is impaired, e.g., static labyrinthine reflexes (Denny-Brown, 1966). If both limbs of the monkey are deafferentated, the use of the limbs is recovered spontaneously (Knapp et al., 1963; Taub and Berman, 1968). In an animal in which the dorsal root afferent nerves are cut to only one limb and the opposite limb is restricted in motion, recovery of the deafferentated limb is enhanced. With this evidence we might conclude that the forced use of the deafferentated asensory limb discouraged disuse and encouraged recovery, or that the intact sensory system in the normal limb selectively inhibited recovery in the deafferentated limb (Taub et al., 1973).

In the motor system similar phenomena have been observed in pyramidal tract lesions; recovery is enhanced by secondary lesions of the contralateral hemisphere (Bard, 1938; Semmes and Chow, 1955) and of the ventrolateral funiculus of the spinal cord (Goldberger, 1969). These findings imply that an inhibitory process exists within the contralateral hemisphere. Amphetamines might improve recovery by suppressing some of these inhibitory cortical areas (Beck and Chambers, 1970).

Classic and operant conditioning methods can achieve near normal function in deafferentated limbs (Taub et al., 1966; Bossom and Ommaya, 1968). Liu and Chambers (1971) demonstrated that monkeys could be trained to perform accurate and complicated maneuvers with their deafferentated limbs without visual guidance.

Further, these maneuvers were performed with little or no feedback from the limb. Thus, training methods "unmasked" latent abilities in the central nervous system.

THERAPEUTIC IMPLICATIONS

Certainly, these findings have therapeutic implications for the child with cerebral palsy. The cautious therapist must note that, although these monkeys performed well under test conditions, in the presence of conditioned stimuli they often exhibited little improvement in spontaneous behavior (Goldberger, 1974). For example, a monkey in which only the pyramidal tract cortex has been preserved may be trained to feed itself or to grasp an object if the conditioned stimulus is applied but is unable to perform the task voluntarily. Conditioned motor behavior is patterned and therefore may be inaccessible to cortical volition in the presence of cortical damage. Hepp-Reymond et al. (1970) showed that conditioned behavior remains unchanged despite extensive cortical and pyramidal tract lesions. Although evidence for the localization of conditioned behavior in the brain is speculative, it is clear that behavior is influenced by lesions in the cerebellum (Growden et al., 1967).

BRAIN STEM SYSTEM ADAPTATION

Eye movements and vestibular reflexes are functions of the brain stem motor system, and recently they have been shown to be capable of a remarkable degree of adaptation. The vestibulo-ocular reflex can be easily altered by chronic visual input training with inverted prisms (Gonshor and Melvill–Jones, 1976). In humans (Gonshor and Melvill–Jones, 1976a and b) and other animals (Miles and Fuller, 1974; Robinson, 1976) eye movements could be induced to change from the normal reflexive direction to the opposite direction after a few days of training with inverted prisms. It has long been known that lesions of the vestibular system that occur with unilateral labyrinthectomies or neuronitis are readily compensated for because symptoms disappear in a few days. As with conditioned motor behavior, the brain stem motor systems are largely independent of cortical control and are influenced by lesions of the cerebellum and cerebellar nuclei (Llinas et al., 1975; Robinson, 1976).

SUMMARY OF NEUROPLASTICITY

Research to date is still at a relatively primitive stage. However, it is clear that regeneration plays a minor role in the recovery of the nervous system from disease or injury (Guth, 1975; Kerr, 1975). Recovery of the nervous system appears to result from compensation by the uninjured parts of the system. Recent experimental studies suggest the following:

1. The immature nervous system, though more adaptive, is no more "plastic" than the adult system.
2. The recovery process may be actively inhibited by the remaining uninjured brain.

3. Behavioral conditioning can restore motor function at the subcortical level.
4. Certain brain stem motor systems, such as the vestibulo-ocular reflexes, are quite malleable.

Motor Behavior

Clinical studies on locomotor prognosis (Crothers and Paine, 1959; Beals, 1966; Bleck, 1975) have hinted that certain kinds of motor behavior, such as walking, are dependent upon a purely central nervous system arrangement. The dominant view well into the 1950's was that locomotion was the result of sensory receptors in the sole of the foot and knee joint capsule that elicited a cross extension response (Kennedy, 1976). This concept has been radically changed. Experimental data strongly suggest that there are certain built-in circuits in the brain that are not dependent upon sensations from the periphery. The first of these experiments was reported by Wilson (1968), who studied the flight control system of the locust. Wilson cut all the sensory nerves to the wings and then stimulated the central nervous system with a noise pattern. With the noise patterns he obtained replicas of the flight pattern from the motor neurons. Thus, for the locust, flight was a "motor score" written in the brain with no need for direct stimulation from the wings. Shik et al. (1966) provided further evidence that sensory input to modulate locomotion in the cat was unnecessary. These workers prepared mesencephalic cats by surgical decerebration and then applied gradations of electrical current to the remaining brain. With varying degrees of electrical stimulation the cats walked, trotted, and ran. Again, this experiment indicates the presence of a center in the brain for locomotion where the "music" has been genetically written and need only be "turned on."

Before we leap into the possible argument of "nature versus nurture," experimental data suggest that environment does play a "fine tuning" role. One example is the experiment of Held and Hein (1963), who placed kittens in a circular room in which the walls were painted with stripes. One kitten was linked to the other by an apparatus in which one kitten walked and pulled the other kitten in a gondola. Thus, there was constant visual stimulation for both, and a comparison between active and passive movement influence was possible. The kittens spent 3 hours per day in the apparatus; the remainder of the day was spent in total darkness. After 30 hours of this trial, the kitten that walked and pulled the gondola showed normal responses to visually guided tasks, blinked when approached by an object, had placing reactions when dropped downward, and avoided the steep side of a cliff. The passive kitten who rode in the gondola at first failed to show any of these normal behaviors but eventually recovered. Other experiments have demonstrated the need for active movement to integrate visual motor control mechanisms. These data demonstrate that self-controlled movement (i.e., active vs. passive exercise) is probably critical in human infant development (Conolly, 1969).

MOTOR PROGNOSIS

Walking Prognosis Tests

In one study (Bleck, 1975) the seven tests for infantile automatism and postural reflexes described in Chapter 2 were performed on non-ambulatory children after the age of 12 months. These tests (Bleck, 1975; Fiorentino, 1963) are: (1) asymmetrical tonic neck reflex (ATNR); (2) neck righting reflex (NR); (3) Moro reflex (MR); (4) symmetrical tonic neck reflex (STNR); (5) parachute reaction (PR); (6) extensor thrust (ET); and (7) foot placement reaction (FPR).

When an infantile automatism or reflex was definitely present (ATNR, NR, MR, STNR, ET) or absent (FPR and PR), a score of one point was recorded. A score of two points or more gave a poor prognosis for walking, a one-point score led to a guarded prognosis, and a zero score indicated a good prognosis.

The results were assessed after the child had passed the seventh year. To qualify as walkers, children had to walk a minimum of 15 meters without falling. Those who could walk only with crutches were also considered functional walkers in the study. Children who walked only with the aid of mobility devices or only in parallel bars were not considered walkers. The accuracy of the predictions was 94.5 per cent.

AGE OF WALKING

In our study we observed that ambulation ability reaches a plateau by the age of 7 years. Crothers and Paine's (1959) data on walking ability are similar (Fig. 3–1). Beals (1966) indicated the same lack of walking ability after the age of 7. Hemiplegic children all walked between the ages of 18 and 21 months. Most spastic diplegic children walked by 48 months. Quadriplegic children (those with total body involvement) had the poorest prognosis.

IMPLICATIONS

The ability to make a reasonably accurate prediction about walking allows the orthopaedist to delay surgery merely to force the child to walk and reduces the role

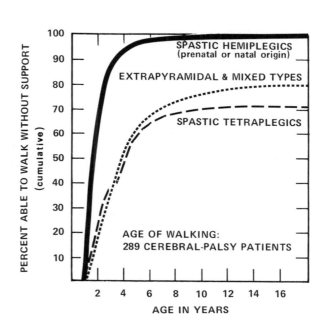

Figure 3–1 Percent of cerebral palsied patients able to walk according to age. Note that ability to begin walking ceases for all groups at about age 7 years. (Redrawn from Crothers, B., and Paine, R. S. [1959] *Natural History of Cerebral Palsy*, Cambridge, Harvard University Press.)

PERCENT ABLE TO WALK WITHOUT SUPPORT (cumulative)

SPASTIC HEMIPLEGICS (prenatal or natal origin)

EXTRAPYRAMIDAL & MIXED TYPES

SPASTIC TETRAPLEGICS

AGE OF WALKING: 289 CEREBRAL-PALSY PATIENTS

AGE IN YEARS

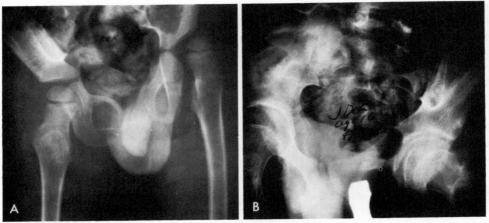

Figure 3-2   A. Radiograph of hips of patient G. D., spastic quadriplegic 2 year old child. Prognosis for walking is poor. Subluxation of hip was treated with bilateral iliopsoas tenotomy, adductor longus and gracilis myotomy, and anterior branch obturator neurotomy. B. Age 16 years. Fourteen years postoperatively, hips have remained located. Patient remains wheelchair dependent.

of surgery in the non-ambulatory patient to that of preventing serious structural change in the hips (Fig. 3-2).

Prognostic testing for walking also benefits the various "therapy" programs because it permits judgments to be made on the efficacy of various treatment programs that use the ability to walk as a criterion of success. If this is the criterion, then it would be possible to have a group of non-ambulatory preschool children with cerebral palsy with a good prognosis (in our study 78 percent walked) and conclude that good results were obtained in 75 to 95 percent of the patients with any treatment method.

Other Prognostic Indicators

Molnar and Gordon (1974), in a study of 233 non-ambulatory cerebral palsied children, found that under the age of 2 years the ability to sit independently was not a good predictor of walking ability, but after the age of 4 the inability to sit did predict non-ambulation.

Beals (1966) devised a motor quotient and a severity index to predict walking in children who had spastic diplegia. The motor age was based upon a standard motor maturity test (see Chapter 2). The motor quotient was derived by division of the chronological age by the motor age in months. The predictions for walking were as follows: If the motor quotient was 30 or above, free ambulation would occur, whereas if the motor quotient was 16 or below, no ambulation would occur. Test results up to the age of 2 years were uniform, but at later ages (up to 5 years) they demonstrated increased variability. A major finding of therapeutic importance was that motor gains reached a plateau or ceased between the ages of 6 and 7 years (Fig. 3-3).

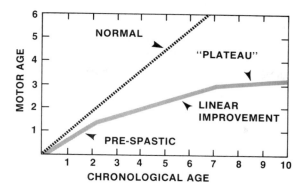

Figure 3–3 Graphic representation of improvement in motor performance of spastic diplegic children. Note plateau (no change in motor performance) beginning at age 7 years. (Redrawn from Beals, 1977.)

In addition, Beals (1966) devised a severity index, which shows the motor age in months at 3 years. Based upon this index, predictions for walking can be determined (Table 3–1). The application of these scores to goal and timing of orthopaedic surgery may be valuable. If the severity index is 0 to 9, surgery should not be done with the goal of achieving free ambulation. If the index is 10 to 11, walking is a reasonable goal, and surgery may be performed to reach that goal. A severity index of 12 to 18 means that free ambulation is possible, and surgery is done only to improve walking.

Bose and Yeo (1975) proposed a cerebral palsy score to determine the severity of gross motor function based upon the status of the patient at any age. Their objective was to select children who would benefit most from treatment and to assess the results of treatment programs. Similar scoring methods have been devised by Forbes and McIntyre (1968) and Reiners (1972). These systems use demerit points, subtracting numbers as deviations from the normal (e.g., sitting impossible, −30; standing impossible, −30; walking impossible, −30; below 25, independent walking was possible). These methods of scoring have no predictive value but only describe numerically the extent of the disability. Because of the growth of the nervous system from birth to about 3 years, functions that were thought to be absent before this age may develop spontaneously as neuronal maturation occurs. These biological facts should be considered when scores are used to assess the results of treatment. Numbers inspire a certain reverence in our culture; however, it seems likely that the reduction of children with cerebral palsy to numbers will always be a limited exercise.

Mental retardation has little if any effect on the ability to walk (Molnar and Gordon, 1974). My own observations of mentally retarded children who were a bit slow in motor development confirm the data of Molnar.

Table 3–1   WALKING PROGNOSIS (Beals, 1966)

Severity Index	
12 or more	Free walking by age 7
10–11	Lowest score consistent with free walking
9	Crutch walking
9–0	No walking

Table 3–2 EQUILIBRIUM REACTIONS AND NEED FOR EXTERNAL SUPPORT

Equilibrium Reactions	Walk without Support	Walk with Crutches	Walk with Walker
side to side	normal	normal	absent
anterior	normal	absent	absent
posterior	absent	absent	absent

EQUILIBRIUM REACTIONS

Equilibrium reactions (methods of testing are described in Chapter 2) determine whether or not the child needs external support in walking. Table 3–2 summarizes findings. Most spastic diplegic children have normal side-to-side and forward equilibrium reactions. Despite absent backward equilibrium reactions they walk freely but fall backward with the slightest push. Some children who have been deficient initially in all equilibrium reactions have graduated from walkers to quad canes. Because the loss of normal equilibrium reactions is due to lesions of the brain, muscle strengthening exercises or corrective surgical procedures cannot be expected to improve these postural controlling mechanisms.

Prognosis for Upper Limb Function

As a generalization, the prognosis for upper limb function is poor when there is a failure to develop limb dominance, lateralization, or ability to cross the midline. When stereognostic sensation in the hand is deficient, function will always be compromised. The child will have to use his eyes (visual feedback) to control his hand. Beals (1966) used his severity index (the motor age at 3 years) to predict upper limb function. The motor test was refined to include the upper limbs (Table 3–3). The most significant finding was that intelligence paralleled the upper limb severity index.

Table 3–3 UPPER LIMB FUNCTION PROGNOSIS (Beals, 1966)

Severity Index	
0–6	Profound disability
7–11	Moderate disability
12–17	Mild disability

STRUCTURAL MUSCULOSKELETAL CHANGES

Structural changes in the muscles, joints, and bones should be appreciated by all who deal with cerebral palsy.

Muscle

The cause of muscular spasticity in cerebral palsy is the effects of brain damage on the gamma nervous system and its control of muscle tone. The gamma nervous system, which innervates the intrafusal fibers of the muscle spindle, has been extensively studied (Granit, 1970). The increased and prolonged hypertonus of muscle in the growing child leads to what has been called "myostatic contracture." In muscle biopsies studied with ordinary stains and light microscopy we have been unable to demonstrate changes in most spastic muscles. We have found a mixture of neurogenic and dystrophic changes in limb muscle biopsies in only three of 279 patients. In patients who have scoliosis and cerebral palsy we have found neuromyopathic changes in the paraspinal muscles on both sides of the curve (Fig. 3–4). Tardieu et al. (1971) studied the effects of immobilization of the triceps sural muscle of the cat in the shortened position. He and his co-workers noted in these muscles a more displaced and abrupt tension-extension curve, less strength, histological evidence of atrophy, and, with electron microscopic examination, a decrease in the number of sarcomeres. Tabary et al. (1971) studied the nature of contracture in spastic gastrocnemius-soleus muscles in 17 patients who had lengthening of these muscles. With light and electron microscopy he and his co-workers found notable increases in the length of the sarcomeres.

Because immobilization of joints and limbs has been so commonly used as a method of treatment to prevent contractures and as a means of postoperative care, the histological effects on muscle fibers as the result of immobilization merit review. Cooper (1972) studied the effects of plaster immobilization in the adult cat soleus, gastrocnemius, and flexor digitorum longus muscles. Within 2 weeks of immobilization, the muscle nuclei became more prominent. In 4 weeks the nuclei were centrally located, muscle fibers were irregular in shape and size, and vacuolar degeneration of fibers was evident. After 6 to 22 weeks of immobilization, hyaline and granular degeneration took place, leaving behind the sarcolemmic tubes. When immobilization was discontinued, regeneration of fibers began in 3 to 5 days. On the basis of data of other experiments, it was concluded that complete regeneration would occur in 3 months. Cooper also noted an increase in the contraction and relaxation times of muscles during immobilization. If these results are clinically applicable, the postoperative immobilization of limbs of patients who have had tendon lengthenings or tenotomies of spastic muscles should be restricted to approximately 3 weeks if at all possible. Moreover, one wonders about the effects of prolonged plaster treatment of dynamic equinus deformity. Is it possible that the good results obtained are due to muscle atrophy and degeneration secondary to immobilization?

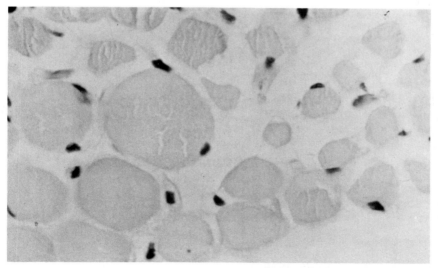

Figure 3–4 Photomicrograph 43×. Biopsy of sacrospinalis muscle from a 12-year-old with spastic quadriplegia and scoliosis. Note variation in size and shape of muscle fibers (hematoxylin-eosin stain).

Joints

The most obvious joint change is subluxation and dislocation of the hip. Cartilage degeneration of the femoral head has been seen in cases of long-standing subluxation of the hip. Complete disappearance of large segments of the articular cartilage has occurred when the femoral head has been out of the acetabulum for several years. Experimental studies have demonstrated that, when cartilage surfaces of a joint are not in contact, joint degeneration occurs (Bennett and Baver, 1937; Hall, 1969). Cartilage needs movement for its nutrition, which is derived from the diffusion of synovial fluid (Ingelmark and Saaf, 1948; Maroudas et al., 1968; Sood, 1971; Freeman, 1972). All experimental evidence indicates that the maintenance of articular cartilage requires movement of the joint — a clinically applicable concept.

If dislocation or subluxation persists, eventually the lateral aspect of the femoral head flattens due to compression by the adjacent gluteus medius and minimus muscles; a deep groove in the femoral head is caused by pressure of the ligamentum teres (Samilson et al., 1972) (Figs. 3–5 and 3–6).

I have seen three adult patients with cerebral palsy who had anterior hip pain and flexion contractures of the hip without subluxation or dislocation. Progressive erosion of the articular cartilage of the femoral head without clear-cut radiographic changes was seen in a young adult athetoid patient. She walked independently but had excessive femoral anteversion and a flexion contracture of the hip (Figs. 3–7 and 3–8).

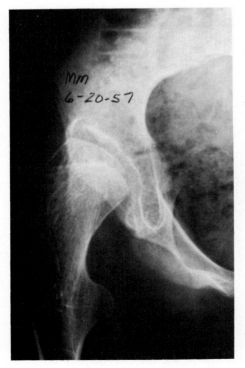

Figure 3–5 Anteroposterior radiograph of hip in a 17-year-old spastic diplegic, crutch-walking young man. Note the flattening of the lateral aspect of the femoral head due to compression by the gluteus medius and minimus muscles.

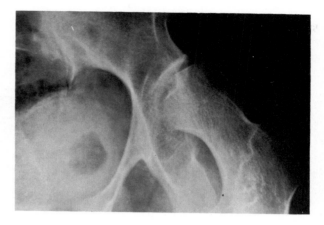

Figure 3–6 Anteroposterior radiograph of hip. Subluxation of the hip in an 18-year-old, crutch-walking spastic diplegic. Note notch in femoral head due to pressure of the ligamentum teres.

Evidence of cartilage degeneration has been observed in long-standing cases of fixed equinus deformity of the ankle (Fig. 3–9). These clinical observations, coupled with experimental data of the effects of compression on articular cartilage, should subdue enthusiasm for forced positioning of joints in plaster casts or orthoses in attemps to correct a contracture. In experimental animals, joints subjected to continuous compressive forces show gross and histological degenerative changes of the articular cartilage (Salter and Field, 1960; Salter and McNeil, 1965).

Patella alta is a common deformity accompanying knee flexion posture in cerebral palsy (Lotman, 1976). In the adult patient who has patella alta, knee pain is the chief complaint. Radiographic and arthroscopic examinations have shown marked fibrillation of the patellar articular cartilage (Fig. 3–10).

Joint capsule contracture is superimposed on the myostatic contracture if the latter is unrelieved for several years. The major joints affected are the elbow, hip, knee, and ankle. The mechanism of contracture is thought to be reorganization of connective tissue so that the collagen fibers fail to glide (Kottke, 1966). Experimental immobilization of rat knee joints demonstrated proliferation of subsynovial intrascapular fibers in the infrapatellar and intercondylar spaces of the knee. Connective tissue extended between joint surfaces to form adhesions, and cartilage degenerated (Evans et al., 1960). Parallel changes in human knee joints that were immobilized for prolonged periods have been described (Enneking and Horowitz, 1972).

In the upper limb the most notable structural change that occurs in cerebral palsy is early deformation of the elbow joint due to posterior subluxation of the radial head, which is apparently secondary to flexion spasticity of the elbow, and pronation spasticity of the forearm.

Bone

The long bones are rarely, if ever, deformed in spastic paralysis. Anterior bowing of the femoral shaft cannot be ascribed to the spasticity of the hip flexors. Measurements of the femoral shaft with lateral radiographic projections of the hip and femur in normal children and in 27 children who had spastic hip flexion deformities failed to demonstrate any significant change from the normal anterior bow of the femur (1 to 20 degrees; mean, 7 degrees) (Bleck, 1968).

Text continued on page 83

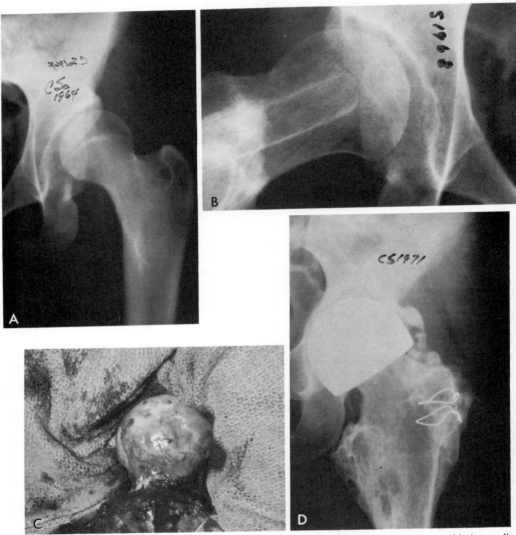

Figure 3-7 A. Patient C. S., age 19 years. Patient is athetoid and ambulatory with internally rotated hip during gait. Complained of pain in anterior hip region. B. One year following femoral rotation osteotomy at which fixation was removed. Hip pain and crepitus persist postoperatively; joint space appears relatively normal. C. Femoral head at operation. Large areas of articular cartilage have been eroded. D. Free of pain at seven years follow-up after cup arthroplasty.

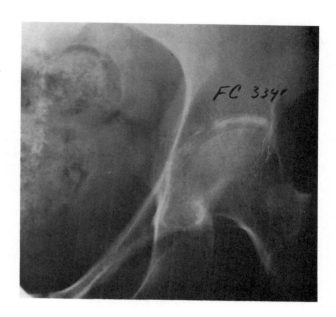

Figure 3–8 Anteroposterior radiograph of hip. Patient 33 years old, crutch-dependent, spastic diplegic. Patient has 60 degrees flexion contracture of hip 18 years after total hamstring transfer and has chronic pain in anterior hip region when walking and at rest.

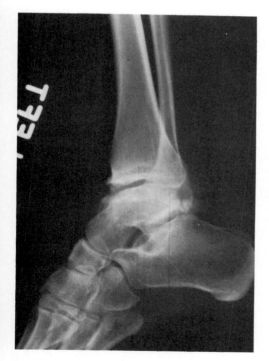

Figure 3–9 Lateral radiograph of ankle with spastic equinus deformity. Patient, 22 years old, had continuous bracing. There is evidence of degenerative arthritis of the ankle; note anterior tibial and talar osteophytes.

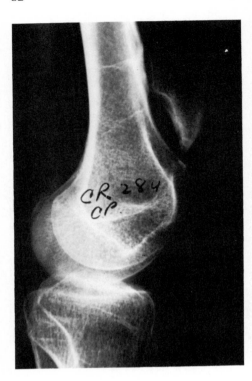

Figure 3–10 Lateral radiograph of knee. Patient 28 years old, spastic triplegic, ambulatory with crutches, had 45 degree flexion deformity of both knees until age 13 years. Fourteen years following hamstring lengthening, has retropatellar pain and crepitus. Patella alta persists.

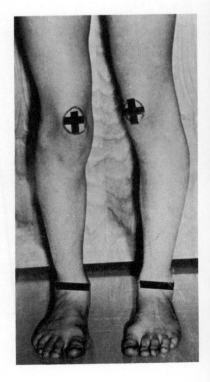

Figure 3–11 Spastic diplegic patient with internally rotated hip gait whose feet are directed straight ahead owing to compensatory external tibial torsion of 40 to 45 degrees.

Excessive femoral anteversion is the major bony structural change. Significant abnormal femoral anteversion in children with spastic hip flexion deformities has been documented (Lewis et al., 1964; Beals, 1969; Bleck, 1971; Baumann, 1972; Fabry et al., 1973).

Another torsional deformity of bone is excessive external tibial-fibular torsion (normal adult mean, 23 degrees) (LeDamany, 1909). This change is often observed in patients who have internally rotated hip walking patterns. External tibial torsion apparently develops as a compensatory change to internal femoral torsion (anteversion) (Sommerville, 1957) (Fig. 3–11).

REFERENCES

Bard, P. (1938) Studies on the cortical representation of somatic sensibility. *Harvey Lectures* 33:143–169.

Baumann, J. V. (1972) Hip operations in children with cerebral palsy. *Reconstructive Surgery and Traumatology* 13:68–82.

Beals, R. K. (1966) Spastic paraplegia and diplegia: an evaluation of non-surgical and surgical factors influencing the prognosis for ambulation. *Journal of Bone and Joint Surgery* 48A:827–846.

Beals, R. K. (1969) Developmental changes in the femur and acetabulum in spastic paraplegia and diplegia. *Developmental Medicine and Child Neurology* 11:303–313.

Beck, C. H., and Chambers, W. W. (1970) Speed, accuracy and strength of forelimb movement after unilateral pyramidotomy in rhesus monkeys. *Journal of Comparative and Physiological Psychology* 70:1–22.

Bennett, G., and Baver, W. (1937) Joint changes resulting from patellar displacement and their relation to degenerative hip disease. *Journal of Bone and Joint Surgery* 19:667–692.

Berman, A. J., and Berman, D. (1973) Fetal deafferentation: the ontogenesis of movement in the absence of peripheral sensory feedback. *Experimental Neurology* 38:170–176.

Bleck, E. E. (1968) Observations and treatment of flexion, internal rotation, and bone deformities of the hip in cerebral palsy. *Thesis,* American Orthopaedic Association.

Bleck, E. E. (1971) The hip in cerebral palsy. *Instructional Course Lectures,* American Academy of Orthopaedic Surgeons, St. Louis, C. V. Mosby Co.

Bleck, E. E. (1975) Locomotor prognosis in cerebral palsy. *Developmental Medicine and Child Neurology* 17:18–25.

Bose, K., and Yeo, K. Q. (1975) The locomotor assessment of cerebral palsy. *Proceedings* (Singapore) 10:21–24.

Bossom, J., and Ommaya, A. K. (1968) Visuo-motor adaptation in prismatic transformation of the retinal image in monkeys with bilateral dorsal rhizotomy. *Brain* 91:161–172.

Brodal, A. (1969) *Neurological Anatomy,* 2nd Ed., New York, Oxford University Press.

Brunner, R. L., and Altman, J. (1974) The effects of interference with the maturation of the cerebellum and hippocampus on the development of adult behavior. *Plasticity and Recovery of Function in the Central Nervous System* (Eds. Stein, P. G., Rosen, J. J., and Butters, N.), New York, Academic Press.

Cajal, R. S. (1928) *Degeneration and Regeneration of the Nervous System* (Transl. May, R. M.), London, Oxford University Press.

Clemente, C. D. (1964) Regeneration in the vertebrate central nervous system. *International Review of Neurobiology* 6:257–301.

Cohen, P., and Kohn, J. G. (1979) Followup study of patients with cerebral palsy. *Western Journal of Medicine* 130:6–11.

Conolly, K. (1969) Sensory motor coordination: mechanism and plans. *Planning for Better Learning* (Eds. Wolff, P. H., and MacKeith, R.), Clinics in Developmental Medicine No. 33, Philadelphia, J. B. Lippincott Co.

Cooper, R. R. (1972) Alterations during immobilization and degeneration of skeletal muscle in cats. *Journal of Bone and Joint Surgery* 54A:919–972.

Crothers, B., and Paine, R. S. (1959) *Natural History of Cerebral Palsy,* Cambridge, Harvard University Press.

Denny-Brown, D. (1966) *The Cerebral Control of Movement,* Liverpool, University of Liverpool Press.

Dobbing, J., and Sands, J. (1973) Quantitative growth and development of the human brain. *Archives of the Diseases in Childhood* 48:757–767.

Edds, M. V. (1953) Collateral nerve degeneration. *Quarterly Review of Biology* 28:260–275.

Enneking, W. F., and Horowitz, M. (1972) The intra-articular effects of immobilization on the human knee. *Journal of Bone and Joint Surgery* 54A:973–985.

Evans, E. B., Eggers, G. N. W., Butler, J. K., and Blumel, D. (1960) Experimental immobilization and remobilization of rat knee joint. *Journal of Bone and Joint Surgery* 42A:737–758.

Fabry, G., MacEwen, G. D., and Shands, A. R. (1973) Torsion of the femur. *Journal of Bone and Joint Surgery* 55A:1726–1738.

Fiorentino, M. R. (1963) *Reflex Testing Methods for Evaluating Central Nervous System Development,* Springfield, Illinois, Charles C Thomas.

Forbes, D. B., and McIntyre, J. M. (1968) A method for evaluating the results of surgery in cerebral palsy. *Canadian Medical Association Journal* 98:646–648.

Freeman, M. A. R. (1972) *Adult Articular Cartilage,* New York, Grune and Stratton.

Geschwind, N. (1974) Late changes in the nervous system: an overview. *Plasticity and Recovery of Function in the Central Nervous System* (Eds. Stein, P. G., Rosen, J. J., and Butters, N.), New York, Academic Press.

Goldberger, M. E. (1969) The extrapyramidal systems of the spinal cord. II. Results of combined pyramidal and extrapyramidal lesions in the macaque. *Journal of Comparative Neurology* 135:1–26.

Goldberger, M. E. (1974) Recovery of movement after central nervous system lesions in monkeys. *Plasticity and Recovery of Function in the Central Nervous System* (Eds. Stein, P. G., Rosen, J. J., and Butters, N.), New York, Academic Press.

Goldman, P. S. (1972) Developmental determinants of cortical plasticity. *Acta Neurobiologiae Experimentalis* 32:495–511.

Goldman, P. S. (1974) An alternative to developmental plasticity: heterology of central nervous system structures in infants and adults. *Plasticity and Recovery of Function in the Central Nervous System,* (Eds. Stein, P. G., Rosen, J. J., and Butters, N.), New York, Academic Press.

Gonshor, A., and Melvill-Jones, G. (1976a) Short term adaptive changes in the human vestibulo-ocular reflex arc. *Journal of Physiology* (London) 256:361–379.

Gonshor, A., and Melvill-Jones, G. (1976b) Extreme vestibulo-ocular adaptation induced by prolonged optical reversal of vision. *Journal of Physiology* (London) 256:381–414.

Granit, R. (1970) *The Basis of Motor Control,* New York, Academic Press.

Growden, J. H., Chambers, W. W., and Liu, C. N. (1967) An experimental study of cerebellar dyskinesia in the rhesus monkey. *Brain* 90:603–632.

Guth, L. (1975) History of central nervous system regeneration research. *Experimental Neurology* 48:3–15.

Hall, M. C. (1969) Cartilage changes after experimental relief of contact in the knee joint of the mature rat. *Clinical Orthopaedics* 64:64–76.

Held, R., and Hein, A. (1963) Movement produced stimulation with development of visually guided behavior. *Journal of Comparative and Physiological Psychology* 56:872.

Hepp–Reymond, M. C., Wiesendanger, M., Brunnert, A., Mackel A., Unger, R., and Wespi, J. (1970) Effects of unilateral pyramidotomy on conditioned finger movement in monkeys. *Brain Research* 24:544.

Ingelmark, B. E., and Saaf, V. (1948) Über die Ernährung des Gelenkknorpels und die Bildung den Gelenkflüssigkeit unter verscheidenen funktionellen Verhältnissin. *Acta Orthopaedica Scandinavica* 17:303.

Kennard, M. D. (1938) Reorganization of motor function in the cerebral cortex of monkeys deprived of motor and premotor areas in infancy. *Journal of Neurophysiology* 1:477–496.

Kennedy, D. (1976) Lecture on neurophysiology in post-graduate course: Basic Science for Clinicians, Stanford University.

Kerr, F. W. L. (1975) Structural and functional evidence of plasticity in the central nervous system. *Experimental Neurology* 48:16–31.

Knapp, H. D., Taub, E., and Berman, A. V. (1963) Movements in monkeys with deafferentated limbs. *Experimental Neurology* 7:305–315.

Kottke, F. J. (1966) The effects of limitation of activity upon the human body. *Journal of the American Medical Association* 196:117–122.

Lashley, K. S. (1938) Factors limiting recovery after central nervous system lesions. *Journal of Nervous and Mental Diseases* 88:733–735.

Lassek, A. M. (1953) Inactivation of voluntary motor function following rhizotomy. *Journal of Neuropathology and Experimental Neurology* 12:83–87.

Lawrence, D. G., and Hopkins, D. A. (1972) Developmental aspects of pyramidal motor control in the rhesus monkey. *Brain Research* 40:117–119.

LeDamany, P. (1909) La torsion du tibia, normal, pathologique, experimental. *Journal of Anatomy and Physiology* 45:598–615.

Lewis, F. R., Samilson, R. L., and Lucas, D. B. (1964) Femoral torsion and coxa valga in cerebral palsy — a preliminary report. *Developmental Medicine and Child Neurology* 6:591–597.

Liu, C. N., and Chambers, N. W. (1958) Intraspinal sprouting of dorsal root axons. *Archives of Neurology and Psychiatry* 79:46–61.

Liu, C. N., and Chambers, W. W. (1971) A study of cerebrellar dyskinesia in bilaterally differentiated forelimbs of the monkey *(Macca mulatta* and *Macca speciosa). Acta Neurobiologiae Experimentalis* 31:263–289.

Llinás, R., Walton, K., and Hillman, D. E. (1975) Inferior olive: its role in motor learning. *Science* 190:1230–1231.

Lotman, D. B. (1976) Knee flexion deformity and patella alta in spastic cerebral palsy. *Developmental Medicine and Child Neurology* 18:315–319.

Maroudas, A., Bullough, P., Swanson, S. A. V., and Freeman, M. A. R. (1968) The permeability of articular cartilage. *Journal of Bone and Joint Surgery* 50B:166–177.

McCouch, C. P. (1961) Factors in the transition to spasticity. *The Spinal Cord* (Ed. Austin, G.), Springfield, Illinois, Charles C Thomas.

Miles, F. A., and Fuller, J. H. (1974) Adaptive plasticity in the vestibulo-ocular responses of the rhesus monkey. *Brain Research* 80:512–516.

Molnar, G. E., and Gordon, S. V. (1974) Predictive value of clinical signs for early prognostication of motor function in cerebral palsy. Albert Einstein College of Medicine of Yeshiva University, Bronx, New York. Paper submitted for the scientific program of the American Academy for Cerebral Palsy, 1975.

Moore, R. Y. (1974) Central regeneration and recovery of functions; the problem of collateral reinnervation. *Plasticity and Recovery of Function in the Central Nervous System* (Eds. Stein, P. G., Rosen, J. J., and Butters, N.), New York, Academic Press.

Mott, F. W., and Sherrington, C. S. (1895) Experiments on the influence of sensory nerves upon movement and nutrition of the limbs. *Proceedings of the Royal Society of London* 57:81–488.

Neligan, G. A. (1974) The human brain growth spurt. *Developmental Medicine and Child Neurology* 16: 677–678.

Oda, M. A. S., and Huttenlocker, P. R., (1974) The effect of corticosteroids in dendritic development in the rat brain. *Yale Journal of Biology and Medicine* 47:155–165.

Reiners, J. (1972) A scoring system for evaluation of ambulation in cerebral palsied patients. *Developmental Medicine and Child Neurology* 14:332–335.

Robinson, D. A. (1976) Adaptive gain control of vestibulo-ocular reflex by the cerebellum. *Journal of Neurophysiology* 39:954–969.

Rosner, B. S. (1974) Recovery of function and localization of function in historical perspective. *Plasticity and Recovery of Function in the Central Nervous System* (Eds. Stein, D. G., Rosen, J. J., and Butters, N.), New York, Academic Press.

Salter, R. B., and Field, P. (1960) The effects of continuous compression in living articular cartilage: an experimental investigation. *Journal of Bone and Joint Surgery* 42A:31–49.

Salter, R. B., and McNeil, R. (1965) Pathological changes in articular cartilage secondary to persistent deformity (abstract). *Journal of Bone and Joint Surgery* 47B:185–186.

Samilson, R. L., Tsou, P., Aamoth, G., and Green, W. (1972) Dislocation and subluxation of the hip in cerebral palsy. *Journal of Bone and Joint Surgery* 54A:863–873.

Schade, J. P., and Von Groenigen, W. B. (1961) Structural organization of the human cerebral cortex. *Acta Anatomica* 47:74–111.

Schneider, G. E., and Jhaveri, S. R. (1974) Neuroanatomical correlates of spared or altered function after brain lesion in the newborn hamster. *Plasticity and Recovery of Function in the Central Nervous System* (Eds. Stein, P. G., Rosen, J. J., and Butters, N.), New York, Academic Press.

Semmes, J., and Chow, K. L. (1955) Motor effects of lesions of the precentral gyrus and of lesions sparing this area in monkeys. *Archives of Neurology and Psychiatry* 73:546–566.

Sharpless, S. (1964) Reorganization of function in the nervous system. *Annual Review of Physiology* 26:357–388.

Shik, M. L., Severin, F. C., and Orlovskii, G. N. (1966) Control of walking and running by means of stimulation of the mid-brain. *Biofizika* 11:756–765.

Sommerville, E. W. (1957) Persistent foetal alignment of the hip. *Journal of Bone and Joint Surgery* 39A:106–113.

Sood, S. C. (1971) A study of the effects of experimental immobilization on rabbit articular cartilage. *Journal of Anatomy* 188:497.

Sperry, R. W. (1947) Effect of crossing nerves to antagonistic limb muscles in the monkey. *Archives of Neurology and Psychiatry* 58:452–473.

Tabary, J. C., Goldspink, G., Tardieu, C., Lombard, M., and Chigot, P. (1971) Nature de la rétraction musculaire des I.M.C. mésure de l'allongement des sarcoméres du muscle étiré. *Revue de Chirurgie Orthopedique et Reparative de l'Appareil Moteur* (Paris) 57:463–470.

Tardieu, G., Tabary, J. C., Tardieu, C., and Lombard, M. (1971) Rétraction, hyperextensibilité et "faiblesse" de l'I.M.C., expressions apparement opposées d'un même trouble musculaire. Conséquences thérapeutiques. *Revue de Chirurgie Orthopedique et Reparative de l'Appareil Moteur* (Paris) 57:505–516.

Taub, E., Parella, P., and Barro, G. (1973) Behavioral development after forelimb deafferentation on day of birth in monkey with and without blinding. *Science* 181:959–960.

Taub, E., Ellman, S. T., and Berman, A. S. (1966) Differentiation in monkeys: effects on conditioned grasp responses. *Science* 151:595–597.

Taub, E., and Berman, A. J. (1968) Movement and learning in the absence of sensory feedback. *Neuropsychology of Spatially Oriented Behavior,* Homewood, Illinois, Dorsey Press.

Teuber, H. L. (1971) Mental retardation after early trauma to the brain: some issues in search of facts. *Physical Trauma as an Etiological Agent in Mental Retardation* (Eds. Angle, C. R., and Bearing, E. A., Jr.), Bethesda, Maryland, National Institutes of Health.

Twitchell, T. E. (1954) Sensory factors in purposive movement. *Journal of Neurophysiology* 17:239–252.

Wall, P. D., and Egger, N. D. (1971) Formation of new connections in adult rat brain after partial differentiation. *Nature* 232:542–545.

Wilson, D. M. (1968) The flight control system of the locust. *Scientific American* 218(5):83–90.

Windle, W. F. (1956) Regeneration of axons in the vertebrate central nervous system. *Physiological Reviews* 36:427–440.

Chapter Four

GOALS AND METHODS OF TREATMENT

GOAL SETTING

When adults with cerebral palsy were questioned about their goals, they reported the following priorities (LeBlanc, 1972): (1) communication, (2) activities of daily living, (3) mobility, and (4) walking. It is significant that walking was the last priority for many of these patients. Walking for quadriplegic persons with total body involvement is generally impractical. The energy needed for walking may be so great that constant fatigue results, precluding effective functioning in the activities of daily living. Even in spastic children who walked independently the energy requirements for walking, as measured by oxygen consumption, increased by 47 to 67 percent (Nakagiri and Tichenor, 1976). We have emphasized mobility for our patients by any means, as the normal population has also used adaptive equipment for mobility, e.g., the horse and the automobile.

Classification of Mobility

When setting goals for cerebral palsied persons we use the same classification of mobility as that devised for those with spina bifida (Hoffer et al., 1973). This classification is as follows:

1. Community walker — can get about the community on his own with or without crutches.
2. Household walker — can get about his own household but needs a wheelchair outside it.
3. Physiological walker — can walk only in a physical therapy department for exercise, usually with the aid of parallel bars. In the household and community this person needs a wheelchair.
4. Nonwalker — no functional walking. Needs a manually operated or powered wheelchair for all mobility.

The nonwalker who uses a wheelchair can be further classified according to his method of transfer:

1. Independent — can get in and out of the wheelchair by himself.
2. Assistive — can get in and out of the chair with the assistance of one person; does not need to be lifted.
3. Dependent — needs to be lifted out of the wheelchair.

Beyond School: Living with Cerebral Palsy

Before discussing treatment methods and their timing, we should first consider the end of treatment and its goals, which should be directed toward the realities of adult life for a span of 50 to 70 years. The objective of management, then, should be the optimum independence of the person in the community. He should not be "captured" by treatment programs, and special schools for the handicapped, although well-intentioned, tend to permanently segregate the handicapped from the community — the antithesis of the integrated approach (Taft, 1972; Milani-Compretti, 1977).

What becomes of the child who has cerebral palsy? A number of follow-up studies have addressed this question, and from these we can obtain a perspective on our management programs. In these studies the following factors appear to be important in helping the patient to gain independence:

1. The more severe the intellectual retardation, the lower the capacity for employment (Ingram et al., 1964; Hassakis, 1974; O'Reilly, 1975).
2. Regular schooling and completion of secondary school is helpful (Bachman, 1972; O'Reilly, 1975).
3. Spastic paralysis is more favorable than athetosis (O'Reilly, 1975), and spastic hemiplegia or diplegia is the most favorable condition for eventual independence (Ingram et al., 1964; Hassakis, 1974).
4. Smaller towns offer better niche employment than cities (Ingram et al., 1964).
5. Independence in mobility and travel is of *major* importance in gaining employmend (p > 0.01) (Bachman, 1972).
6. Hand skills make employment more feasible (p. > 0.05) (Bachman, 1972).
7. Orthopaedic surgery was performed in 45 percent of 119 patients in O'Reilly's study (1975).
8. Prolonged treatment programs have not been demonstrated to improve the chances for independence (Cohen and Kohn, 1979).
9. Competitive employment cannot be the *only* goal of management and treatment. Sheltered employment was needed for over 50 percent of those who had cerebral palsy (Moed and Sitwin, 1963).

Next to employment a prime goal of treatment should be independent living and the prevention of institutionalization. A life with a modicum of happiness and minimum dependence upon other people for ordinary living is not only human (in Milani-Compretti's phrase [1977] it is "humanization versus medicalization") but also economically sound. The elimination of the need to finance institutional care for one person for half a century should be an economic incentive to those who pay taxes to foster rational management.

PRESCRIPTION AND TIMING OF PHYSICAL AND OCCUPATIONAL THERAPY

Infancy

In the infant, motor development is the primary goal of management. The question of whether physical therapy influences motor development or merely parallels it consistent with the extent of brain damage and maturation of the nervous system is unclear at present. Only a few studies that attempt to answer this question have been reported (Wright and Nicholson, 1973; Scherzer et al., 1976).

However, physical therapy services are valuable in teaching the mother how to place her child in positions that inhibit abnormal posture and tone so that sitting, feeding, and hand use are facilitated. Parents are encouraged to touch and hold their child. Occupational therapy per se is probably not required, although the principles of stimulation (occupational therapists have been the leading advocates of sensory input) are incorporated into the therapy program. Whether a physical therapist or an occupational therapist conducts the program depends upon the interests and talents of the therapist and the particular organization of the therapy unit. Programs for infants usually consist of one to three weekly 1-hour visits with the therapist. These visits should not be considered "treatment" or a magical attempt to cure but should be presented as instructional periods much like a piano lesson. The therapist defines the extent of the motor problem, notes the emergence of normal posture, delineates the presence of persistent abnormal reflexes, and watches for structural changes — mainly in the hip, knee, and ankle.

Preschool Age

At this age most children with cerebral palsy will begin to walk, depending upon the extent of cerebral damage. When the child begins to get up on his knees, stand, and then move about erect by holding onto furniture ("cruising"), the therapist curbs the desire of the parents to help the child walk by holding onto his hands and attempting to force development. Premature forced walking is thought to exaggerate the flexion posture of the hips (Bobath and Bobath, 1958). If, however, by the age of 4 or 5 years when the child is ready to attend school walking has not been achieved despite good prognostic signs, standing equilibrium tests should be given to determine what kind of external support is necessary. If the side-to-side equilibrium reactions are normal, but the anterior and posterior reactions are deficient, it is practical to teach the child how to use crutches (usually the forearm type).

If the prognosis for walking is poor and the child has reached school age, mobility and transportation to school are essential. Therefore, at this time a mobility program using a wheelchair with special seating (see Chapter 7) should be initiated. The therapist's role shifts to teaching the child how to transfer himself to and from the wheelchair and how to perform activities of daily living.

With the total body involved child the occupational therapist concentrates on teaching the child how to use his arms, beginning with feeding. To facilitate chewing and swallowing, oral stimulation methods can be tried. To use his hands optimally, the child must be comfortably and securely seated; special seat inserts for the wheelchair may be indicated (see Chapter 7). Head control, if not complete, may be reinforced with adaptive head-holding equipment or biofeedback devices (see Chapter 7).

School Age: 5 to 8 Years

By the age of 6 years the child should be free of contractures, have stable hips, and have reached the goals of the sensory-motor training program (Baumann, 1975). Baumann confirms my own observations that by school age and thereafter (6 to 18 years), children become "bored with endless remedial exercises." Furthermore, some neurodevelopmental techniques become difficult for the therapist to perform because of the weight of the patient. Nor do school-age children accept daily exercises guided by parents. Consequently, the best "therapy" program is one that makes use of sports with therapeutic goals, e.g., swimming, riding, skiing. From sports the child derives pleasure and emotional rewards. The ambulatory child also needs to concentrate on achieving mobility, a sense of direction, and competence in performing the activities of daily living — dressing, using the toilet, bathing, grooming, getting in and out of automobiles, using public transportation, and learning the monetary system. Adaptive equipment should be used for the compensation of disability rather than overdoing remediation training. For severely involved children some therapists (Cotton, 1977) have claimed success with a 2-year structured repetitive in-patient training program for living called "conductive education" devised by Petou in Budapest.

During the school age years, the occupational therapist is often asked to reinforce the educational process, first by analyzing what might be perceptual and/or visual-motor deficits and then by beginning remedial training. It seems prudent to control such remediation attempts by pre- and post-"treatment" testing. It may be advisable for the teacher and therapist to consider compensatory methods of education rather than to strive to overcome what may be permanent cerebral deficits in specific intellectual processes, e.g., abstract thinking.

An important study by Bell, Abrahamson, and McRae (1977) should temper our zeal for currently popular methods of perceptual, visual-motor, and "sensory integration" training in the attempt to improve reading skills. This 12-year prospective study found no evidence that deficits in visual perception or motor skills had any relationship to reading retardation. Furthermore, it is questionable whether remedial work in fine or gross motor skills is effective in helping children to learn to read (Robinson and Schwartz, 1973). Yule (1976) criticized the currently fashionable approach to the teaching of reading when he noted that children should be taught reading "rather than receiv[ing] perceptual-motor skills training, music and movement drama, counselling and a whole host of other perhaps irrelevant matters."

Because "sensory integrative" therapy appears to be the most popular type of treatment today, a very brief explanation of its basis seems indicated here. Sensory therapists emphasize the importance of the tactile and vestibular senses (equilibrium), the principle that sensory input always precedes motor response, and the sensory feedback that informs the neural system of the accuracy of its responses. Integration refers to the process of reception and delineation that is required to organize sensory information for use (Vezie, 1975). The presumption is that although the cells of the central nervous system cannot regenerate, there is evidence that the neurological system has a "remarkable plasticity" that allows it to "reroute, compensate, and respond to therapeutic methods that will facilitate change" (Vezie, 1975). The therapist chooses a variety of positions, postures, and activities, including games. For example, the child may be swung in a hammock with his arms and legs free, and as he swings forward toward the therapist he claps hands with the therapist. The goal is to provide vestibular stimulation in the transverse plane. For more detailed description of the indications, methods, and results of this therapy, consult the references listed (Ayeres, 1971, 1972; McKibbin, 1973).

In my experience, the most sensible type of physical therapy at this age is the development of better balance by equilibrium training. In view of the experimental data on the adaptability of the vestibular-ocular system, balance training (including sports) seems rational. Furthermore, experience suggests that advanced motor skills, such as tightrope walking, roller skating, gymnastics, dancing, and skiing must be learned and practiced. All of these skills require practice in postural control.

Physical Therapy "Methods"

Thompson (1977) reported the results of a questionnaire sent to 233 cerebral palsy therapy units. The responses indicated that most therapists used a combination of "methods." The Ayeres (1971, 1972) and Bobath systems (1954, 1958, 1966) were used most often, followed by those of Rood (1954), Phelps, Deaver, and Fay, Daman, and Delecato (1958, 1960). What is the orthopaedist to make of this variety of "therapies"? Herman (1976) probably offered the best critique. He emphasized that continuous feedback on performance is essential for the sense of magnitude of position, force, and movement. Based upon clinical and experimental data Herman listed four factors that are necessary for optimal training and learning. The information given to the patient must be: "(1) delivered without delay, (2) shaped spatially, (3) augmented, and (4) reinforced."* He concluded that current therapy techniques fail to accomplish this objective. It is probable that recently described biofeedback techniques for motor control have more to offer (Harrison, 1975, 1977). Herman makes the point that motor learning is dependent upon the ability to compensate for the sensory disturbance. However, one has to learn, and this is where the emphasis should be. The patient learns not only by "doing" (motor learning) but because the "doing" is necessary to compensate.

WHEN TO STOP THERAPY

As a general rule the time to stop therapy is when the child is 6 to 8 years old and is playing with his peers in school, in the playground, and after school in his neighborhood. If the child's level of intelligence can cope with the normal educational process, regular school is in order. If we accept the follow-up data of the studies summarized in this chapter, the integration of the cerebral palsied child into a normal school environment is important. Thus, it is essential that physicians and therapists state that the optimum benefits of therapy have been obtained.

Data supplied by Beals (1966) (see Chapter 3) confirm that improvement in

---

*Murdoch, G. (Ed.): *Advances in Orthotics*, London, Edward Arnold, 1976, p. 497.

motor performance of children who have spastic paraplegia or diplegia reaches a plateau at about the age of 7 years (Fig. 3–4). Also, walking patterns are fixed at an early age. The study of Burnett and Johnson (1971) showed that the adult walking pattern in children was achieved 55 weeks after walking began at the latest. These observations on motor development correlate well with the anatomical studies of cerebral and cerebellar development referred to in Chapter 3. It has been my observation that by the age of 7 years, the gait patterns of cerebral palsied children are fixed, and the adult pattern will therefore be the same unless it is altered by surgery of the limbs.

More severely handicapped children need adaptive equipment to compensate for the loss of a particular function. The management program for these children entails the cooperation of the rehabilitation engineer and the orthotist to implement non-verbal communication, self-feeding, and mobility. Much of this program can be accomplished by the age of 8 years.

To summarize, the goal of the therapeutic program should be the development of the child as a person, not as a permanent patient.

EVALUATING THERAPEUTIC METHODS

All too often the zeal for cure by professionals and parents has led to excessive dependency on professionals and unrealistic expectations and goals by both parent and child. Medical and paramedical workers in the field of cerebral palsy might do well to recognize that a treatment system can become a religion. As with many religious beliefs, the number of variant systems of therapy tends to multiply. When therapy is viewed as a religion, it is not surprising that each practitioner tends to promote his own beliefs. These comments should not detract from the enthusiastic and loving care shown by so many therapists who must deal day by day with the child and his parents. It is only when therapy, like truth, becomes exaggerated that it becomes heresy. The role of the therapist is now changing to include that of a consultant, research associate, orthopaedic assistant, and diagnostician (Goldberg, 1975).

Therapy programs in cerebral palsy have not been evaluated because it is claimed that there are too many variables in the patient population. Furthermore, controls are difficult to impose. To solve this problem, Martin and Epstein (1976) suggested some methods of evaluation of the single patient. Figures 4–1 to 4–6 explain their methods.

Studies of the efficacy of physical therapy in cerebral palsy are rare. The few studies reported have cast doubt on what often has been presented as certainty (Pless, 1976). Wright and Nicholson (1973) conducted two prospective controlled studies, one of 42 children for 6 months and one of 25 children for 1 year. They divided the patients into three treatment groups: (1) those receiving Bobath therapy for 12 months; (2) those receiving no physical therapy for 12 months; and (3) those receiving no therapy for 6 months followed by 6 months of treatment. They found no significant differences after 12 months between treated and untreated children when the children were analyzed with regard to motor function, range of movement of joints, and loss of primitive reflexes. They concluded that the Bobath treatment (Bobath and Bobath, 1958) was of no value.

Scherzer et al. (1976) conducted a double blind study of 24 children under the

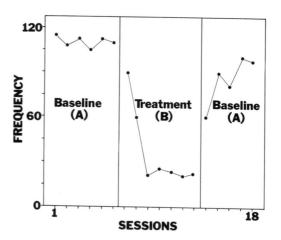

Figure 4–1 Treatment withdrawal design (A-B-A). Stable motor activity at baseline (A) is followed by treatment (B). Following withdrawal of treatment, there is a return to baseline (A). (Reproduced courtesy of Leonard Epstein, Auburn University, Auburn, Texas, from Martin, J. E., and Epstein, L. H. (1976). Evaluating treatment effectiveness in cerebral palsy, *Physical Therapy* 56:285–294.)

age of 18 months. The control group received only minimum therapy to extend the range of motion of their limbs at school twice a week. The experimental group had a neurophysiological program of physical therapy designed to stimulate motor milestones on an individual basis supplemented by a program carried on at home by parents. This study reported a trend toward positive change in children with higher intelligence. Older children who had less treatment improved more. The experimental group who had neurophysiological therapy showed greater improvement in motor and social functions, but there was little difference between the control and experimental groups in behavior at home. Scherzer concluded that more studies must be done over a longer period of time.

Paine (1962) was able to compare a group of 74 patients who had no therapy with 103 children who had intensive physical therapy, bracing, and orthopaedic surgery.

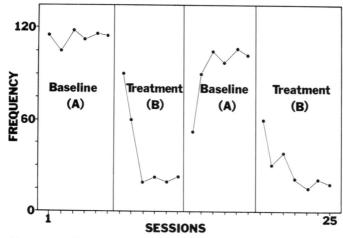

Figure 4–2 Treatment withdrawal-reinstatement design (A-B-A-B). After baseline (A), treatment (B) is given and then withdrawn with motor stability at baseline (A). Treatment can be reinstituted and behavior remains stable. Therefore, treatment was not effective. (Reproduced courtesy of Leonard Epstein, Auburn University, Auburn, Texas, from Martin, J. E., and Epstein, L. H. (1976). Evaluating treatment effectiveness in cerebral palsy, *Physical Therapy* 56:285–294.)

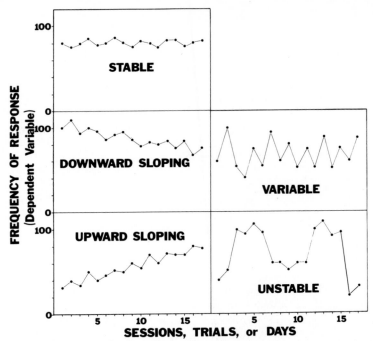

Figure 4–3 Five examples of measurement of various responses to treatment. A. Stable. B. Downward sloping. C. Variable. D. Upward sloping. E. Unstable. (Reproduced courtesy of Leonard Epstein, Auburn University, Auburn, Texas, from Martin, J. E., and Epstein, L. H. (1976). Evaluating treatment effectiveness in cerebral palsy, *Physical Therapy* 56:285–294.)

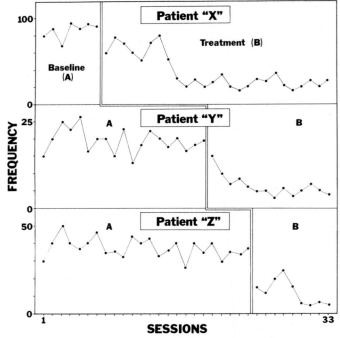

Figure 4–4 Various baseline designs of three children with cerebral palsy. Baseline measures are obtained for the same type of motor behavior in each patient (A), and treatments are applied sequentially (B). (Reproduced courtesy of Leonard Epstein, Auburn University, Auburn, Texas, from Martin, J. E., and Epstein, L. H. (1976). Evaluating treatment effectiveness in cerebral palsy, *Physical Therapy* 56:285–294.)

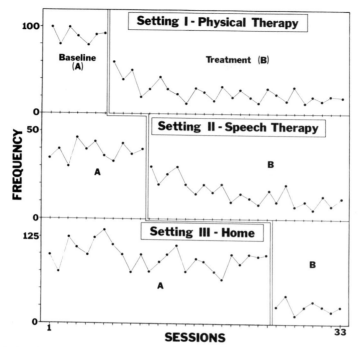

Figure 4–5 Various baseline designs in different settings for treatment of the child. After a baseline for a given response is established in all settings (A), treatment is begun and the same response is recorded (B). (Reproduced courtesy of Leonard Epstein, Auburn University, Auburn, Texas, from Martin, J. E., and Epstein, L. H. (1976). Evaluating treatment effectiveness in cerebral palsy, *Physical Therapy* 56:285–294.)

He found that those who had mild spastic hemiplegia improved with and without treatment. More severely involved spastic patients who had various forms of treatment did have a better gait and fewer contractures. Physical therapy did not reduce the need for orthopaedic surgery and made no difference in patients with athetosis.

A small controlled study on the effects of presumed vestibular stimulation was reported by Kanter et al. (1976). The children receiving treatment were spun in a swivel chair for 1 minute a day. The experimental group consisted of two children with Down's syndrome aged 6 and 24 months. The controls were three normal infants between the ages of 6 and 9 months and two children with Down's syndrome. Assessment of the motor ability of all the children revealed that the two with Down's syndrome who had no treatment did not increase their motor performance. One normal child and one Down's child who had the treatment increased their motor abilities 21.5 and 16 points, respectively. The authors suggested that the improvement in motor ability shown after vestibular stimulation was due to advancement of vestibular inhibitory mechanisms.

PLASTER CASTING

Plaster casts have been used consistently as a method of therapy only in patients with spastic equinus deformity. Yates and Mott (1977) have published preliminary

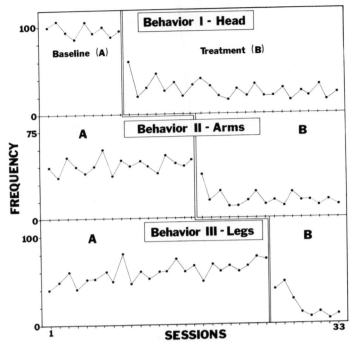

Figure 4–6 The various baseline designs of behavior in three different areas (A). Treatment was instituted at different times in an attempt to reduce extraneous movements of the head, arms, and legs (B). (Reproduced courtesy of Leonard Epstein, Auburn University, Auburn, Texas, from Martin, J. E., and Epstein, L. H. (1976). Evaluating treatment effectiveness in cerebral palsy, *Physical Therapy* 56:285–294.)

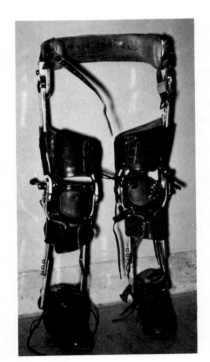

Figure 4–7 "Full control" lower limb bracing typically used for children with cerebral palsy 20 to 25 years ago.

results in the application of bilateral short leg walking plasters in 49 children. Their patients were selected for treatment only if they had dynamic equinus deformity and the ankle could be dorsiflexed to the neutral positive position. These plaster casts were termed "inhibitive." A prefabricated wooden footplate built-up to provide pressure under the metatarsal heads and extend the toes was applied first. Then a short leg walking plastic (Zoroc) was applied. The casts were then bivalved and Velcro fastening straps affixed. The average duration of treatment with the cast was 10 months. Yates and Mott stated that 100 percent of the patients exhibited changes in "tone," and all but four walking patients improved their gait; the posture and movement of non-walkers also improved. The reason for the change in muscle "tone" toward more relaxation, even in the upper limbs, may be found in an unexplained mechanism called neurological "inhibition."

I have not used this method except in a few patients. The use of plaster is tedious and time-consuming and presents the usual risks of skin pressure sores and blisters. Instead, I prefer to use rigid plastic ankle-foot orthoses in patients with dynamic equinus deformity (i.e., no contracture); if the orthosis cannot resist the degree of spasticity, myoneural blocks of the gastrocnemius muscle using 45 percent alcohol may be helpful.

ORTHOTICS AND REHABILITATION ENGINEERING

Limb Orthoses

Even though "full control" lower limb and trunk metal orthoses were abandoned 17 years ago (Figs. 4–7 and 4–8) (the Bobaths demonstrated how useless these were), selective use of orthoses still has a place in patient management. Plastic orthoses are used for the specific conditions described in Chapters 4 and 5. I have not

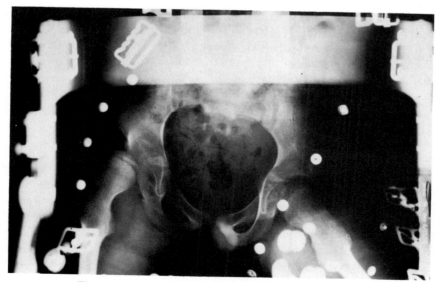

Figure 4–8 Hip dislocation, that occurred despite bracing.

used night splinting in an attempt to prevent structural change. Our analysis of the incidence of recurrence of gastrocnemius-soleus contracture after lengthening of the Achilles tendon indicates that absence of night splinting has not increased the recurrence of equinus deformity in any greater percentage than reported by others who have been devoted to nighttime orthotics (Lee, 1977). With a recurrence rate of only 9 per cent with Achilles tendon lengthening, we would have wasted 90 percent of the orthoses if we had applied them to all patients. In addition, we have observed that night splints are not well tolerated during sleep, and patients use them at home irregularly.

Rehabilitation Engineering

The contribution of the engineer to that of the orthotist in solving the needs of patients for communication, mobility and seating, and activities of daily living is a new concept. How these needs can be met is discussed in Chapter 6 on the management of the total body involved patient.

ORTHOPAEDIC SURGERY

Role and Timing

Orthopaedic surgery appears to have established a permanent and important place in the management of cerebral palsy. The progression of structural changes in joints, despite assiduous "therapy" and "bracing," has been evident when patients have been followed for long periods. If a child receives follow-up observation only to the age of 15 or 16 years, the physician may develop an illusion that structural changes make no difference. For example, painful degenerative arthritis as a result of subluxation of the hips in a crutch-walking spastic paraplegic may not jeopardize the patient's mobility until *after* the age of 18 years (Fig. 4–9). A dislocated hip may not become painful until after the age of 18. Furthermore, orthopaedic surgery in late adolescence is more difficult, has more complications, and causes an increased incidence of postoperative psychological problems (Williams, 1977). Consequently, orthopaedic surgery to prevent and correct serious structural change ought to be performed *before* the age of 15 years.

THE PRESCHOOL CHILD

I prefer to defer surgery for functional or cosmetic improvement of gait until the child has learned to walk. It is impossible to analyze the possible gait pattern either clinically or electromyographically until the child is actually walking, with or without crutches. If a child has a good prognosis for walking, surgery will not hasten the development of ambulation. Although my data are not statistically significant, I have observed that surgery, particularly on the feeet, may even delay walking (Bleck, 1975). Surgery is sometimes given credit as the one therapy that allowed the child to walk. In such dramatic therapeutic triumphs it is likely that surgery was unconsciously timed to coincide with the developmental onset of independent walking.

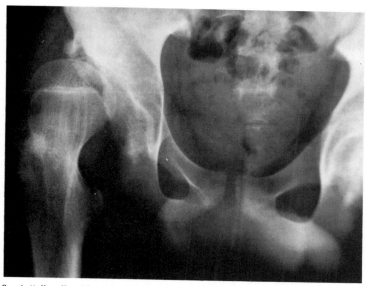

Figure 4–9 A "silent" subluxation of the hip that pain made evident in an 18-year-old, ambulatory man with cerebral palsy.

Providing there are no structural changes (e.g., hip subluxation or contracture of the gastrocnemius-soleus muscle or of the knee joint), there is no harm in deferring surgery until the child can walk. The exception to this rule in the preschool child occurs when prevention of subluxation and dislocation of the hips is necessary. In all children who have spastic hip muscles radiographs of the hips should be made in infancy and repeated every 6 to 8 months. If subluxation of the hip is occurring, surgical release of the spastic muscles is indicated. The locomotor prognosis determines the type of surgery required. If, for example, the child has subluxation of the hips and a poor prognosis for walking, we perform a myatomy of the adductor longus and gracilis muscles, a neurectomy of the anterior branch of the obturator nerve, and an iliopsoas tenotomy. If, however, the child has a good prognosis for walking, we do not wish to risk the permanent weakness of hip flexion that sometimes occurs after iliopsoas tenotomy of a very spastic iliopsoas muscle. In such a child we would recommend lengthening or recession of the iliopsoas muscle (see Chapter 5).

THE SCHOOL AGE CHILD

The optimum time for lower limb surgery in the ambulatory child appears to be between the ages of 5 and 7 years. At this time the gait pattern can be analyzed. Surgery need not be staged over a period of years. With repeated examinations, careful analysis of the gait problem, and recognition of potential skeletal changes, all surgery can be performed at one time and at as many joint levels as necessary. Longer anesthesia times are required for one-stage surgery, but the actual duration of anesthesia is not as important as induction and recovery from it (as in an airplane trip it is the taking off and landing that present the greater risk). With a postoperative regimen that entails a limited time in a plaster cast and early mobilization, most children do not require an unduly prolonged period of postoperative rehabilitation (usually a maximum of 6 months of postoperative physical therapy supervision is all that is necessary).

ADOLESCENT AND ADULT

In the adolescent and adult, fixed contractures and permanent skeletal changes are often present. Consequently, surgery for functional improvement is not as satisfying. In the late adolescent years (over age 15) surgery is usually performed to correct deformities that cause pain and discomfort in the hip, knee, ankle, and foot. In the adult, most surgery is performed for painful degenerative arthritis of the hip secondary to subluxation and dislocation.

Preparation of the Child and Parent for Surgery

Above all, the child and parents must feel secure with the surgeon. Ideally, the child and parents should become familiar with a physical therapist for 3 to 4 months before surgery. The therapist will need the full cooperation of the child in the period of postoperative rehabilitation. If the child is inordinately fearful or anxious, surgery should be postponed until he gains confidence, is able to accept the reality of hospitalization, recognizes the need to take medications for postoperative discomfort, and understands the need to follow through with a postoperative program supervised by a physical therapist for an estimated period of time.

Before entering the hospital the child should be told what to expect from the surgeon and the surgery:

1. It is going to hurt but medications will keep him comfortable.
2. Ordinarily the first two postoperative days are the most difficult.
3. Incisions will be made, but the "stitches" will not have to be removed because absorbable suture material is used.
4. A plaster cast extending to a certain point on the limb will be applied.
5. The length of time the cast will be on and when the child will be permitted to stand and then walk should be explained.

The surgeon must have patience with seemingly hostile parents. When they attack the surgeon, parents (and sometimes older children) are displacing their resentment that this disaster has occurred to them. Their hostility is directed against the one who confronts them with the painful realities they would rather not face (Steinhauer, 1974).

In addition, the child and his parents should be told what to expect of the hospital organization and of the hospital services, including the operating room. Ideally, for the optimum psychological benefit and to enhance a smooth recovery, a child ought to be admitted for surgery 2 or 3 days in advance. In this way he will be able to integrate the many radical changes in his life, particularly those presented by the modern and highly complex hospital (Sylvester, 1977). With the current costs of hospitalization the tendency is toward short stays (our mean hospital stay in 1975–

1976 for cerebral palsy reconstructive limb surgery was 4.83 days*). I wonder, however, if we are concerned about the "whole" child and his limited ability to adjust to the hospital environment and personnel (nurses, interns, students, residents, laboratory technicians, radiographic technicians, and clerks) within 8 to 10 hours preoperatively. If so, and if we recognize the great importance of decreased anxiety and patient cooperation for a smooth recovery and a good result, we might question the present fashionable "in and out" policies of utilization review agencies. Are they really so "cost-effective"?

To assist children and parents in understanding the day by day and hour by hour complexities of the modern hospital and its hordes of personnel, every child needs a "best friend" in the hospital (Sylvester, 1977). Busy doctors, nurses in teams and shifts, unknowledgeable volunteers, and efficient technicians do not usually have time to establish such a relationship. In answer to this obvious need the Newcomen Center of Guys' Hospital, London, has employed this kind of person. Such a worker is not a professional but has the intellect to understand hospital procedures and the human concern to be a "best friend." In the surgical management of a chronic neuromuscular disease like cerebral palsy, I could not recommend any one staff position more highly (Parks, 1977).

DRUG THERAPY

Although alcohol has been declared to be the best drug available for muscle relaxation, it is not really practical nor in the best interests of a patient's general health to merit recommendation. Alcoholism is simply too prevalent to deliberately encourage it.

Diazepem (Valium) is widely used for presumed control of spasticity and athetosis. Its action appears to affect mainly the central nervous system, and it does lessen anxiety and startle reactions of some patients. Ambulatory patients, particularly children, do not respond well to this drug because it seems to interfere with their ability to concentrate. Diazepam has been and continues to be a valuable drug for total body involved patients, especially adults who have athetosis. Diazepam given postoperatively (5 to 10 mg intramuscularly every 4 to 6 hours) helps to control discomfort due to muscle spasm.

Dantrolene sodium (Dantrium) was released for use in 1974. In our experience (Ford et al., 1976) its use is limited. Ambulatory children with spastic hemiplegia or diplegia have not been continued on the drug, even though we reported some objective improvement in various measurements of gait and balance. The side effects — some mental dullness and the need to check liver function by serum SGOT levels every 3 to 4 months — outweighed the possible functional gains attributed to dantrolene sodium. We have recommended a trial of dantrolene sodium for those quadriplegics who are total body involved. The initial dose is 0.5 mg per kilogram of body weight four times a day. Depending upon the response, the dose may be increased to 3 mg per kilogram four times a day. Soboloff (1977) conducted a 5-year study of 58 children and adults with cerebral palsy who received dantrolene sodium regularly. Ranges of joint motion, joint function, and oral testimony of patients and parents were used to assess its efficacy. The results indicated that this drug works best in children under the age of 10 years. There was no evidence of liver disease in any patient.

---

*Children's Hospital at Stanford.

REFERENCES

Ayeres, A. J. (1971) Characteristics of types of sensory integrative dysfunction. *American Journal of Occupational Therapy* 7:329–334.

Ayeres, A. J. (1972) Improving academic scores through sensory integration. *Journal of Learning Disabilities* 5:336–343.

Bachman, W. H. (1972) Variables affecting post–school economic adaptation of orthopaedically handicapped and other health impaired students. *Rehabilitation Literature* 3:98–114.

Baumann, J. (1975) The Swiss approach to cerebral palsy. *Instructional Course Lectures,* American Academy for Cerebral Palsy, St. Louis, C. V. Mosby Co.

Bell, A. E., Abrahamson, D. S., and McRae, K. N. (1977) Reading retardation: A twelve year prospective study. *Journal of Pediatrics* 91:363–370.

Beals, R. K. (1966) Spastic paraplegia and diplegia: an evaluation of non-surgical and surgical factors influencing the prognosis for ambulation. *Journal of Bone and Joint Surgery* 48A:827–846.

Beals, R. K. (1977) *Prognosis in Spastic Diplegia.* First William C. Duncan Seminar on Cerebral Palsy, University of Washington, Seattle.

Bobath, B. (1954) A study of abnormal postural reflex activity in patients with lesions of the central nervous system. *Physiotherapy* 40:9–12.

Bobath, K., and Bobath, B. (1958) An assessment of motor handicap of children with cerebral palsy and their response to treatment. *Occupational Therapy Journal* 27:1–16.

Bobath, K. (1966) *The Motor Deficit in Patients with Cerebral Palsy.* Clinics in Developmental Medicine No. 23, Philadelphia, J. B. Lippincott Co.

Burnett, C. N., and Johnson, E. W. (1971) Development of gait in childhood, Parts I and II. *Developmental Medicine and Child Neurology* 13:196–206, 297–215.

Capute, A. J., Accordes, P. J., Vining, E. P. O., Rubenstein, J. E., Walcher, J. R., Harryman, S., and Ross, A. (1976) Primitive reflex profile predictor of independent ambulation. Baltimore, John F. Kennedy Institute, Department of Pediatrics, Johns Hopkins University.

Cohen, P., and Kohn, J. G. (1979) Followup study of patients with cerebral palsy. *Western Journal of Medicine* 130:6–11.

Cotton, E. (1977) A bedroom routine for the cerebral palsied child. Study Group on Integrating Multiply Handicapped Children, St. Mary's College, Durham, England. London, The Spastics Society Medical Education and Information Unit.

Daman, G., and Delecato, C. (1960) Children with severe brain injuries. *Journal of the American Medical Association* 74:257–262.

Fay, T. (1958) Neuromuscular reflex therapy for spastic disorders. *Journal of Florida Medical Association* 44:1234–1240.

Ford, L. F., Bleck, E. E., Collins, F. J., and Stevick, D. (1976) Efficacy of dantrolene sodium in the treatment of spastic cerebral palsy. *Developmental Medicine and Child Neurology* 18:770–783.

Goldberg, K. (1975) The high-risk infant. *Physical Therapy* 55:1092–1096.

Harrison, H. C. (1975) Training spastic individuals to achieve better neuromuscular control using electromyographic feedback. *Movement and Child Development* (Ed. Holt, K. S.), Clinics in Developmental Medicine No. 55, Philadelphia, J. B. Lippincott Co.

Harrison, H. (1977) Augmented feedback training of motor control in cerebral palsy. *Developmental Medicine and Child Neurology* 19:75–78.

Hassakis, P. C. (1974) Outcomes of cerebral palsy patients. Annual Meeting of the American Academy for Cerebral Palsy, Denver, Colorado.

Held, R., and Hein, A., in Conolly, K. (1969) *Planning for Better Learning* (Eds. Wolff, P. H., and MacKeith, R.), Clinics in Developmental Medicine No. 33, Philadelphia, J. B. Lippincott Co.

Herman, R. (1976) Postural control and therapeutic implications. *Advances in Orthotics* (Ed. Murdoch, G.), London, Edward Arnold.

Hoffer, M. M., Feiwell, E., Perry, R., Perry, J., and Bonnett, C. (1973) Functional ambulation in patients with myelomeningocele. *Journal of Bone and Joint Surgery* 55A:137–148.

Ingram, T. T. S., Jameson, S., Errington, J., and Mitchell, R. G. (1964) *Living with Cerebral Palsy.* Clinics in Developmental Medicine No. 14, Philadelphia, J. B. Lippincott Co.

Kanter, R. M., Clark, D. C., Allen, L. C., and Chase, M. A. (1976) Effects of vestibular stimulation on nystagmus response and motor performance in the developmentally disabled infant. *Physical Therapy* 156:414–421.

LeBlanc, M. (1972) Personal communication.

Martin, J. E., and Epstein, L. H. (1976) Evaluating treatment effectiveness in cerebral palsy. *Physical Therapy* 56:285–294.

McKibbin, E. H. (1973) The effect of additional tactile stimulation in a perceptual-motor treatment program for school children. *American Journal of Occupational Therapy* 27:191–197.

Milani–Compretti, A., and Gidoni, E. A. (1967) Routine developmental examination in normal and retarded children. *Developmental Medicine and Child Neurology* 9:631–638.

Milani–Compretti, A., and Gidoni, E. A. (1967) Pattern analysis of motor development and its disorders. *Developmental Medicine and Child Neurology* 9:625–630.

Milani–Compretti, A. (1977) *In* Study Group in Integrating the Care of Multiply Handicapped Children, St. Mary's College, Durham, England. London, The Spastics Society Medical Education and Information Unit.

Mitchell, R. G. (1962) The Landau reaction (reflex). *Developmental Medicine and Child Neurology* 4:65–70.

Moed, M., and Litwin, D. (1963) The employability of the cerebral palsied. A summary of two related studies. *Rehabilitation Literature* 24:266–271.

Nakagiri, K. K., and Tichenor, C. J. C. (1976) Energy cost of hour walking in static encephalopathy children with and without their plastic ankle-foot orthosis (Master's thesis). Palo Alto, Stanford University School of Medicine, Division of Physical Therapy.

O'Reilly, D. E. (1975) Care of the cerebral palsied: outcome of the past and needs of the future. *Developmental Medicine and Child Neurology* 17:141–149.

Paine, R. S. (1962) On the treatment of cerebral palsy — the outcome of 177 patients. *Pediatrics* 29:605.

Parks, L. (1977) The need for "someone with nothing to do." Study Group on Integrating the Care of Multiply Handicapped Children, St. Mary's College, Durham, England. London, The Spastics Society Medical Education and Information Unit.

Pless, B. I. (1976) On doubting and certainty. *Pediatrics* 58:7–9.

Robinson, M. E., and Schwartz, L. B. (1973) Visuo-motor skills and reading ability. *Developmental Medicine and Child Neurology* 51:281.

Rood, M. S. (1954) Neurophysiologic reactions as a basis for physical therapy. *Physical Therapy Review* 34:444–449.

Scherzer, A. L., Mike, V., and Ilson, J. (1976) Physical therapy as a determinant of change in the cerebral palsied infant. *Pediatrics* 58:47–51.

Soboloff, H. (1977) A five year study of cerebral palsied children with the use of dantrolene sodium. Paper read at the annual meeting of the American Academy of Cerebral Palsy and Developmental Medicine, Atlanta.

Steinhauer, P. D., Muskin, D. N., and Rae-Grant, Q. (1974) Psychological aspects of chronic illness. *Pediatric Clinics of North America* 21:825–840.

Sylvester, E. (1977) Lecture on psychological problems in pediatric orthopaedic patients. Children's Hospital at Stanford University, Palo Alto.

Taft, L. T. (1972) Are we handicapping the handicapped? *Developmental Medicine and Child Neurology* 14:703–704.

Tauber, H. L. (1971) Mental retardation after early trauma to the brain: Some issues in search of facts. *Physical Trauma as an Etiological Agent in Mental Retardation* (Eds. Angle, G. R., and Bering, E. A.), Bethesda, Maryland, National Institutes of Health.

Thompson, S. (1977) Results of questionnaire on therapy. American Academy for Cerebral Palsy and Developmental Medicine. Regional Course, New Orleans.

Vezie, M. B. (1975) Sensory integration: A foundation for learning. *Academic Therapy* 10(3).

Williams, I. (1977) The consequences of orthopaedic surgery in the adolescent cerebral palsied: medical educational and parental attitudes. Study Group on Integrating the Care of Multiply Handicapped Children, St. Mary's College, Durham, England. London, The Spastics Society Medical Education and Information Unit.

Wright, T., and Nicholson, J. (1973) Physiotherapy for the spastic child: an evaluation. *Developmental Medicine and Child Neurology* 15:146–163.

Yates, H., and Mott, D. H. (1977) *Inhibitive Casting*. First William C. Duncan Seminar on Cerebral Palsy, University of Washington, Seattle.

Yule, W. (1976) Issues and problems in remedial education. *Developmental Medicine and Child Neurology* 18:674.

Chapter Five

SPASTIC HEMIPLEGIA

GENERAL CHARACTERISTICS

The typical posture of the child with spastic hemiplegia consists of an equinus inclination of the foot and ankle and flexion of the elbow, wrist, and fingers, with an adducted thumb (Fig. 5–1). Many mild cases exist. These can be discerned when examination of the central nervous system is stressed. For example, in a child with a mild spastic equinovalgus foot, running will bring out flexion of the elbow on the involved side.

Because these children have an intact unilateral sensorimotor system in their upper and lower limbs, the management of their motor problem is not very difficult. Most of them walk at an early age (18 to 21 months), gain independence in activities

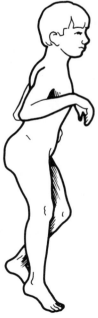

Figure 5–1 Typical posture, spastic hemiplegia.

of daily living, can participate in peer group activities, and can attend regular school. Their greatest handicap (which often has a late onset) is apt to be a convulsive disorder with concomitant mental retardation and behavior problems (Perlstein and Hood, 1956; Jones, 1976).

The details of the assessment and physical and occupational therapies have been discussed in Chapters 2 and 3. Long-term physical and occupational therapeutic programs are not necessary. Surgery is only an incidental event in their care.

UPPER LIMB MANAGEMENT

Orthotics

Because orthoses usually preclude naturally attempted bimanual hand functions, children often discard them during the day. In very young children whose nervous system is still maturing, we have used plastic opponens type splints to keep the thumb out of the palm for part of the day. Similar use can be made of plastic volar wrist extension splints. We have not been successful in splinting a flexed elbow or a pronated forearm.

Surgery

Goals and Perspectives. Everyone now recognizes the common proprioceptive and stereognostic sensory deficits in the hands of children who have spastic hemiplegia (Hohman et al. [1958] found them in 72 percent; Tachdjian and Minear [1958] found deficits in 41 percent). There are no reports that any form of treatment or the passage of time has restored this lost sensation. If "the key to muscle action is sensory feedback" (Perry, 1975), then perfectly normal hand function is impossible after surgery.

The surgical goals in the arm and hand of spastic hemiplegic children are limited to (1) improved function as a helping hand that acts as a stabilizer for objects to be manipulated by the normal hand; (2) improvement of gross function — grasp, release, and pinch; and (3) improved appearance. With regard to appearance, a severe flexion deformity of the wrist and fingers is a grotesque sight. In a hemiplegic person who has a normal opposite upper limb and is walking well, the gross deformity of the wrist and hand highlights the disability. The deformed hand can act as a barrier to employment and easy social acceptance. Consequently, surgery is indicated to correct the deformity solely on a cosmetic basis.

Timing of Surgery. Most surgeons would probably agree that surgery should be deferred until the motor pattern is established and the child is old enough to cooperate, generally after the age of 4 years. An exception to this general rule should be made in treating the child with severe pronator spasticity that can lead to posterior subluxation of the head of the radius.

Several different surgical procedures can be done at one time, and operations in many separate stages are not necessary. The deformities of the thumb and wrist can be corrected simultaneously.

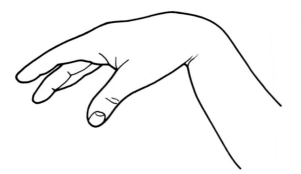

Figure 5–2 Spastic hand, pattern 2. To open the fingers, the wrist must flex.

PATTERNS OF PARALYSIS

Goldner (1976) classified spastic paralytic deformities of the hand in order to delineate a scheme of treatment. However, it is not possible and is probably tedious to give specific formulas for each hand problem in every possible spastic hand pattern. Surgical decisions must be made on the basis of careful repetitive examinations, functional testing and analysis by an occupational therapist, and occasionally the results of diagnostic peripheral nerve and myoneural blocks. With these reservations, knowledge of a general grouping of spastic hand patterns may be useful:

1. Mimimal involvement. The patient has pinch, grasp, and release functions but lacks dexterity and speed. No surgery is required.
2. Thumb-in-palm, wrist flexed moderately; to extend the fingers the wrist must be dropped into full flexion (this has the effect of tenodesis on the finger extensors) (Fig. 5–2). Surgery is indicated to improve function.
3. Thumb-in-palm, wrist and fingers flexed completely; the patient is unable to extend the fingers even when the wrist is flexed. Surgery is indicated at least to improve appearance and hand hygiene (Fig. 5–3).

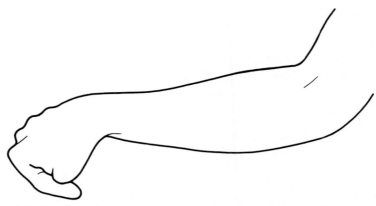

Figure 5–3 Spastic hand, pattern 3. Complete flexion of wrist and fingers, thumb in palm.

A classification by functional patterns may be given as follows:

1. Voluntary control.
2. No voluntary control; "mirror" movements by the opposite hand are the controlling mechanisms.
3. No voluntary or "mirror" movement control.

Surgery is indicated for functional improvement in the first two patterns. In pattern 3, surgery is indicated for appearance, comfort, and hygiene; restoration of function cannot be promised.

Surgery produces the best results in hands with spastic paralysis. Hands that are deformed due to athetosis can be helped occasionally (Goldner, 1976). In athetosis tendon transfers may result in the opposite and at times more disabling deformity. The dystonic hand may appear very deformed but has no contractures or skeletal changes; it is afflicted by an intermittent abnormal posturing that readily relaxes to normal with sleep and sedation, and sometimes voluntarily. Therefore, no peripheral surgery is likely to be successful.

Thumb-in-Palm Deformity. The goal of surgery is to get the thumb out of the palm so that grasp and pinch functions can occur. True opposition is not often obtained; "key" pinch will suffice (Figs. 5–4 and 5–5).

Although the following procedures are described separately for clarity, they must be combined in practice to correct the thumb deformity as required by the preoperative analysis of the problem.

ADDUCTOR POLLICIS SPASTICITY. In young children and in those who have mild to moderate spasticity and passively correctable abduction, tenotomy of the adductor pollicis insertion through a web space incision is adequate. In addition, most experienced surgeons advise release of the origin of the first dorsal interosseous muscle from the first and second metacarpals (Goldner, 1955, 1975, 1976; House, 1975; Silver et al., 1976).

More severe adduction deformities require the Matev procedure (Matev, 1963; Silver et al., 1976). This entails a palmar incision to strip the origin of the adductor pollicis muscle from the shafts of the second and third metacarpals and to detach the origins of the flexor pollicis brevis and the distal two thirds of the adductor pollicis brevis. This procedure includes the detachment of the origins of the first dorsal interosseous muscle. Contracture of the thumb web skin necessitates a Z-plasty (but rarely in children).

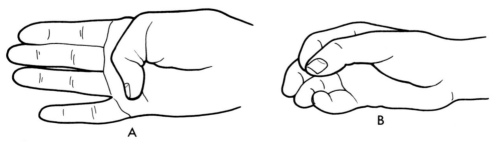

A   B

Figure 5–4 A. Thumb-in-palm deformity; spastic adductor pollicis, and, at times, spastic flexor longus. B. Normal pinch.

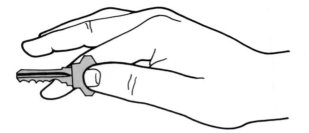

Figure 5–5 Key pinch: opposition of the thumb with the radial side of the index finger.

Spasticity of the flexor pollicis longus, although not common, should be relieved by lengthening the tendon in the distal one third of the forearm. Silver et al. (1976) lengthened this tendon in only two of their patients.

INSTABILITY OF THE METACARPOPHALANGEAL JOINT OF THE THUMB. Of all procedures that will make the difference between success and failure in indwelling thumb reconstruction, the assurance of stability of the metacarpophalangeal joint of the thumb is the most important. If this joint is hypermobile in flexion or extension, stabilization is necessary (Fig. 5–6). To accomplish this one of two procedures may be chosen: arthrodesis or capsulorrhaphy.

Arthrodesis: This procedure can be performed in children who have open epiphyses (Goldner, 1975, 1976). Through a midlateral radial or ulnar incision over the joint, the lateral band is retracted dorsally, the capsule and collateral ligaments are incised, the joint is dislocated, and the articular cartilage is removed to expose subchondral bone. "Nibbling" away the articular cartilage is safer in growing children. The joint surfaces are coapted manually in 5 to 10 degrees of flexion and 10 degrees of internal rotation. Bone chips can fill the intervening spaces. In children, fine smooth crossed Kirschner wires secure the fixed joint (Fig. 5–7). To accomplish the fixation, a power drill is almost essential. The wires are cut off under the

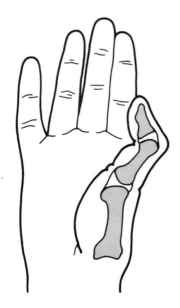

Figure 5–6 Common instability of the metacarpophalangeal joint.

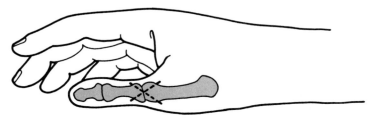

Figure 5–7   Arthrodesis of the metacarpophalangeal joint of the thumb. Crossed pin fixation.

skin and removed when fusion is solid in 6 to 10 weeks. A plaster cast holds the thumb and wrist in the corrected position while healing occurs.

In patients with closed epiphyses, I prefer a small ($3/32$ inch) screw for fixation. After the joint surfaces are denuded and shaped, the joint is manually compressed. A small hole of the same diameter as the screw is bored with an air-powered dental burr in the distal end of the dorsal surface of the metacarpal neck. This hole is drilled obliquely into the center of the proximal phalanx. The dental burr is used to enlarge the opening for the screw head so that it can be countersunk slightly. The screw is inserted to effect compression of the joint surfaces (Fig. 5–8). With this rigid fixation, it is possible to remove the postoperative plaster cast in 3 to 4 weeks so that early motion of the hand and wrist can commence. If the screw hole breaks during the procedure, all is not lost. The joint can always be fixed with multiple crossed threaded Kirschner wires.

Capsulorrhaphy (Zancolli, 1968; Filler et al., 1976).   This alternative to arthrodesis consists of detachment of the volar capsule of the metacarpophalangeal joint from the metacarpal bone and advancement of the capsular attachment proximally into a groove in the bone. Fixation is accomplished by a pullout suture that is threaded first through the capsule and then through two drill holes directed dorsally in the neck of the metacarpal and tied over a button on the dorsum of the thumb (Fig. 5–9). Thirty degrees of flexion are recommended by advocates of this procedure. Plaster cast immobilization for 6 weeks is usually necessary.

Of the two procedures, I prefer arthrodesis. With capsulorrhaphy there is a risk of an increasing flexion deformity.

WEAKNESS OF THUMB EXTENSION AND ABDUCTION.   There are almost unlimited possibilities for surgically reinforcing active abduction and extension of the thumb (Goldner, 1955, 1975, 1976; Samilson and Morris, 1964; Keats, 1965; House, 1975; Silver et al., 1976). Such reinforcement is usually necessary for success. The extensor and/or abductor pollicis longus muscle is rarely active or strong.

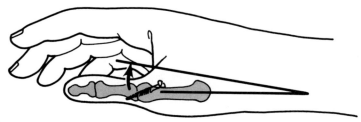

Figure 5–8   Arthrodesis of the metacarpophalangeal joint of the thumb. Fixation with a screw. The joint is fused in a 5 to 10 degree flexed position.

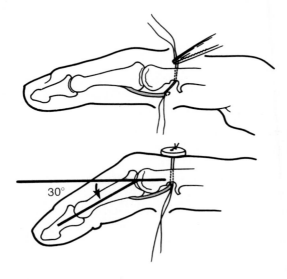

Figure 5-9 Technique for volar capsule advancement to stabilize metacarpophalangeal joint of the thumb.

In most cases I prefer re-routing of the extensor pollicis longus tendon. This permits reinforcement of both abduction and extension of the thumb with one transfer. There is no need to separate the two functions. Three muscles are preferred for reinforcement:

1. The brachioradialis — when there is no need to remove finger or wrist flexors to obtain a balanced hand.
2. The flexor carpi radialis — when there is concomitant wrist flexion deformity.
3. The flexor digitorum superficialis — when there is a need to relieve a finger flexion deformity.

Re-routing of the Extensor Pollicis Longus Tendon. Through a lazy-S incision made from the metacarpophalangeal joint of the thumb to about 4 centimeters proximal to the wrist, the extensor is dissected to free it from its dorsal hood insertion to its musculotendinous junction. The tendon is brought out of its fibro-osseous tunnel on the radial styloid and shifted in a radial direction. It is held in this direction by overlapping it with subcutaneous fat and fascia to make an anchoring tunnel 3 or 4 centimeters long.

Techniques for reinforcement of the re-routed thumb extensor are:

Brachioradialis transfer. After its insertion on the radial styloid is cut, the tendon is stripped from the radius to its musculotendinous junction to insure maximal excursion. The extensor pollicis longus is cut at its musculotendinous junction and interwoven under appropriate tension into the brachioradialis tendon (Fig. 5-10).

Flexor carpal radialis transfer. This tendon is cut at its insertion in the volar aspect of the wrist and brought out through a separate incision 8 to 10 centimeters proximal to the wrist; it is then re-routed subcutaneously and sutured under proper tension by interweaving it through the cut end of the re-routed thumb extensor.

Flexor digitorum superficialis transfer. The tendon is cut at the proximal phalanx. It is a good idea to leave the distal ends of the tendon in the finger so that they

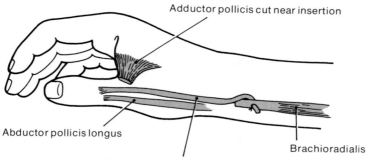

Adductor pollicis cut near insertion

Abductor pollicis longus

Brachioradialis

Re-routed extensor pollicis longus

Figure 5–10 Technique for reinforcement of thumb abduction by transfer of brachioradialis to re-routed extensor pollicis longus. The abductor pollicis longus is shortened and advanced (see text).

may form scar tissue and prevent hyperextension at the proximal interphalangeal joint. The tendon is pulled out 8 to 10 centimeters above the wrist and sutured under proper tension to the cut end of the re-routed thumb extensor (Fig. 5–11).

"Proper" tension in these transfers is hard to describe. A practical guide is that there should be enough tension so that the thumb remains extended and abducted when the wrist is in the neutral position but can be passively placed opposite the index finger and 2 centimeters radial to it; also, it should be possible to adduct the thumb so that its tip is within 1 to 1.5 centimeters of the palm (Goldner, 1976).

Postoperative plaster immobilization of the thumbs and wrist is continued for 3 to 4 weeks, and the transfer is protected for an additional month with a removal splint. Immobilization time will depend upon the status of the associated arthrodesis of the thumb.

INSTABILITY OF THE CARPOMETACARPAL JOINT OF THE THUMB. This can be recognized by hyperflexion of this joint. Shortening of the abductor pollicis longus and extensor pollicis brevis tendons is an added refinement of the thumb reconstruction. The annular ligament that covers these two tendons is incised; the tendons are Z-lengthened and resutured under maximal tension by advancement of the proximal ends of the Z to the base of the first metacarpal.

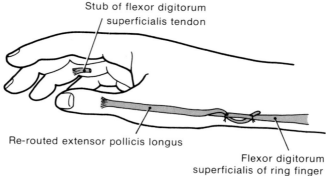

Stub of flexor digitorum superficialis tendon

Re-routed extensor pollicis longus

Flexor digitorum superficialis of ring finger

Figure 5–11 Technique for reinforcement of thumb abduction by transfer of the flexor digitorum superficialis to re-routed extensor pollicis longus.

If the carpometacarpal joint is stable, the tendons of both the abductor pollicis longus and the extensor pollicis brevis should be shortened by cutting each tendon 1 centimeter distal to its musculotendinous junction. A hole is made in the proximal end of the tendon, and the cut distal end of the tendon is pulled through the hole to obtain sufficient tension and then sutured. Tension is correct when the first metacarpal is extended and externally rotated.

DISTAL INTERPHALANGEAL JOINT OF THE THUMB. Arthrodesis of the distal interphalangeal joint of the thumb is advisable if the joint is deviated, hyperflexed, or hyperextended. After the cartilage surfaces are removed, the joint is fixed in 5 to 10 degrees of flexion with threaded pins that are then cut off beneath the skin.

If the extensor pollicis longus is active and strong (a rarity), no reinforcement is necessary.

If the distal interphalangeal joint is hyperextended, the extensor pollicis longus tendon may need to be lengthened.

The thumb-in-palm deformity may be the most difficult to correct. Samilson and Morris (1964) reported that in 128 operative procedures in hands of patients who had cerebral palsy, the least satisfactory results were obtained in the thumb deformity. If one procedure fails, an intermetacarpal bone block should not be done in desperation. The immobile abducted thumb is more bothersome to the patient than the presumed improvement in function.

In summary, the one-stage reconstruction of the thumb-in-palm deformity usually requires (1) release of adductor pollicis; (2) arthrodesis of the metacarpophalangeal joint; (3) shortening of the abductor pollicis longus and extensor pollicis brevis tendons; (4) re-routing of the extensor pollicis longus tendon; and (5) reinforcement of the re-routed extensor pollicis longus by transfer of the brachioradialis, flexor carpi radialis, or flexor digitorum superficialis tendon.

Wrist Flexion Deformity. The most common cause of the wrist flexion deformity is a spastic flexor carpi ulnaris muscle, and possibly the most overused transfer is that of its tendon. A transfer procedure should be done if the wrist extensors are nonfunctional.

Lengthening of the flexor carpi ulnaris tendon is recommended in children 4 to 6 years old if wrist extensors are present. A Z-lengthening of the tendon in the distal forearm is comparable to lengthening the Achilles tendon in the leg—a procedure done without hesitation.

Transfer of the flexor carpi ulnaris tendon is advisable when the wrist extensors are weak (the muscle test grade is less than fair — 3 or less). After the tendon is cut at its pisiform insertion, it is pulled out through a separate proximal incision at the junction of the middle and distal thirds of the forearm to the tendon of the extensor carpi radialis *brevis*. Since the flexor carpi ulnaris tendon is usually too short, it is necessary to suture it to the tendon of the extensor carpi radialis brevis rather than to its insertion on the metacarpal. (For straight wrist extension it is sutured to the extensor carpi radialis brevis; the radialis longus deviates the wrist.) Of all wrist tendon transfers, this one seems to be the most satisfying (Samilson and Morris, 1964; Keats, 1965; Filler, 1974).

Note: Do not rob the wrist of both flexor tendons, as grasp stability will be lost. If wrist extension power is in the fair to normal range (muscle test grade 3 to 5), do not transfer a spastic wrist flexor to the wrist extensor. Lengthening of the tendon is preferred in such cases.

WRIST ARTHRODESIS

Indications.   Although wrist arthrodesis seems to be an attractive once and for all procedure, it is not often necessary. Arthrodesis should *not* be done if:

1. the fingers can extend only by flexing the wrist;
2. the fingers can flex only by extending the wrist;
3. tendon transfers are feasible to improve the wrist position.

Wrist arthrodesis is a satisfactory solution for a severe wrist flexion deformity if:

1. there is generalized poor muscle control and strength that precludes reasonable active flexion and extension of the fingers;
2. there is a severe fixed deformity that precludes correction with tendon lengthening and transfer alone;
3. tendon transfers have been done and the wrist position either has not been corrected or is hyperextended.

To test the effects of wrist arthrodesis on hand function, a preoperative trial of immobilization in a short arm plaster cast is a help but is only feasible if the wrist can be passively extended to the neutral position.

Arthrodesis can be performed in growing children. However, I have used this procedure in children only when the patient's wrists and fingers are severely flexed and show no evidence of voluntary control.

Operative Technique.   The technique is practically the same in children and adults. A longitudinal dorsal incision exposes the extensor tendons, which are then retracted. The dorsal capsule of the joint is opened, and the navicular and lunate bones are excised; the articular surfaces of the carpal bones and distal radius are denuded of cartilage. The denuded articular surface of the capitate is fixed to the saucer-like depression in the denuded surface of the radius. A Steinmann pin is introduced at the distal end of the third metacarpal in the web space between the third and fourth metacarpal heads. The pin is driven straight through the base of the third metacarpal, across the carpal bones, through the capitate, and into the center of the distal radial epiphysis into the shaft of the radius (epiphyseal arrest is not likely if the pin is driven through the central portion of the epiphysis). Iliac bone grafts are added.

A plaster cast is used until fusion is solid. If finger and wrist flexor tendons are contracted at the time of arthrodesis, they may need to be lengthened.

The wrist should be placed in a neutral position. To achieve the best position the wrist should be extended to the point where the first metacarpal is in alignment with the shaft of the radius (Figs. 5–7 and 5–8).

Finger Flexion Deformities.   A finger flexion deformity may be caused by spastic flexor digitorum superficialis muscles, spastic flexor digitorum profundus muscles, or both. Tests that determine which muscles are spastic and which are contracted are described in Chapter 2.

Legthening of these contracted muscles is best done by the Z-method at their tendons in the distal half of the forearm. Overlengthening of the profundus muscle causes severe weakness. The profundus should be lengthened only to the point where when the wrist is in the neutral dorsiflexed position, the finger joints will be pulled into about 45 degrees of flexion.

Transfer of the contracted flexor digitorum superficialis tendons can be done to reinforce (1) a weak extensor pollicis longus, (2) a weak extensor carpi radialis brevis, or (3) weak extensor digitorum communis muscles. To reinforce the latter two muscles, the superficialis tendons should be pulled through a large opening in the pronator quadratus muscle (Goldner, 1976).

Note: An important general rule is that the profundus muscles should never be removed from the fingers. Lengthening of the profundus tendons must be done judiciously.

A relatively new procedure has been proposed to correct contracture of both finger flexor tendons. The profundus tendons are cut above the wrist, and their proximal ends are sutured to the distal ends of the extracted superficialis tendons (Braun et al., 1974). This procedure can result in pronounced weakness of finger flexion. We have seen two patients who had severe intrinsic-plus hands after such a procedure. The fingers were virtually fixed in extension. Perhaps insufficient tension was applied at the time of suture of the tendons in these two patients. Braun, who had this same postoperative result initially, recommended splinting the fingers in 45 degrees flexion for 6 weeks postoperatively.

The "flexor slide" operation, in which the origins of the flexors are detached from the humerus and allowed to slide distally, has been successful at times (Inglis and Cooper, 1966; White, 1972). White (1972) reported 11 failures with this operation out of 21 cases. To ensure complete relief of contracture extensive release of the origin of the profundus muscle is required (Hadad, 1977). The problem with extensive (and non-selective) release of the muscle origin is loss of flexion power; with more limited release, failure of correction may result. Selective lengthening of tendons is probably a better solution.

Finger Hyperextension Deformity. In this deformity, hyperextension occurs at the proximal interphalangeal joint and flexion at the distal interphalangeal joint. The deformity appears to be associated most often with a wrist flexion position that continuously stretches the extensor tendons across the dorsum of the proximal joints. If there is excessive elasticity of the ligaments, the volar capsule of the proximal joint is stretched as well. In this case the proximal joints are hyperextended. In a few cases the cause may be spastic intrinsic muscles.

INDICATIONS FOR SURGERY. If the fingers lock in hyperextension at the proximal joints and voluntary flexion does not unlock them, surgery is necessary to correct the deformity.

The surgical procedures are designed to produce a permanent flexion contracture of the joint. Two procedures have been described. I perform both procedures to ensure against recurrence. The wrist flexion deformity must also be corrected.

Volar Capsulorrhaphy (Goldner, 1976). Radial and ulnar midlateral incisions over the proximal interphalangeal joint expose the retinacula, which are incised. The volar joint capsule is detached from the distal end of the proximal phalanx and then pulled proximally to flex the joint. The capsule is anchored to its new attachment with sutures passed through the bone and tied to a dorsal button. The retinacula are sutured by overlapping the dorsal leaf distally and the volar leaf proximally (Fig. 5–12).

Superficialis Tenodesis (Swanson et al., 1966). The flexor tendons are exposed through a midlateral incision over the proximal joint, and the sheath is then opened and retracted volar-ward. The volar aspect of the proximal phalanx is stripped to its periosteum. The superficialis tendon is then anchored to the distal end of the

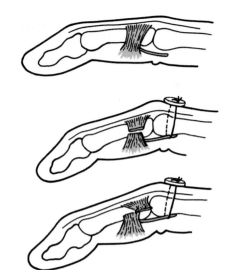

Figure 5–12 Technique for volar capsule advancement of proximal interphalangeal joint, and retinacular overlap to correct hyperextension locking of the proximal joint; can be combined with superficialis tenodesis.

proximal phalanx with a suture that passes through two drill holes in the phalanx and is tied over a dorsal button (Fig. 5–13).

In the postoperative immobilization the wrist is placed in the neutral position, and the fingers are flexed 30 degrees at the proximal interphalangeal joints. The position is maintained with a plaster cast and aluminum splints for 5 to 6 weeks.

Pronation Deformity. Pronation spasticity and early contracture are common. Posterior subluxation of the radial head occurs early in life and accounts for a fixed deformity that limits elbow extension. In some children dislocation of the radial head occurs later. Although Keats (1974) reported success with a bilateral radial head

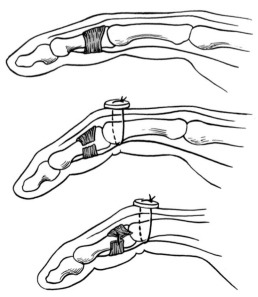

Figure 5–13 Technique for tenodesis of flexor digitorum superficialis to correct locked hyperextension of the proximal joint. Can be combined with volar capsule advancement.

excision in a 7-year-old child with cerebral palsy, I have had disappointing results with radial head excision in children with closed epiphyses.

INDICATIONS FOR PRONATOR TERES TENOTOMY. Prevention of subluxation of the radial head seems possible if the pronation contracture is released early enough. In older children who have a pronation contracture and some active voluntary supination, pronator teres tenotomy may restore better supination.

Pronator teres tenotomy can be performed alone or in combination with a flexor carpi ulnaris transfer to the distal radius (Green and Bank, 1962). In my own experience, simple tenotomy of the pronator teres is sufficient. House (1975) is of the same opinion. More complex procedures such as reversing the insertion of the pronator teres to act as a supinator have failed to restore active function.

The operative technique of pronator teres tenotomy is simple. A straight incision is made over the insertion of the pronator teres on the proximal radius. The tendon is detached from its radial insertion and excised up to its muscle. The forearm is immobilized in the supine position for 3 weeks; then active supination activities are begun.

Elbow Flexion Deformity. This has been the most difficult upper limb problem to treat. Some surgeons have reported only failure (Samilson and Hoffer, 1976), while others now report success (Mital, 1977; Goldner et al., 1977). I have not performed enough elbow flexion releases to make a personal judgment, but I will recommend the procedure when it is indicated.

INDICATIONS FOR SURGERY. If elbow extension lacks only 30 to 40 degrees, the problem is probably not worth treating. However, greater degrees of limitation cause restrictions in function, and are not cosmetically acceptable in the hemiplegic person who otherwise appears almost normal. Another type of candidate for surgery might be a child who might be able to walk with crutches if his elbows were extended.

OPERATIVE TECHNIQUES. Mital's procedure consists of excision of the lacertus fibrosis, Z-lengthening of the biceps tendon, and incision of the brachialis aponeurosis. To these procedures, Goldner adds the following as necessary to obtain correction: (1) myotomy of the brachialis and reinforcement of the lengthened biceps with the proximal and distal segments of the cut brachialis; (2) detachment of the origins of the wrist flexors and sometimes the origin of the brachioradialis; (3) anterior transfer of the ulnar nerve; and (4) anterior capsulotomy of the joint.

In both procedures, the postoperative management is the same. It entails the splinting of the elbow in extension for 3 weeks, graduated supervised exercises, and prolonged night splinting.

Mital reported good results in 32 cases. Goldner also reported 32 cases that were followed for 1 to 22 years. There were only three recurrences in Goldner's series, and four cases had a slow recovery of flexion strength. Thus, the procedure appears worthwhile if the elbow is severely flexed.

ELBOW FLEXION DEFORMITY IN HEMIDYSTONIA. Dystonic posturing of the upper limb does not involve contractures or skeletal deformities. Some of these patients have severe hyperflexion posturing of the elbow, which is uncomfortable and disabling.

To assess the effects of surgery in such patients, a 1 percent lidocaine solution can be injected into the muscle belly of the biceps; this may produce considerable relief of the hyperflexed position. If so, a neurectomy of the musculocutaneous nerve may alleviate the severely flexed posture in such patients, as demonstrated in two of my own patients who were followed for 3 and 4 years.

LOWER LIMB MANAGEMENT

Orthotics

ANKLE-FOOT ORTHOSIS FOR EQUINUS DEFORMITY

Orthotic management is preferred for dynamic equinus deformity. I do not recommend lengthening of the Achilles tendon or gastrocnemius muscle for a dynamic equinus abnormality, especially in the preschool years when the child's central nervous system is still maturing.

We have used the rigid plastic ankle-foot orthosis for dynamic equinus deformity since 1972 (Staros and LeBlanc, 1975). The orthosis forces the heel to contact the ground and thus may stimulate the dorsiflexor area on the plantar surface of the heel (Duncan, 1960). The advantages of the plastic ankle-foot orthosis are its light weight and the ability of the patient to wear ordinary shoes (see Fig. 6–2).

If the spasticity of the gastrocnemius-soleus muscle is strong, the orthosis may not keep the heel down. If this occurs, a myoneural block of 45 percent alcohol of the gastrocnemius muscle bellies may enable the orthosis to be worn effectively (for technique see Chapter 2).

If the gastrocnemius-soleus muscle is contracted, the orthosis will fail. When bilateral or unilateral metal upright 90-degree equinus stop orthoses are used, the high top shoe merely hides the equinus abnormality. The heel rides up inside the shoe. As with all other foot deformities, the theory of high top shoe prescriptions seems to be "if you don't see it, it's not there" (Perry, 1974).

BIOFEEDBACK DEVICES FOR DYNAMIC EQUINUS DEFORMITY

In patients with dynamic equinus deformity or very mild contracture, an auditory biofeedback device has proved to be a simple and sometimes effective method of correction (Conrad and Bleck, 1977). This inexpensive system consists of a pressure-sensitive on/off electronic switch inside the shoe under the heel. The switch is connected to a battery-powered "beeper" (a microbuzzer manufactured by Citizens America Corp., Santa Monica, California). When the "beep" is heard, heel contact occurs. The child and his parents are instructed in the use of the device by the physical therapist. The device should be worn by the child 3 hours per day for 3 months at home. This appears to be a more effective therapeutic regimen than the commonly prescribed "gait training" in a physical therapy department for 30 to 60 minutes one, two, or three times per week.

Based upon the results achieved, we recommend this method of treatment for a child over the age of 4 years who has a dynamic equinus deformity and a passive range of dorsiflexion of the ankle to at least the neutral postion (zero degrees).

ANKLE-FOOT ORTHOSES FOR DYNAMIC VARUS OR VALGUS DEFORMITY

In the preschool child, a valgus inclination can shift to a varus one. This phenomenon is due possibly to the persistence or dominance of the tonic reflex areas on the plantar skin of the foot and to the lack of uniformity in their disappearance. The inversion reflex area is located on the medial distal border of the plantar skin; the eversion reflex area is on the distal lateral border of the plantar skin (Duncan, 1960). The tonic reflexes of the foot are spinal reflexes mediated through the skin; they should disappear by the end of the first year. Persistence of these reflexes indicates delayed cortical maturation, a characteristic of cerebral palsy.

Foot equilibrium reactions may also explain the shift from a valgus to a varus position of the foot. In children with cerebral palsy, the normal early shift from the foot eversion standing posture to the foot inversion posture ("medial arch reaction") is delayed (Gunsolus et al., 1975). As a consequence, a flexible valgus position may shift to a varus position as maturation occurs in the preschool child.

For these neurological reasons it seems prudent to avoid surgical treatment of a flexible foot deformity in the child until the central nervous system is completely matured. During this period, orthotics are useful. The rigid plastic ankle-foot orthosis (see Fig. 6–2) can be used to hold a valgus or varus foot in the correct position. The orthosis is fabricated from a plaster mold of the foot and leg in the corrected position.

We have had no success with the UCBL (University of California Biomechanics Laboratory) shoe insert in holding or correcting pes valgus when the peroneal muscles are spastic (Bleck and Verzins, 1977). Similarly, the plastic ankle-foot orthosis also fails to give effective control of the valgus foot with severe peroneal muscle spasticity. In these cases we use a single *medial* upright metal ankle-foot orthosis. The lateral T-strap merely holds the upright in the shoe channel. Figure 5–14 shows the mechanics of this orthosis. If the foot is in the varus position, the unilateral lateral metal upright orthosis with a medial T-strap can be effective.

Surgery

EQUINUS DEFORMITY

Indications for Surgery. Contracture of the gastrocnemius-soleus muscle requires surgery. There is no evidence that manual stretching, exercises, plaster casts, or orthoses have ever effected a release of the contracture.

If the foot is capable of dorsiflexion to a neutral (zero) position when measured with the plantar surface of the heel and the foot in varus position (to lock the midtarsal joints), surgery is not indicated in most patients.

The choice of surgical procedures for correction of an equinus deformity includes neurectomy, gastrocnemius lengthening, gastrocnemius origin recession, Achilles tendon lengthening, and Achilles tendon translocation. All procedures are designed to reduce the stretch reflex and to lengthen the muscle. All weaken the muscle. Too much weakness causes overdorsiflexion; a calcaneus deformity is functionally worse than the equinus abnormality.

Gait studies have demonstrated that the gastrocnemius muscle becomes active at heel contact and continues its activity through the mid-stance phase of gait. The function of the gastrocnemius is to reduce the forward acceleration of the tibia during the stance phase. The muscle does not "push off" at toe contact. Instead, the terminal stance of gait is mechanical; the foot action consists of a "roll-off" motion (Perry, 1976). If the patient has a fixed equinus deformity, this "roll-off" action is not possible; the patient vaults over his foot, raises the center of gravity, and expends more energy than normal during level walking.

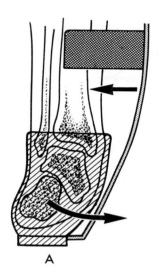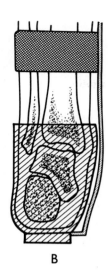

Figure 5–14 Unilateral *medial* upright ankle foot orthosis to correct severe spastic pes valgus. A. The mechanism of the brace is demonstrated. As the medial upright (which can be bent more medially for more correction) approximates the calf, a valgus force is exerted on the heel through the brace channel in the shoe. A lateral T-strap merely holds the upright in the shoe channel and exerts no correction. A lateral upright is used for a varus foot. B. Orthosis in corrected position.

A   B

Denervation of the gastrocnemius (and at times the soleus) no longer seems to be popular. Neurectomy may increase the risk of a postoperative calcaneus deformity and does not lengthen the muscle. Silver and Simon (1959) have had continued success (Silver, 1977) with neurectomy of the gastrocnemius combined with recession of its origins.

The choice between gastrocnemius lengthening only and Achilles tendon lengthening is supposed to be based upon the Silfverskiöld test. If the foot dorsiflexes *easily* beyond the zero position when the knee is flexed 90 degrees, and if dorsiflexion does not correct the equinus abnormality when the knee is extended, midcalf lengthening of the gastrocnemius muscle is thought to be advisable. This phenomenon of isolated gastrocnemius contracture is rare.

Perry and his co-workers (1974) showed with electromyograms that the Silfverskiöld test is unreliable. When the ankle was dorsiflexed 90 degrees, electrical activity was recorded in *both* the gastrocnemius and soleus muscles. Furthermore, in three of eight cases when the Silfverskiöld test was positive—i.e., indicative of soleus spasticity — the electromyograms recorded no soleus activity during walking.

Craig and VanVoren (1976) measured the proximal migration of the gastrocnemius muscle bellies after gastrocnemius muscle lengthening and Achilles tendon lengthening. Metallic markers and radiographic examinations were used. The postoperative radiographs showed a proximal shift a mere 0.8 cm of the gastrocnemius muscle after Achilles tendon lengthening, but there was a 4.7 cm shift after gastrocnemius muscle lengthening. Based upon these data, they recommended both operations at the same time. The equinus deformity recurred in 9 percent of their cases.

Lee and Bleck (1977) studied the results of 117 operations for equinus abnormality; 59 were of the Strayer-Baker type of gastrocnemius lengthening, and 65 were of the Hoke type of Achilles tendon lengthening. The recurrence rate after the Strayer-Baker lengthening was 30 percent; after the Hoke Achilles tendon lengthening, it was

9 percent. Schwartz et al. (1977) also reported a high recurrence rate (41 percent) after the Strayer-Baker lengthening.

Our data and those of others (Banks and Green, 1958; Sharrard, 1972) support my recommendation for Achilles tendon lengthening in practically all cases of equinus deformity.

Throop et al. (1975) reported their experience with translocation of the Achilles tendon to a more anterior insertion on the calcaneus. Their reason for performing this procedure in 79 cases was to preserve the "push-off" strength of the gastrocnemius. They estimated that the procedure reduced plantar flexion strength by 50 percent. Their success rate of correction was 89.9 percent. These results are not appreciably different from those reported with Achilles tendon lengthening. The translocation procedure is more complicated than lengthening. The tendon must be detached from its insertion on the calceneus, moved anteriorly, and reattached to bone. Although the authors reported no increased morbidity with this procedure, the simplest procedure that works is probably the best.

The postoperative functional result of Achilles tendon lengthening can be ascertained preoperatively. If the patient can voluntarily dorsiflex the foot with the range permitted by the equinus position with the knee fully extended, the postoperative gait may be almost normal. If, however, the foot can be dorsiflexed only when the knee is flexed 90 degrees and when hip flexion is resisted (an automatic motion caused by the flexor withdrawal reflex), then the postoperative gait will be improved, but a steppage gait (hip and knee flexed) will persist so that the toe can clear the floor during swing phase.

HOKE ACHILLES TENDON LENGTHENING OPERATIVE TECHNIQUE.   Through a longitudinal 5 to 7 cm posterior medial incision, the posterior portion of the Achilles tendon is exposed and its sheath preserved. Three cuts are made in the tendon: (1) one half of the tendon is cut medially and distally; (2) one half medially and proximally; and (3) one half is cut laterally between the two medial cuts. The foot is dorsiflexed just to neutral (zero degrees). The tendon ends slide apart, leaving a lateral splice in between. No tendon sutures are necessary (Fig. 5–15). If the contracture is mild, the procedure can be done through a single transverse incision. The postoperative skin scar is almost invisible.

A postoperative long leg plaster with the knee slightly flexed (5 degrees) and the ankle dorsiflexed at zero degrees (or at 1 or 2 degrees) is worn for 6 weeks. Walking is permitted as soon as the plaster is dry. If convenient, the long leg plaster can be cut down to a short leg plaster in 3 weeks. After removal of the plaster, ordinary low quarter shoes or sneakers (tennis shoes) are worn.

A similar sliding lengthening procedure can be done by the two-cut method of White; this is used by Banks and Green (1958). One half the tendon is cut proximally in its posterior-lateral segment and one half distally in its anterior-medial segment. Others have used a subcutaneous approach with this technique. I have found that in a teaching program the Hoke method is most reliable, almost never produces overcorrection, has few complications, and gives good end results.

GASTROCNEMIUS LENGTHENING (STRAYER, 1950; BAKER, 1956) OPERATIVE TECHNIQUE.   A 5 to 7 cm longitudinal incision is made at the junction of the proximal and middle thirds of the calf where the muscle bellies of the gastrocnemius join to form the broad gastrocnemius aponeurosis overlying the soleus. The sural vein and nerve are retracted. One edge of the gastrocnemius aponeurosis is identified and separated from the underlying soleus. The aponeurosis is cut transversely

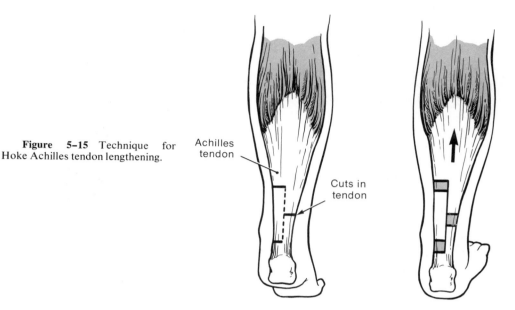

Figure 5–15 Technique for Hoke Achilles tendon lengthening.

Achilles tendon

Cuts in tendon

(a 1 to 2 cm segment can be removed). The muscle bellies of the gastrocnemius are easily separated from the soleus. The knee is extended and the foot dorsiflexed. A long leg walking plaster is used for 6 weeks postoperatively.

The Baker modification of the Strayer procedure consists of a proximally directed "tongue" cut in the aponeurosis. The base of the tongue is distal. When the foot is dorsiflexed with the knee extended, this tongue slides distally to effect lengthening. Often a section of the median fibrous raphe of the soleus is included, and some surgeons also strip the soleus muscle fibers from the emerging Achilles tendon. This extensive muscle stripping has possibly caused more scar tissue and accounted for the high recurrence rate of contracture reported with this procedure.

Postoperative Calcaneus Deformity. Although rare in our series of cases (0.85 percent) and not too frequent in Schwartz's (Schwartz et al., 1977) series (4 percent), calcaneus deformity is a major complication. It is most important to avoid *overlengthening* of the tendon. The sliding methods of lengthening allow control of the tension in the muscle, whereas with a complete Z-lengthening and resuture procedure, it is almost impossible to restore the proper tension.

Operative shortening of the overlengthened Achilles tendon has not been successful in correcting this distressing postoperative complication. If the anterior tibial muscle is spastic, it may be transferred through the interosseous membrane to the calcaneus. The most satisfactory solution (with or without anterior tibial tendon transfer) has been to stop all ankle motion with a rigid plastic ankle-foot orthosis which holds the foot in a slight equinus position. Foot-ankle function is restored by the addition of a rocker-sole and cushion heel to the shoe. The principle applied is the same one used in prosthetics with the SACH (solid ankle cushion heel) foot.

Equinus Deformity in Hemidystonia. I have performed neurectomy of both gastrocnemius muscle heads in three patients who had severe and disabling dystonic equinus deformity. All three patients had a full range of passive dorsiflexion of the ankle well above the neutral position. All patients were over 13 years old and had

had extensive trials of various therapeutic methods, muscle-relaxing drugs, and restrictive ankle orthoses.

Preoperative assessment was made with a 45 percent alcohol myoneural block of both gastrocnemius muscle heads. This block resulted in considerable improvement of the equinus abnormality over a period of 2 to 6 weeks. No "athetoid shift" to a new dystonic pattern occurred.

In all three patients, a neurectomy of the medial and lateral heads of the gastrocnemius was performed through a transverse incision just distal to the popliteal crease. Postoperatively, a long leg walking plaster was used for 3 weeks to assist wound healing.

Follow-up observation has been pursued for 5 years in one patient and 4 years in two patients. There have been no recurrences of the severe equinus posturing. One patient who had dystonic varus posturing of the foot successfully wears a rigid plastic ankle-foot orthosis.

In contrast to patients with spastic equinus deformity who have undergone neurectomies plus lengthenings, none of these three patients has developed a calcaneus deformity. The reason is probably the absence of any coexistent spasticity of the anterior tibial muscle, a condition that may be present in patients with spastic equinus.

PES VARUS

The causes of pes varus are spasticity of the posterior tibial muscle, which produces hindfoot varus, and weakness of the peroneal muscles, which results in midfoot varus. Occasionally, the anterior tibial muscle may be spastic.

Electromyograms during walking have shown continuous dysphasic activity of the posterior tibial muscle in patients with pes varus (Hoffer, 1976). Electromyographic examination may be helpful in deciding on the proper surgical treatment in puzzling cases. A varus inclination often accompanies equinus deformity. In this type of problem, the gait electromyogram may demonstrate either phasic or dysphasic activity of the posterior tibial muscle. If the muscle is dysphasic, posterior tibial tendon lengthening should be done in addition to Achilles tendon lengthening.

Surgical treatment is indicated in a child older than 4 years who has a dynamic pes varus deformity. When the deforming force of the spastic muscle persists, skeletal changes in the direction of the deforming force can be anticipated. Early surgery can prevent skeletal deformities.

The surgical procedures to be described are those I have found to be the simplest, most effective, and associated with the least number of late postoperative complications.

Operative Technique for Passively Correctable Hindfoot Varus and Posterior Tibial Tendon Lengthening. With this procedure, Bank and Panagakos (1966) reported good results, confirming my preference for this simple operation. Through a 3 to 5 cm longitudinal incision directly over the posterior tibial tendon *proximal to the medial malleolus,* the tendon is Z-lengthened. The foot is placed in the neutral position, and the tendon is sutured side-to-side with non-absorbable sutures. A short leg walking plaster is worn for 6 weeks. The procedure can be combined with Achilles tendon lengthening.

Intramuscular tenotomy of the posterior tibial tendon has been described by

Ruda and Frost (1971). Their procedure consisted of a tenotomy of the posterior tibial tendon in the middle third of the calf. No plaster immobilization was used; the patients walked soon after surgery. Of 29 cases, no failures and only two recurrences were reported. Ruda and Frost recommended that this intramuscular tenotomy be performed before the age of 6 years.

I have not performed intramuscular tenotomy because the operative dissection is more complex than the supramalleolar Z-lengthening of the tendon. No doubt Ruda and Frost's method is effective most of the time; however, I would be cautious in performing this operation (or any other lengthening of tendons) in patients under the age of 4 years because it presents a risk of a shift from a varus to a valgus foot in a child whose central nervous system is still maturing.

Procedures not recommended for correction of posterior tibial muscle spasticity include:

1. Tenotomy of the tendon at its insertion on the navicular. This attractively simple operation presents a frequent risk of collapse of the talonavicular joint with resultant valgus deformity of the midfoot within 6 to 12 months postoperatively. It is impossible to reattach the tendon.

2. Transfer of the posterior tibial tendon. This procedure has its adherents and detractors. Bisla et al. (1976) reported good results in 13 of 19 cases, whereas Turner and Cooper (1972) had poor results in 10 of 14 patients; reversal from varus to valgus deformity occurred. Banks (1976) had only moderate success. Schneider and Balon (1977) reported poor results with posterior tibial tendon transfer; within 1 year, 68 percent of the feet were in either the valgus or the calcaneus position.

The weight of the evidence plus my own experience has convinced me not to recommend this procedure. Moreover, the transfer of the spastic posterior tibial muscle is not physiological. In normal persons, the posterior tibial muscle is active only in the stance phase of walking and does not readily convert to a swing phase muscle when transferred anteriorly. In addition, when a spastic muscle is transferred, tension is increased and spasticity is likely to be aggravated.

3. Anterior re-routing of the posterior tibial tendon. Baker and Hill (1964) reported good results in 27 feet when the tendon was removed from its sheath and slipped anterior to the medial malleolus. Many of the apparently good results deteriorated owing to late calcaneus deformities as the spastic posterior tibial muscle continuously acted as a strong dorsiflexor of the ankle.

Passively Correctable Midfoot Varus Deformity and Anterior Tibial Tendon Transfer. INDICATIONS. When the peroneal muscles are weak but are phasically contracting on gait electromyograms, this transfer is the logical choice. It is easy to create a valgus deformity by anchoring the tendon too far laterally. The tendon insertion should be moved no further lateral than the second cuneiform bone.

To obviate valgus deformity as the result of transfer, a split anterior tibial tendon transfer was devised (Hoffer, 1974). One half of the tendon is transferred laterally. This split transfer (named "SPLATT" by its originators) has been successful in correcting spastic equinovarus deformities in adults who had cerebral vascular accidents. In children with cerebral palsy, the medial limb of the anterior tibial tendon that remains attached to its insertion may continue to act as an inverter of the midfoot.

In children the split anterior tibial tendon transfer seems indicated if gait electromyograms show phasic anterior tibial activity and dysphasic peroneal activity and clinical examination indicates "weak" peroneals. In this situation transfer of the entire anterior tibial tendon may produce a late pes valgus deformity.

The *operative technique* of anterior tibial tendon transfer consists of the following steps: (1) detach the anterior tibial tendon from its insertion on the first meta-tarsal-cuneiform bones; (2) pull the tendon out through a separate incision at the junction of the middle and distal thirds of the leg over the anterior muscular compartment; (3) re-route the tendon subcutaneously; and (4) anchor it in a drill hole in the second cuneiform bone with a pull-out wire suture. In order to avoid pressure necrosis of the plantar skin when securing the wire suture through the tendon, I use (instead of a button) a plastic foam-padded aluminum splint (1.5 cm × 3 cm with two holes for the wire) over a piece of sterile felt.

A postoperative short leg walking plaster is used for 6 weeks. After plaster removal, only ordinary (low quarter) shoes are necessary.

Hindfoot Varus Deformity, Not Passively Correctable: Closed Wedge Osteotomy of the Calcaneus (Silver et al., 1967).   INDICATIONS.   If passive correction of a hindfoot varus deformity is not possible, a closed wedge osteotomy of the calcaneus is an effective and simple procedure. It must be accompanied by lengthening of the posterior tibial tendon and, if required, Achilles tendon lengthening.

OPERATIVE TECHNIQUE.   Through a lateral oblique incision coursing from a point anterior to the Achilles tendon to a distal point almost parallel to the peroneal tendons, the lateral aspect of the calcaneus is exposed subperiosteally. A wedge of bone with a lateral base is removed from the calcaneus. Sufficient bone is removed to correct the heel varus deformity when the wedge is closed. A staple maintains the closure (Fig. 5–16).

Hindfoot and Midfoot Varus Deformity, Not Passively Correctable: Triple Arthrodesis.   INDICATIONS.   If the hind- and midfoot cannot be passively corrected, triple arthrodesis is the best procedure to use in children over the age of 12 years. The deforming force of the spastic muscles should be relieved as required by lengthening the Achilles tendon and the posterior tibial tendon. If the peroneal muscles are non-functional, the anterior tibial tendon should be transferred to the middle of the foot into the tarsal bones.

Triple arthrodesis is a standard operative procedure, but its use in patients with cerebral palsy is not common. Horstman (1977) reported the use of triple arthrodesis in only 37 patients from a pool of 899 who had cerebral palsy. Only 20 of these patients had equinovarus deformities. Varus deformities were more successfully corrected than valgus deformities.

Orthopaedic surgeons have been reluctant to use triple arthrodesis because of the risk of the "ball and socket" ankle joint that occasionally develops many years later (Fig. 5–17). This late complication is thought to be due to the removal of the torque absorption function of the subtalar joint by arthrodesis. The subtalar joint absorbs the torques generated by rotation of the foot on the ground during walking. If these rotational forces cannot be absorbed at the subtalar joint, the next proximal joint that may do so is the ankle (Inman, 1976). Not every patient who has a triple arthrodesis will develop a "ball and socket" ankle joint. This inconsistency may be explained by the great individual variations that occur in the axis of the ankle joint. This axis is oblique, and it corresponds almost exactly to a line drawn just below the tips of the malleoli. When a second line is drawn through the midline of the tibia, the

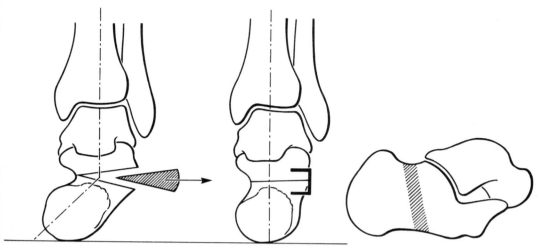

Figure 5–16 Technique of lateral closing wedge osteotomy for varus deformity of the hindfoot.

mean axis of the joint is 82.7 degrees (S.D. ± 3.7 degrees, with a range of 74 to 94 degrees) (Inman, 1976). It is possible that ankle joint axes that are more horizontal will rotate more, and such patients are more likely to develop a late "ball and socket" ankle joint after a triple arthrodesis.

The *operative technique* of triple arthrodesis is so well known and is described in so many surgical orthopaedic textbooks that the details need not be repeated here. Excessive valgus position of the foot created by overgenerous, laterally based wedges of bone from the three joints should be avoided.

I do not use staples or any other form of internal fixation. Two Steinmann pins, one through the heel across the subtalar joint and one dorsally across the talonavicular joint, permit the application of a heavily padded postoperative plaster. We

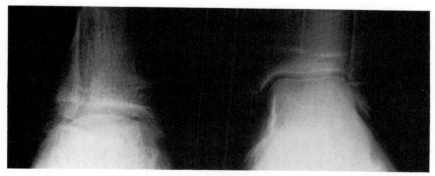

Figure 5–17 Anteroposterior radiograph of ankle joints of a spastic hemiplegic 18-year-old male; post-triple arthrodesis on left side of radiograph shows "ball and socket" ankle joint. Note that if a line is drawn between the tips of the malleoli to delineate the ankle axis, the axis is almost horizontal on the ball and socket side, and oblique on the normal side (see text for explanation).

sandwich the foot and ankle between dorsal and plantar ABD pads that are secured with rolled cast padding (technique of W. M. Roberts, M.D., North Carolina Orthopaedic Hospital). This padding accommodates the considerable postoperative swelling that occurs. The plaster needs splitting infrequently. This long leg plaster and pins are removed 4 weeks postoperatively. A short leg walking plaster is then used for 4 to 6 weeks.

Continuous suction drainage of the wound up to 48 hours postoperatively has been a useful added technical feature that helps to prevent wound breakdown.

PES VALGUS

Although pes valgus occurs in patients with spastic hemiplegia, it is more common with spastic diplegia. It is a difficult deformity to treat. The problems and various surgical treatments of pes valgus are discussed in Chapter 6.

PES CAVUS

Causes.   Pes cavus is only occasionally seen in spastic hemiplegia. It is probably caused by spasticity of the intrinsic muscles of the foot. Pes cavus can be defined as a forefoot equinus deformity beyond the normal range of plantar flexion of the tarsal and metatarsal bones (Fig. 5–18). Ankle equinus inclination is not often present and should not be confused with the primary problem of forefoot equinus deformity.

The normal weight-bearing foot has approximately 20 degrees of plantar flexion of the first metatarsal measured from the horizontal plane. I use this measurement at the time of correction of the deformity. Barenfed et al. (1971) measured the degree of

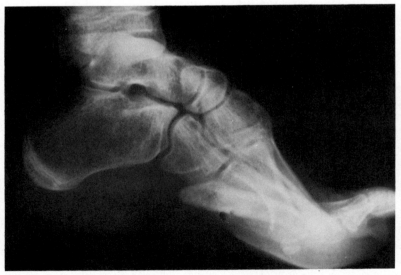

Figure 5–18   Pes cavus in a spastic hemiplegic shown in a lateral radiograph. Note equinus position of forefoot.

forefoot equinus inclination on standing lateral radiographs of normal children's feet. The obtuse angle between the horizontal plane of the calcaneus and a line along the shaft of the first metatarsal varied from 140 to 160 degrees. If the angle of the ankle joint was less than 140 degrees, the foot was defined as cavus. In 75 percent of the children with pes cavus, the angle was less than 125 degrees.

Operative Procedures.   Various procedures have been used for correction of the cavus abnormality. Before it is established as a bony deformity, it may be possible to correct and prevent its progression with plantar fasciotomy, release of the origins of the toe flexors from the calcaneus, and neurectomy of the intrinsic foot musculature (Burman, 1938). I have not performed any of these procedures. The problem is timing. Usually by the time the cavus abnormality produces symptoms of foot discomfort (midtarsal joint pain and painful calluses on the plantar surfaces of the metatarsal heads), the deformity is definitely skeletal. At this stage, soft tissue procedures are likely to fail.

Midtarsal closed dorsal wedge osteotomies correct the cavus deformity but shorten the foot considerably. Goldner (1976) performed closed dorsal wedge osteotomies through the cuneiform bones. Japas (1968) described a V osteotomy in the coronal plane with the apex of the V in the middle cuneiform bones.

If the deformity is not too severe (45 to 50 degrees of the forefoot equinus angle), I prefer an osteotomy of the V type through the bases of the metatarsal shafts, with the apex of the V proximal (Swanson, 1966). The metatarsals are dorsiflexed through the osteotomy to the 20 to 25 degree plantar flexion angle measured against the plantar aspect of the heel. The foot has the contour of a gentle ski slope, but this is not troublesome to the patient. No joints are fused, and little shortening of the foot results. Plantar fasciotomy and correction of claw toe deformities, if present, are done at the same time as the osteotomy.

Metatarsal or other tarsal osteotomies will not correct a "drop foot" caused by weak ankle dorsiflexor muscles. This type of problem will also require a triple arthrodesis and tendon transfers of the peroneus longus or the posterior tibial tendon if their muscles are strong enough and are functional.

METATARSUS ADDUCTUS

Causes.   In spastic hemiplegia, a unilateral bunion with hallux valgus has been seen in several patients (Fig. 5–19). The major deforming force appears to be the spastic abductor hallucis muscle (Bleck, 1967). The intrinsic muscles of the foot are active during the stance phase of gait, and the abductor hallucis is a major intrinsic muscle. Metatarsus adductus appears to develop after Achilles tendon or gastrocnemius muscle lengthening, probably because the intrinsic muscles are substituted for the weakened gastrocnemius and soleus muscles during walking.

Indications for Surgery.   In dynamic metatarsus adductus, the role of the abductor hallucis can be ascertained by infiltrating its muscle belly with 5 to 10 ml of 1 percent lidocaine. If the metatarsus adductus can be passively corrected, as demonstrated by an anteroposterior radiograph taken with the forefoot manually abducted, abductor hallucis release is indicated. If the deformity is marked and is not passively correctable, a capsulotomy of the metatarsal-tarsal joints is advisable in children under the age of 4 years; a metatarsal osteotomy may be done in older children. With either of these procedures, the abductor hallucis should be released.

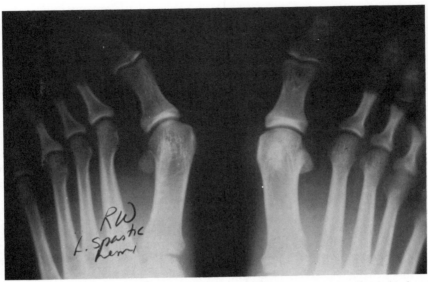

Figure 5–19 Left spastic hemiplegia, patient 16 years old. Anteroposterior radiographs show greater adduction of the first metatarsal on the hemiplegic side and the secondary hallux valgus.

Operative Technique of Abductor Hallucis Release.   A 2.5 cm longitudinal incision is made over the medial aspect of the first metatarsal, and the tendon of the abductor hallucis is found and grasped with a Kocher hemostat (Fig. 5–20). The tendon is cut distal to the hemostat, which is used to pull the tendon out of the wound so that a 1 cm piece can be removed. With the forefoot in abduction and the heel in the neutral position, a short leg walking plaster is applied and is used for 6 weeks. After removal of the plaster, no special shoes or splints are necessary.

The results of abductor hallucis release have been excellent (Bleck, 1967), except in two patients who had fixed adduction of the first metatarsal. In these two patients, hallux valgus developed later.

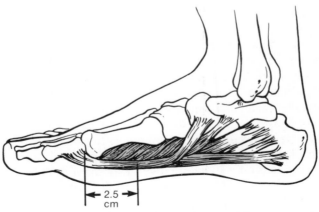

Figure 5–20 Through a 2.5 cm incision over medial aspect of first metatarsal neck, the abductor hallucis tendon is readily found, and is easily released.

HALLUX VALGUS

Causes.   The deformity can be due to a spastic adductor hallucis muscle alone or in association with adduction of the first metatarsal, and it occurs commonly in pes valgus deformities in which excessive pressure on the medial border of the foot and great toes forces the great toe into abduction.

Indications for Surgery.   Discomfort due to the secondary bunion or to calluses on the medial aspect of the great toe is an indication for surgery. If the hallux valgus is dynamic only, tenotomy of the adductor hallucis insertion may be successful. Usually, more extensive surgery is required.

If the first metatarsal is adducted, the Mitchell osteotomy through the neck of the metatarsal may give good results.

If hallux valgus is not completely passively correctable (particularly in older children and adolescents), closed wedge osteotomy of the base of the proximal phalanx may correct the deformity. With all surgical procedures on bone, an adductor hallucis tenotomy is performed. Sequist (1977) reported successful results in the treatment of spastic hallux valgus in 20 of 26 patients. He performed an adductor hallucis tenotomy, a lateral capsulotomy of the metatarsal-phalangeal joint, and pin fixation. I have had better results, with less metatarsal-phalangeal joint stiffness, with the osteotomy of the proximal phalanx and adductor hallucis tenotomy than with procedures that entail opening the joint capsule and using intra-articular pin fixation.

Operative Technique.   The Mitchell first metatarsal osteotomy is so well known that the operative technique need not be described here (Mitchell, 1958; Boyd, 1966).

The osteotomy of the base of the proximal phalanx begins with a longitudinal medial incision that exposes the proximal half of the proximal phalanx. After the periosteum is stripped from the base of the entire phalanx, a small-bladed sagittal power saw is used to remove from the base of the phalanx a wedge of bone with its base medial. Two small holes are drilled through the medial cortex proximal and distal to the osteotomy. A suture is drawn through the holes and tied securely to close the wedge.

Postoperative care consists of use of a short leg walking plaster for 4 weeks followed by a wood-soled postoperative orthopaedic shoe for an additional 4 weeks.

Risks.   There have been three main problems with metatarsal neck osteomy:

1. Failure to allow slight plantar flexion in the distal fragment (the head of the metatarsal). To accomplish a few degrees of plantar flexion of the metatarsal head, the saw cut should be inclined slightly posterior.
2. Reported failure of union of the osteotomy and aseptic necrosis of the metatarsal head. This can be avoided by not detaching the lateral capsule from the head.
3. Failure to correct residual hallux valgus. This deformity can be recognized at the time of metatarsal osteotomy and can be corrected by the closed wedge proximal phalangeal osteotomy.

TOE DEFORMITIES

Flexion deformities of the toes are more common in adolescents and adults than in children. When flexion contractures of the toes cause discomfort, a tenotomy of the toe flexor will usually solve the problem.

KNEE FLEXION AND HYPERTENSION DEFORMITIES

In hemiplegia, knee flexion deformities are managed as described in the following chapter on spastic diplegia. The results of therapy in patients with spastic hemiplegia are often better than in those with diplegia because there is a normal opposite limb.

Hypertension of the knee is due to spasticity of the quadriceps and is best left alone unless it is very severe. A rectus femoris proximal tenotomy will allow slightly more knee flexion in swing phase.

A non-surgical solution for knee hyperextension may be found in the plastic ankle-foot orthosis with the ankle dorsiflexed above the neutral position (Rosenthal, 1975). This orthosis can be successful only if the ankle can be dorsiflexed above the neutral position. The possible effect of the orthosis on the knee can be estimated by observation of the patient's knee as he walks up an inclined ramp.

HIP FLEXION AND INTERNAL ROTATION DEFORMITY

As with knee flexion, the management of this abnormality is the same as that in the child who has spastic diplegia. Iliopsoas recession and derotation subtrochanteric femoral osteotomy have corrected the gait of practically all such hemiplegic children to almost normal in function and appearance.

The most common pitfall of femoral derotation osteotomy in the child with spastic hemiplegia is failure to recognize and treat simultaneously the concomitant excessive external tibial-fibular torsion (greater than 30 degrees) that frequently occurs in such children. Untreated, this torsional deformity of the leg becomes glaringly evident after correction of the femoral torsion. To prevent this unhappy result the abnormality must be recognized preoperatively by examination, and derotation osteotomy of the proximal tibia and fibula must be done. External rotation of the leg is satisfactory when, with the knee extended, the foot is externally rotated 10 degrees from the midsagittal plane.

LEG LENGTH DISCREPANCY

Stunting of linear growth in the hemiplegic limb is common, but the discrepancy rarely exceeds 1.5 cm. If it exceeds 2 cm, leg length should be equalized by distal femoral epiphyseal arrest or stapling of the normal limb. No shoe lifts are ordinarily required for a mild leg length discrepancy. A short leg does not cause scoliosis; spinal curvature results from unknown forces that act on the spinal mechanism independently from the leg length discrepancy. The hemiplegic child is already burdened with an abnormal gait; shoe lifts merely add to the disability.

SCOLIOSIS

The incidence of scoliosis is higher in children with cerebral palsy than in the normal population (normal, 1.9 percent; cerebral palsy, 6 percent [Balmer and

MacEwen, 1970]). In hemiplegia, the spinal curve patterns are identical with and indistinguishable from those in idiopathic scoliosis. Management is the same as that of idiopathic scoliosis: a spinal orthosis is used to treat curves under 45 degrees, and surgery is used for those over 45 degrees.

REFERENCES

Baker, L. D. (1956) A rational approach to the surgical needs of the cerebral palsy patient. *Journal of Bone and Joint Surgery* 38A:313–323.

Baker, L. D., and Hill, L. M. (1964) Foot alignment in cerebral palsy. *Journal of Bone and Joint Surgery* 46A: 1–15.

Balmer, G. A., and MacEwen, G. D. (1970) The incidence and treatment of scoliosis in cerebral palsy. *Journal of Bone and Joint Surgery* 52B:134–137.

Banks, H. H., and Green, W. T. (1958) Correction of equinus deformity in cerebral palsy. *Journal of Bone and Joint Surgery* 40A:1359–1379.

Banks, H. H., and Panagakos, P. (1966) Orthopaedic evaluation in the lower extremity in cerebral palsy. *Clinical Orthopaedics and Related Research* 47:117–125.

Banks, H. H. (1976) The foot and ankle in cerebral palsy. *Orthopaedic Aspects of Cerebral Palsy* (Ed. Samilson, R. L.), Philadelphia, J. B. Lippincott Co.

Barenfed, P. A., Weseley, M. S., and Shea, J. M. (1971) The congenital cavus foot. *Clinical Orthopaedics and Related Research* 79:119–126.

Bisla, R. S., Lovis, H. J., and Albano, P. S. (1976) Transfer of the tibialis posterior tendon in cerebral palsy. *Journal of Bone and Joint Surgery* 58A:497–500.

Bleck, E. E. (1967) Deformities of the spine and pelvis in cerebral palsy. *Orthopaedic Aspects of Cerebral Palsy* (Ed. Samilson, R. L.), Philadelphia, J. B. Lippincott Co.

Bleck, E. E., and Berzins, U. J. (1977) Conservative management of pes valgus with plantar flexed talus, flexible. *Clinical Orthopaedics and Related Research* 122:85–94.

Boyd, B. M., and Carr, C. R. (1966) Correctional osteotomy for metatarsus primus varus and hallux valgus. *Journal of Bone and Joint Surgery* 48A:1649.

Braun, R. M., Vise, G. T., and Roper, B. (1974) Preliminary experience with superficialis-to-profundus tendon transfer in the hemiplegic upper extremity. *Journal of Bone and Joint Surgery* 56A:466–472.

Burman, M. S. (1938) Spastic intrinsic muscle imbalance of the foot. *Journal of Bone and Joint Surgery* 20:145–148.

Conrad, L., and Bleck, E. E. (1977) Biofeedback training for correction of equinus. Paper read at annual meeting of the American Academy for Cerebral Palsy and Developmental Medicine, Atlanta.

Craig, J. J., and VanVoren, J. (1976) The importance of gastrocnemius recession in the correction of equinus deformity in cerebral palsy. *Journal of Bone and Joint Surgery* 58B:84–87.

Duncan, W. R. (1960) Tonic reflexes of the foot. *Journal of Bone and Joint Surgery* 42A:859–868.

Filler, B. C., Stark, N. H., and Boyes, J. H. (1976) Capsulodesis of the metacarpophalangeal joint of the thumb in children with cerebral palsy. *Journal of Bone and Joint Surgery* 58A:667–670.

Goldner, J. L. (1955) Reconstructive surgery on the upper extremity in cerebral palsy and spastic paralysis. *Journal of Bone and Joint Surgery* 37A:1141–1155.

Goldner, J. L. (1975) Cerebral palsy: upper extremity reconstructive surgery. *Instructional Course Syllabus,* American Academy for Cerebral Palsy.

Goldner, J. L. (1976) The upper extremity in cerebral palsy. *Orthopaedic Aspects of Cerebral Palsy* (Ed. Samilson, R. L.), Philadelphia, J. B. Lippincott Co.

Goldner, J. L. (1977) Surgical treatment of cavo varus. Paper read at the annual meeting of American Orthopaedic Association.

Goldner, J. L., Goodman, W. B., and Bookman, M. (1977) The long term results of soft tissue elbow releases for improved elbow and forearm function in children with cerebral palsy. Paper read at annual meeting of American Academy for Cerebral Palsy and Developmental Medicine, Atlanta.

Green, W. T., and Banks, H. H. (1962) The flexor carpi ulnaris transplant and its use in cerebral palsy. *Journal of Bone and Joint Surgery* 44A:1343–1352.

Gunsolus, P., Welsh, C., and Houser, C. E. (1975) Equilibrium reactions in the feet of children with spastic cerebral palsy and of normal children. *Developmental Medicine and Child Neurology* 17: 580–591.

Hadad, R. J. (1977) Upper limb surgery in cerebral palsy. *Regional Course,* American Academy for Cerebral Palsy and Developmental Medicine, New Orleans.

Hohman, L. B., Baker, L., and Reed, R. (1958) Sensory disturbances in children with infantile hemiplegia, triplegia and quadriplegia. *American Journal of Physical Medicine* 37:1–6.

Hoffer, M. M., Reswig, J. A., Garrett, A. M., and Perry, J. (1974) The split anterior tibial tendon transfer in treatment of spastic varus of the hindfoot in childhood. *Orthopaedic Clinics of North America* 5:31–38.

Hoffer, M. M. (1976) Basic considerations and classification of cerebral palsy. *Instructional Course Lectures* 25:96–106, American Academy of Orthopaedic Surgeons, St. Louis, C. V. Mosby Co.

Horstmann, H. M., and Eilert, R. E. (1977) Triple arthrodesis in cerebral palsy. Paper read at the annual meeting of the American Academy of Orthopaedic Surgeons, Las Vegas.

House, J. H. (1975) A dynamic approach to the "thumb-in-palm" deformity in cerebral palsy. *Instructional Course Syllabus,* American Academy for Cerebral Palsy.

Inglis, A. E., and Cooper, W. (1966) Release of flexor-pronator origin for flexion deformities of the hand and wrist in spastic paralysis: a study of eighteen cases. *Journal of Bone and Joint Surgery* 48A:847–857.

Inman, V. T. (1976) *The Joints of the Ankle,* Baltimore, The Williams & Wilkins Co.

Japas, L. H. (1968) Surgical treatment of pes cavus by tarsal V osteotomy. *Journal of Bone and Joint Surgery* 50A:927–944.

Jones, M. (1976) Differential diagnosis and natural history of the cerebral palsied child. *Orthopaedic Aspects of Cerebral Palsy* (Ed. Samilson, R. L.), Philadelphia, J. B. Lippincott Co.

Keats, S. (1965) Surgical treatment of the hand in cerebral palsy: correction of the thumb-in-palm and other deformities. *Journal of Bone and Joint Surgery* 47A:274–284.

Keats, S. (1974) Congenital bilateral dislocation of head of radius in a seven year old child. *Orthopaedic Review* 111:33–36.

Lee, C. L., and Bleck, E. E. (1977) Surgical correction of equinus deformity in cerebral palsy. Paper read at the annual meeting of the American Academy for Cerebral Palsy and Developmental Medicine, Atlanta.

Matev, I. (1963) Surgical treatment of spastic "thumb-in-palm" deformity. *Journal of Bone and Joint Surgery* 45B:703–708.

Mital, M. H. (1977) Flexion contractures and involuntary bias in upper extremities at the elbow: its surgical management. *Developmental Medicine and Child Neurology* 19:116 (Abstract).

Mitchell, C. L., Fleming, J. L., Allen, R., Glenney, C., and Sanford, G. A. (1958) Osteotomy–bunionectomy for hallux valgus. *Journal of Bone and Joint Surgery* 40A:41–60.

Perlstein, M. A., and Hood, P. M. (1956) Infantile spastic hemiplegia, intelligence, oral language and motor development. *Courrier* 6:567.

Perry, J. (1974) Personal communication.

Perry, J., Hoffer, M. M., Giovan, P., Antonelli, D., and Greenberg, R. (1974) Gait analysis of the triceps surae in cerebral palsy. *Journal of Bone and Joint Surgery* 56A:511–520.

Perry, J. (1975) Pathomechanics. *Atlas of Orthotics — Biomechanical Principles and Applications* (Ed. American Academy of Orthopaedic Surgeons), St. Louis, C. V. Mosby Co.

Perry, J. (1976) Cerebral palsy gait. *Orthopaedic Aspects of Cerebral Palsy* (Ed. Samilson, R. L.), Philadelphia, J. B. Lippincott Co.

Rosenthal, R. K. (1975) A fixed ankle below-the-knee orthosis for the management of genu recurvatum in spastic cerebral palsy. *Journal of Bone and Joint Surgery* 57A:545–549.

Ruda, R., and Frost, H. M. (1971) Cerebral palsy spastic varus and forefoot adductus, treated by intramuscular posterior tibial tendon lengthening. *Clinical Orthopaedics and Related Research* 79:61–70.

Samilson, R. L., and Morris, J. M. (1964) Surgical improvement of the cerebral palsied upper limb: electromyographic studies and results in 128 operations. *Journal of Bone and Joint Surgery* 46A:1203–1216.

Samilson, R. L., and Bechard, R. (1973) Scoliosis in cerebral palsy. *Current Practice in Orthopaedic Surgery* (Ed. Adams, J. P.), St. Louis, C. V. Mosby Co.

Samilson, R. L., and Hoffer, M. M. (1976) Problems and complications in orthopaedic management of cerebral palsy. *Orthopaedic Aspects of Cerebral Palsy* (Ed. Samilson, R. L.), Philadelphia, J. B. Lippincott Co.

Schneider, M., and Balon, K. (1977) Deformity of the foot following anterior transfer of the posterior tibial tendon and lengthening of the achilles tendon for spastic equinovarus. *Clinical Orthopaedics and Related Research* 125:113–117.

Schwartz, J. R., Cau, W., Bassett, F. H., and Coonrad, R. W. (1977) Lessons learned in the treatment of equinus deformity in ambulatory spastic children. *Orthopaedic Transactions* 1:84.

Sequist, J. L. (1977) Surgical correction of hallux valgus in cerebral palsy. Paper submitted to program committee of American Academy for Cerebral Palsy and Developmental Medicine (unpublished).

Sharrard, W. J. W., and Bernstein, S. (1972) Equinus deformity in cerebral palsy. *Journal of Bone and Joint Surgery* 54B:272–276.

Silver, C. M., and Simon, S. D. (1959) Gastrocnemius muscle recession (Silfverskiöld operation) for spastic equinus deformity in cerebral palsy. *Journal of Bone and Joint Surgery* 41A: 1021–1028.

Silver, C. M., Simon, S. D., Spindell, E., Lichtman, H. M., and Scala, M. (1967) Calcaneal osteotomy for valgus and varus deformities of the foot in cerebral palsy. *Journal of Bone and Joint Surgery* 49A:232–246.

Silver, C. M., Simon, S. D., Lichtman, H. M., and Motamed, M. (1976) Surgical correction of spastic thumb-in-palm deformity. *Developmental Medicine and Child Neurology* 18:632–639.

Silver, C. M. (1977) *Instructional Course on Management of Spastic Hemiplegia,* American Academy of Orthopaedic Surgeons, Las Vegas.

Staros, A., and LeBlanc, M., (1975) Orthotic components and systems. *Atlas of Orthotics — Biomechanical Principles and Applications* (Ed. American Academy of Orthopaedic Surgeons), St. Louis, C. V. Mosby Co.

Strayer, L. M. (1950) Recession of the gastrocnemius. *Journal of Bone and Joint Surgery* 32A:671–676.

Swanson, A. B. (1960) Surgery of the hand in cerebral palsy in the swan-neck deformity. *Journal of Bone and Joint Surgery* 42A:951–964.

Swanson, A. B., Browne, H. S., and Coleman, J. D. (1966) The cavus foot: concepts of production and treatment by metatarsal osteotomy. *Journal of Bone and Joint Surgery* 48A:1019.

Tachdjian, M. O., and Minear, W. L. (1958) Sensory disturbances in the hands of children with cerebral palsy. *Journal of Bone and Joint Surgery* 40A:85–90.

Throop, F. B., DeRosa, G. P., Reech, C., and Waterman, J. (1975) Correction of equinus in cerebral palsy by the Murphy procedure of tendo-calcaneus advancement — a preliminary communication. *Developmental Medicine and Child Neurology* 17:182–185.

Turner, J. W., and Cooper, R. R. (1972) Anterior transfer of the tibialis posterior through the interosseous membrane. *Clinical Orthopaedics and Related Research* 83:241–244.

White, W. F. (1972) Flexor muscle slide in the spastic hand. *Journal of Bone and Joint Surgery* 54B:453–459.

Zancolli, E. (1958) *The Structural and Dynamic Bases of Hand Surgery,* Philadelphia, J. B. Lippincott Co.

Chapter Six

DIPLEGIA AND PARAPLEGIA

GENERAL CHARACTERISTICS

Spastic diplegia is the most common type of cerebral palsy in the United States. In 1965, in an unpublished survey of the type of cerebral palsy in our case load, we found that 47.5 percent of all patients with cerebral palsy had spastic diplegia associated with premature birth. In 1977 my estimate is that this type of cerebral palsy accounts for 60 percent of our patients.

Diplegia, according to accepted terminology, is defined as spastic involvement of the lower limbs with minor motor deficits in the upper limbs. Paraplegia, in contrast, involves the lower limbs only with no deficits in the upper limbs. Paraplegia is rare. If it is encountered, high spinal cord lesions should be ruled out (bladder problems coexist with spastic paralysis of the lower limbs), and a hereditary basis should be considered as the cause.

The general characteristics of spastic diplegia include the following points:

1. Upper limb function is good with only minor incoordination of the fingers on fine motor skill testing (e.g., approximating each finger tip to the thumb in sequence).
2. The lower limbs are definitely spastic with the following typical pattern (Fig. 6–1):
    a. Hip flexion spasm and contracture.
    b. Hip internal rotation with excessive femoral anteversion.
    c. Hip adduction spasm and contracture.
    d. Knee flexor or extensor spasticity predominates.
    e. Equinus ankle.
    f. Valgus foot with flexible plantar-flexed talus.
3. Speech and intellect are usually normal or only slightly impaired.
4. Esotropia and perceptual and visual-motor deficits may be associated.
5. Neurological examination shows hyperactive lower limb reflexes, positive Babinski signs, no infantile automatisms, and deficient posterior equilibrium reactions.
6. Most patients can walk independently (only 5 to 10 percent need crutches) but tend to fall backward easily owing to deficient equilibrium reactions (see Chapters 2 and 3 for assessment and interpretation of equilibrium reactions).

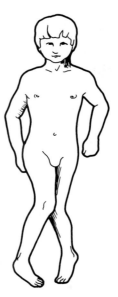

Figure 6–1 Typical posture of spastic diplegia.

NATURAL HISTORY

Most patients walk by the age of 48 months. The deficient posterior equilibrium reaction seems to persist throughout life but is not a serious disability.

Almost all of these children can be "integrated" into regular school by the age of 7 or 8 years (some never need attend a special school). Almost all should be able to lead useful and independent lives provided that they have not been conditioned or segregated into the "handicapped" population through well-intentioned "medicalization" and overtreatment of their neurological deficits. In adolescents, the one predominant disability that blocks development of adult independence has been an anxiety neurosis that, in some cases, appears to have been generated by parental and professional overtreatment and excessive striving to remedy deficits rather than to compensate for them. Examples of such remedial efforts include (1) to "practice walking better"; (2) to attempt schooling in philosophy when the grasp of abstractions is not possible; (3) to improve handwriting when typewriting is easier to learn.

ORTHOTICS

Shoes

Sneakers (tennis shoes) provide good ground contact and probably better sensory input. Hiking boots with crepe soles help stabilize the ankle by decreasing the possible range of plantar and dorsiflexion so that postural adaptation and control by the anterior tibial and gastrocnemius-soleus muscles need not be as great; boots also add a bit of weight that probably helps to control balance.

I have found no use for special or corrective orthopaedic shoes (Bleck, 1971a).

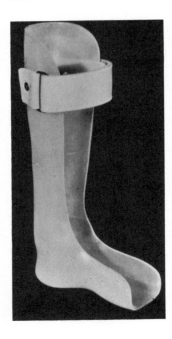

Figure 6-2 Rigid plastic ankle-foot orthosis for dynamic equinus deformity, pes valgus, or both.

Dynamic Equinus Deformity

With this deformity the biofeedback device described in Chapter 4 can be tried. We frequently use the rigid plastic ankle-foot orthosis (Fig. 6-2) or, if the spasm is too great, we use 45 percent alcohol myoneural blocks of the gastrocnemius muscle (Chapter 2).

When the equinus position is fixed the customary 90 degree ankle-stop orthosis with a high shoe merely hides the deformity. Achilles tendon lengthening is indicated when contracture is present to this degree (Fig. 6-4).

Pes Valgus

Pes valgus is common in spastic diplegia. I do not recommend surgical correction until the child is 7 years of age or older. In the interim, a rigid plastic ankle-foot orthosis (AFO) made from a mold of the foot in the corrected position will usually suffice (Fig. 6-2).

If the peroneal muscles are too spastic for the restraining capability of the plastic orthosis, unilateral medial upright orthoses as described in Chapter 4 may be effective.

Hip Adduction

Garrett's hip abduction orthosis may be helpful in a preschool child who has adductor spasm (but no contracture) and a developing central nervous system (Garrett et al., 1966).

Hip Flexion and Internal Rotation

No orthosis has been satisfactory in treating this combination of defects. The cable twister orthosis appears to affect only the external rotation of the tibia and fibula; thus, another deformity is created as a compensation for the internal rotation of the hip.

Knee Flexion

If the knee is flexed over 15 degrees in stance phase after hamstring lengthening (due to quadriceps weakness and little or no quadriceps spasticity), a knee-ankle-foot orthosis with adjustable knee joints can help until sufficient quadriceps strength is gained.

Knee Hyperextension

The rigid plastic ankle-foot orthosis with the ankle dorsiflexed can be used providing the ankle has a satisfactory range of passive dorsiflexion (Rosenthal 1975).

TIMING OF ORTHOPAEDIC SURGERY

Surgery should not be performed for gait improvement until the child has been walking independently for a year. Exceptions to this general rule may be made in patients with structural changes: hip subluxation, knee-joint contracture, and contracture of the gastrocnemius-soleus muscles.

The optimum age for surgery appears to be between the ages of 4 and 8 years. I try to finish most of the treatment program by the age of 7 to 8 years. The increased incidence of postoperative psychological problems in the adolescent (Williams, 1977) reinforces the recommendation to correct and prevent structural deformities reasonably early in life. Surgery should not be regarded as a last resort or as "something that can always be done when all other methods have failed." Neither should it be unduly staged so that with each birthday the gift is another hospitalization and another period of immobilization in a plaster (Fig. 6–3). The goal of treatment is a healthy functionally independent person, not a permanent patient.

ORTHOPAEDIC SURGERY, LOWER LIMB

In order to understand the complex functional and structural abnormalities in the lower limb, it is necessary to regard each as a separate entity even though they almost always coexist. The surgeon must carefully examine and re-examine the patient's gait, joints, and muscles so that the appropriate surgical procedures can be combined and excessive "staging" can be avoided (for examination methods see Chapter 2).

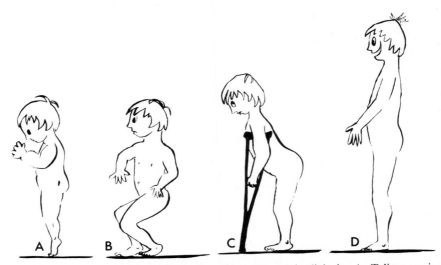

Figure 6–3 Usual "staging" of orthopaedic surgery in spastic diplegia: A. Talipes equinus. B. Crouch after heel cord lengthening. C. Crouch corrected by hamstring lengthening. D. Final erect posture after hip flexion contracture corrected. It may be possible to combine surgery at three levels to get directly from A to D. (Drawing courtesy of Mercer Rang, M.D., Toronto.)

Hip

ADDUCTION DEFORMITY

Anatomy, Physiology, and Biomechanics. The adductor muscles of the hip originate from the pubis anteriorly and insert on the femur medially. Strange (1965) has pointed out that anatomically the hip adductors function as external rotators. Their innervation comes from the obturator nerve except that one half of the adductor magnus is supplied by the tibial division of the sciatic nerve.

Electromyograms of the adductors during level gait in normal persons show that the adductor muscles contract at the end of the stance phase. The exact function of the adductors has been a subject of controversy. Murray (1968) has shown that the maximum mean electrical output of the gluteus and medius muscles (hip abductors) occurs when the hip is in 5 degrees of adduction. It appears that the adductors stabilize the pelvis so that the abductors can function optimally. As the hip abducts, the strength of the abductors is diminished. Consequently, for maximum efficiency and smoothness of walking, the femora should be kept in slight adduction. Over-abduction should be avoided.

The function of the hip abductors during gait has been well-established (Inman, 1947; Saunders et al., 1953); these are the muscles that are essential for energy conservation in preventing excessive lateral shift of the trunk during single limb balance by keeping the pelvis level. The pelvis is pulled down on the weight-bearing limb. This shift of the trunk (about 2 cm) occurs very quickly from limb to limb. Without good functioning hip abductors, a lurching gait that consumes high levels of energy occurs.

The base of the gait is correlated with the necessity of keeping the femora in slight adduction during gait. The base measures 5 to 10 cm from heel to heel in normal subjects, although close analysis shows that it varies considerably between

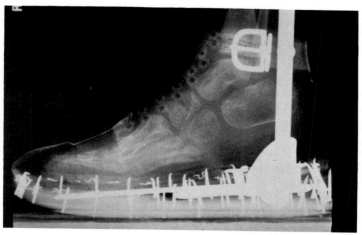

Figure 6–4 Radiograph of foot and ankle in typical 90 degree talipes equinus–stop orthosis, and shoe. The talipes equinus is conveniently hidden.

persons; some normal persons have a base from heel to heel of only 1 centimeter (mean in children: 7.6 cm [Scrutton, 1969]). Consequently, in cerebral palsy patients who have adductor spasticity, the goal of treatment should be to keep the base of the gait between 5 and 10 cm.

Another controversy concerning the adductors is whether or not they are the main cause of the internal rotation gait patterns seen so commonly in spastic diplegia. Possibly the controversy arises because perception of internal rotation during gait varies. By this I mean that the adduction of the femur during the stance phase of gait may appear to be internal rotation to some observers, while to others the amount of internal rotation is not noticeable (Fig. 6–5). Furthermore, adduction

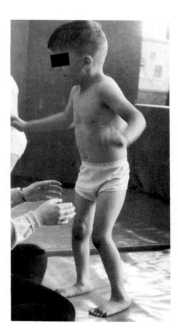

Figure 6–5 Spastic diplegia, patient age 6 years. Does he have hip internal rotation, adduction, or both? Range of motion of each hip: abduction 30 degrees, internal rotation 90 degrees, external rotation 10 degrees. Hip flexion contracture is 35 degrees.

spasticity occurs simultaneously with flexion spasticity and internal rotation during gait. We can make clinical observations on minimally involved patients such as the spastic hemiplegic child who has internal rotation during gait. In these children, no contracture or spasticity of the adductors can be demonstrated. As will be discussed in the later secton on internal rotation, the major deforming force appears to be excessive femoral anteversion.

Banks and Green (1960) described their experience with surgical treatment of adduction spasticity in cerebral palsy. They reported that of 89 patients, 15 continued to rotate internally even after adductor myotomy and anterior branch obturator neurectomy. I have seen persistent internal rotation of the hip even after bilateral intrapelvic obturator neurectomy.

It is true that motion pictures made by surgeons in the operating room after exposure and stimulation of the anterior branch of the obturator nerve show the limb internally rotating. However, I believe we can demonstrate that when the patient has a slight flexion deformity of the knee, the heel, as it rests on the table, acts merely as a pivot point. As a consequence, when adduction occurs, the force of gravity causes internal rotation of the hip when the adductors are stimulated. If the unanesthetized patient who has no knee flexion contracture is asked to adduct — i.e., bring his feet together — no internal rotation of the femur occurs. It does occur, however, in a normal patient with excessive femoral anteversion when the knees are held in flexion by posterior splints, so that the limb rotates on the heel as a pivot point. It is thus not surprising that surgeons have concluded honestly, but erroneously, that the adductors are the major internal rotating force.

Clinical Examination. When the child walks, adduction spasticity is manifested by the knees knocking together and a short stride length. Children with marked adduction spasticity who walk with crutches may use a swing-through or swing-to gait to conserve energy and to go faster. Scissoring of the lower limbs is present when one limb crosses over the other during walking. In the nonambulatory patient with severe adduction spasticity both knees are clamped tightly together and one limb may cross over the other. Scissoring can also be brought out by holding the child by the axillae and swinging him from side to side.

With the child lying supine, the range of abduction of the hip should be tested with the hips in extension and in flexion. Because the adductors are also flexors of the hip axillae (up to 70 degrees of flexion), a modest flexion contracture of the hip (up to 20 degrees) can be elicited by the Thomas test. More flexion deformity than this indicates a concomitant spasticity and contracture of the iliopsoas muscle.

The strength of the hip abductors can be determined with the side-lying hip abduction test. Because of the limited range of abduction caused by adduction spasticity and, in some patients, the lack of direct central control of the hip abductor muscle, this test is not reliable. The child should also be tested to differentiate dystonic posturing in cases of tension athetosis. If a patient has only dystonic posturing and abduction can be accomplished beyond 20 degrees with relaxation or repetitive movements, then surgery designed to relieve adduction spasticity may result in an abducted position of the hip postoperatively.

Indications for Surgery. In the ambulatory patient, surgery to relieve adduction spasticity is indicated when there is abduction of each hip limited to 20 degrees or less and/or scissoring (Sharrard, 1975). In the non-ambulatory patient, indications for surgery are abduction of each hip limited to 20 degrees or less with the hip extended, scissoring, and radiographic evidence of subluxation of the hip. In the non-ambulatory patient, surgery for adductor spasticity usually must be combined with iliopsoas tenotomy.

When in doubt about the effects of surgery to relieve adductor spasticity in ambulatory patients, myoneural blocks of the adductor longus can help in making a decision. In young children, myoneural blocks of the belly of the adductor longus muscle in three or four locations with 3 ml of 45 percent alcohol under brief general anesthesia provide help in analyzing the problem. The block will last between 2 and 6 weeks. This gives the child, the parents, the physical therapist, and the surgeon a chance to observe the effect of the block. In older cooperative children, a myoneural block can be achieved with 1 percent lidocaine. I have found, however, that in many patients lidocaine causes dizziness; by the time the patient has recovered from it, the block has worn off and there is little opportunity to observe its effects.

TYPES OF ADDUCTOR SURGERY. *Adductor longus myotomy and anterior branch obturator neurectomy* can be done when indicated in the ambulatory or non-ambulatory patient. Posterior branch obturator neurectomies are not recommended because overabduction of the hip can result. If an error has to be made in treating adductor spasticity, it should be on the side of not doing quite enough. If after anterior branch obturator neurectomy and adductor longus myotomy, the child still has scissoring, an intrapelvic obturator neurectomy can always be done. In the non-ambulatory patient with subluxation of the hip, the operative approach used for adductor myotomy and anterior branch obturator neurectomy can also be used for iliopsoas tenotomy.

Adductor origin transfer to the ischium (Fig. 6–6). This operation has become

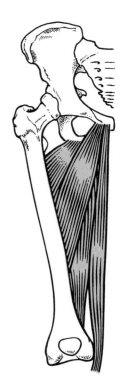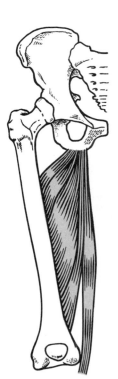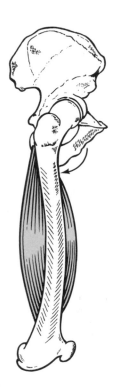

Figure 6–6   Adductor origin transfer.

popular. Jacqueline Perry (Garrett, 1976) originated adductor transfer in patients who had poliomyelitis. Since then, other surgeons have reported good results in patients with cerebral palsy (Stephenson and Donovan, 1971; Baumann, 1972; Griffin et al., 1976; Couch et al., 1977). Other surgeons have modified the procedure by limiting the number of adductor origins transferred. Whereas Couch et al. (1977) transferred the origins of the adductor longus and brevis and the gracilis plus release of the origins of the adductor magnus, Evans (1977) transfers *only* the adductor longus and gracilis. Hoffer (1977) transfers the adductor longus and brevis and gracilis to the fascia overlying the adductor magnus; he does limit the transfer to the longus and gracilis in less severe cases.

In the reported series, one criterion of success appears to be improvement of the internal rotation of the hip. Krom (1969) found that in 10 of 20 patients, the hip rotation posture was converted to neutral or external rotation postoperatively (in this series 14 of the 20 patients also had iliopsoas tenotomy). Of the 35 patients reported by Couch et al. (1977), failure to correct internal rotation occurred in only five. In my own observations as a visitor to a number of clinics, correction of hip internal rotation during gait after adductor transfer does not always result.

Another criterion for success has been the measurement of the base of the gait. Couch et al. (1977) found a mean preoperative measurement of 13.5 cm and a postoperative mean of 24 cm (range, 12 to 37 cm). Is a broad-based gait a goal?

Two questions should be posed. Is there any difference between transfer of the adductor origins and adductor longus and gracilis myotomy with anterior branch obturator neurectomy? Also, is the additional operative complexity, time, and postoperative immobilization required for adductor transfer worthwhile when compared with the easier adductor myotomy and neurectomy? Table 6–1 summarizes what I perceive as the advantages and disadvantages of each procedure.

In conclusion, I would reserve the adductor transfer procedure for the independent walking patient who has hip abduction limited to 20 degrees or less and who does not require an iliopsoas lengthening or recession procedure. In the patient who

Table 6–1 ADVANTAGES AND DISADVANTAGES OF ADDUCTOR MYOTOMY WITH ANTERIOR BRANCH OBTURATOR NEURECTOMY AND ADDUCTOR ORIGIN TRANSFER

	Advantages	Disadvantages
Adductor transfer	(1) Preserves adductor strength for pelvic stability during stance (?) (2) May correct the internal rotation deformity (?)	(1) Longer operation; technically more demanding (2) Theoretically should require a longer immobilization period (but in practice this is not done)
Adductor myotomy and anterior branch obturator neurectomy	(1) Easier and shorter operation (2) Short immobilization period (3) Quicker recovery (4) Can do other procedures at the hip at the same time (e.g., iliopsoas recession or lengthening)	(1) Weakens adduction; but if adductor brevis and magnus are preserved, this does not seem to be significant (2) Does not correct hip internal rotation with assurance

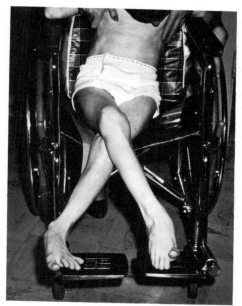

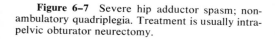

Figure 6–7 Severe hip adductor spasm; non-ambulatory quadriplegia. Treatment is usually intrapelvic obturator neurectomy.

depends on crutches, it probably does not make much difference which procedure is done. In the non-ambulatory patient who has poor prognostic signs for walking (see Chapters 2 and 3), adductor transfer does not offer enough advantages to outweigh the more extensive surgery and postoperative care required.

Intrapelvic obturator neurectomy is indicated in those patients in whom anterior branch obturator neurectomy has failed to relieve a sufficient amount of the adductor spasticity. It is indicated in the non-ambulatory patient in whom one leg is actually crossed over the other or who has severe adduction spasticity and contracture (Fig. 6–7). It can be combined with adductor myotomy to correct contracture. The postoperative course of intrapelvic obturator neurectomy is much easier for the patient because the abdominal wound is less painful and usually heals with fewer complications than the groin wounds.

Operative Technique for Adductor Myotomy and Anterior Branch Obturator Neurectomy. The linear incision begins about 2 cm distal to the origin of the adductor longus and continues along the longus for 5 cm. The deep fascia is incised, and the adductor longus is carefully freed and defined posteriorly with a curved Mayo hemostat. Cutting electrocoagulation severs the adductor longus near its musculotendinous junction. Bleeding points should be coagulated so that the wound is dry. With blunt dissection, the two branches of the anterior branch of the obturator nerve are located in the connective tissue overlying the adductor brevis. The branches are stimulated either by pinching with the hemostat or by an electric stimulus to make sure that these are indeed the nerves. Then with a hemostat the nerves are isolated, picked up and cut distal to the hemostat, and dissected proximally for about 2 cm to the point where the nerve is cut. I do not cut the adductor brevis unless there is a marked contracture. The gracilis muscle is routinely sectioned with the cutting electrocoagulation knife. In older children with deep wounds, closed suction irrigation drainage is instituted. The subcutaneous tissues are closed with absorbable sutures, and the skin is closed with absorbable synthetic sutures reinforced with sterile adhesive closures.

Postoperative immobilization with long leg plasters with each hip held in 30 to 40 degrees abduction for 3 weeks is sufficient. Forced overabduction can lead to an excessive compression of the articular surfaces of the hip joints and may result in postoperative stiffness. After the plasters are removed, the patient should be exercised in parallel bars if he has the ability or potential to walk. If not, the usual bed-sitting routine or wheelchair transfer routine is instituted. I have not used side-lying hip abductor exercises but instead have taught the patient weight-shifting exercises in order to bring out, if possible, the true function of the gluteus medius and minimus muscles.

ERRORS IN ADDUCTOR LONGUS MYOTOMY AND ANTERIOR BRANCH OBTURATOR NEURECTOMY

1. Failure to find the anterior branches of the obturator nerve. This is due to excessive bleeding in the wound or, more commonly, to failure to carefully isolate the posterior surface of the adductor longus and separate it from the connective tissue overlying the adductor brevis before the muscle or tendon is cut. If the cutting extends into the adductor brevis before the branches of the nerve are identified, it may be very difficult to locate them, and in haste to get the operation completed, the wound is closed. When the deformity recurs, it is claimed that the nerves regenerated. Recurrence may also be caused by more severe adductor spasticity than was appreciated preoperatively. In this situation, intrapelvic obturator neurectomy can be done.

2. Failure to correct the internal rotation deformity of the hip. This "failure" is caused by overexpectation on the part of the surgeon, the parents, and the patient. It must be appreciated that internal rotation during gait is a complex activity and depends not only on muscle but on structural changes in the femur.

3. Failure to correct the subluxation of the hip or, more commonly, to prevent its further development. We have documented cases of subluxation and even dislocation of the hip that occurred 8 years after presumed success with the operation to prevent subluxation and dislocation of the hip and despite assiduous bracing and exercise. In these cases there was an underlying iliopsoas spasticity and contracture that required release in addition to the adductor surgery.

4. A broad-based gait with marked trunk lurch may result after adductor release surgery. This can be avoided by not overdoing the adductor surgery — that is, by leaving the posterior branch of the obturator nerve alone or by not performing adductor myotomy and anterior branch obturator neurectomy just because the adductors feel spastic, even though the passive range of motion of the hip is 30 to 40 degrees. The worst lurching gaits have been observed in patients who had intrapelvic obturator neurectomy. The base of the gait in these patients may be 12 to 18 inches.

5. A permanent postoperative "frog-leg" or abduction deformity. This can be avoided by immobilizing the limbs no longer than 3 weeks and by avoiding exaggerated forced abduction of the hips during plaster immobilization. Forced abduction can cause pressure necrosis of the articular cartilage of the hip joint (Salter and Field, 1960).

6. Wound infection. Samilson et al. (1967) reported an increased infection rate with a transverse incision (of 14 patients who had wound infections in a series of 189

operations, 12 had a transverse incision). The longitudinal incision is preferred. In addition, careful hemostasis by the use of electrocautery and closed suction drainage of the wound for 24 to 48 hours should help to reduce the infection rate.

7. A dynamic postoperative abduction posture of the hips. This occurs postoperatively in patients who have, not spastic paralysis but athetosis or dystonia without contracture. Careful preoperative assessment should assist in obviating this complication.

Adductor myotomy with anterior branch obturator neurectomy and other adductor release surgery is probably the most overutilized operation in cerebral palsy patients. Critical studies of this operation have been published (Banks and Green, 1960; Silver et al, 1966; Samilson et al., 1967).

Operative Technique of Adductor Origin Transfer (Couch et al., 1977). The hips are flexed 90 degrees and abducted the maximum amount, and the lower limbs are supported on gynecological leg rests. A transverse incision is made from the pubic tubercle to the ischium. The origins of the adductor longus, adductor brevis, and gracilis are detached from the pubic ramus (if desired, only the adductor longus and gracilis need be detached). The adductor longus is extensively dissected free from the enveloping soft tissue distally. The ischial tuberosity is exposed. The hips are then put into extension and abduction, and the muscle origins are sutured to the periosteum of the ischium and the tendinous origin of the adductor magnus.

Postoperatively, bilateral metal knee-ankle-foot orthoses with a drop lock at the knee and a pelvic band are applied. The patient begins weight bearing on a tilting frame a few days postoperatively. The knees are unlocked at intervals during the day for passive range of motion exercises. This immobilization is continued for 4 weeks.

This postoperative regimen of Couch et al. seems to obviate the pitfalls of prolonged immobilization and overabduction of the hips.

HIP FLEXION DEFORMITY

Anatomy, Physiology, and Biomechanics. The following muscles are considered to be flexors of the hip: sartorius, tensor fascia femoris, rectus femoris, adductors, and iliopsoas (Duchenne, 1959; Brunnstrom, 1962). Although these muscles act synergistically and vary with joint position, a consideration of their probable isolated function helps to determine the specific muscle or muscles that might produce flexion deformities in spastic paralysis.

The *sartorius* and *rectus femoris* flex the hip up to 90 degrees; they are weak hip flexors. The rectus femoris is more effective if the knee flexes simultaneously. Spasticity of the rectus femoris usually occurs in conjunction with spasticity of the entire quadriceps femoris. Electromyography has demonstrated spasticity of the quadriceps preoperatively and postoperatively after rectus femoris release (Bleck et al., 1975).

In addition to adducting the hip, the *pectineus* flexes it in all positions but not beyond 90 degrees. The *adductor longus, adductor brevis,* and *adductor magnus* act as flexors from the hyperextended position but not beyond 50 to 70 degrees. After these ranges, the adductors become extensors. In the erect position, the lower portion of the adductor magnus is an extensor, and the extensor function of the adductor magnus increases as the joint is flexed. In the extended position, the adductor longus is a weak internal rotator. The *gracilis* muscle acts as a flexor for up to 20 to 40 degrees of flexion and then becomes an extensor.

Pure adductor spasticity has been observed in only four patients. In these patients the amount of hip flexion deformity was no greater than 10 degrees. Furthermore, in three patients with a preoperative hip flexion deformity of greater than 15 degrees I noted no decrease in the hip flexion deformity following adductor myotomy and anterior branch obturator neurectomy. Two patients with severe hip flexion deformities who had bilateral intrapelvic obturator neurectomies showed no improvement of the flexion deformity.

The *tensor-fascia femoris* is a weak hip flexor and abductor and also a weak hip internal rotator. Almost pure spasticity of the tensor fascia femoris has been seen in only three patients, all of whom had a flexion and abduction deformity of the hips. Release of the tensor fascia femoris corrected the abduction deformity but not the hip flexion deformity.

The *iliopsoas* is the main flexor of the hip. It is composed of fibers that arise from the medial wall of the ilium and the psoas portion, which originates from the transverse process of the lumbar vertebrae; the two muscles form a conjoined tendon that inserts on the lesser trochanter of the femur. This large muscle is so deeply seated that palpation and inspection are impossible; therefore, for many years it was overlooked as the major deforming force in spastic paralysis. It appears that the iliopsoas muscle, by reason of its high insertion on the lumbar spine, may bring the trunk forward over the forward-thrusting head of the femur at the beginning of swing phase of level gait (Strange, 1965). It is clinically evident that level walking is possible without iliopsoas function. Brunnstrom (1962) had a patient with bilateral flaccid paralysis of the iliopsoas. This patient was able to walk but had a forward tilt of the pelvis and lumbar lordosis, and his gait lacked speed and smoothness.

Electromyographic analysis of the iliopsoas demonstrated electrical silence of the iliacus portion of the muscle during level walking in normal persons (Close, 1964). Basmajian (1972) reported continuous slight electrical activity of the iliacus during standing; he also recorded action potentials in all degrees of flexion. Keagy et al. (1966) and Morinaga (1973) demonstrated electrical activity of the psoas major muscle during heel rise and the initial 40 percent of the swing phase (Fig. 6–8).

The *sartorius* is electrically active during flexion, abduction, and lateral rotation of the femur. The rectus femoris and the vasti muscles show maximum electrical activity during thrusting movements such as bicycle pedaling but produce no electrical signs during flexion of the hips (Basmajian, 1962). During level gait, the rectus femoris and the vasti show short bursts of activity at the beginning of stance, during the transition from stance to swing, and at the very end of the stance phase. The adductors trigger electrical activity at the end of stance phase before the iliopsoas (Fig. 6–8).

In cerebral palsy patients with hip flexion spasticity, Perry et al. (1976) found definite dysphasic activity and prolonged activity of the iliopsoas on gait electromyograms.

Biomechanical adaptation to the hip flexion deformity occurs as compensation in two ways, depending upon the status of the knee musculature.

1. Posterior inclination of the pelvis. When the knees are flexed owing to spastic hamstrings, the pelvis inclines posteriorly and the lumbar spine flattens (Fig. 6–9). The patient assumes a sitting position while standing up.

If the patient also has an equinus deformity and the gastrocnemius-soleus

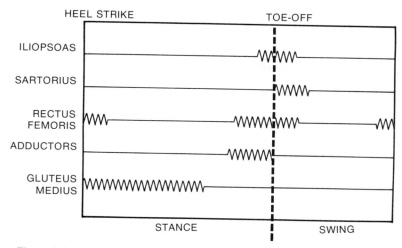

HEEL STRIKE   TOE-OFF

ILIOPSOAS

SARTORIUS

RECTUS
FEMORIS

ADDUCTORS

GLUTEUS
MEDIUS

STANCE   SWING

Figure 6–8   Electrical activity of major hip muscles during normal level gait.

muscle has been weakened too much by lengthening and/or neurectomy, the crouch becomes worse (Fig. 6–10).

If the patient has had an operation lengthening or transferring *only* the hamstrings, the compensating effect of knee flexion is lost; the pelvis then inclines anteriorly and lumbar lordosis increases. Because extension of the lumbar spine is

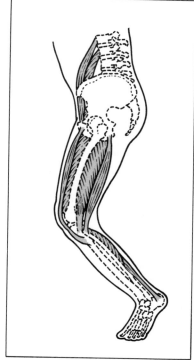

Figure 6–9   Hip flexion deformity; compensation by posterior pelvic inclination, flat lumbar spine, flexed knees.

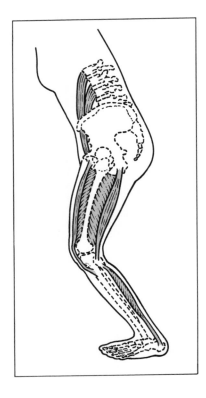

Figure 6–10   If gastrocnemius-soleus is weakened excessively, crouch will become worse.

limited, this patient may have to lean his trunk forward to bring the center of gravity of his trunk anterior to the ankle joint between the bases of support (Fig. 6–11).

2. Anterior inclination of the pelvis. When the knees cannot be flexed owing to quadriceps muscle spasticity, the pelvis increases its anterior inclination and the lumbar spine becomes more lordotic (Figs. 6–12 and 6–13).

Radiographic analyses of the pelvic and spinal compensatory mechanisms have been done using standing lateral radiographs of the lumbar spine, pelvis, and proximal femur (Bleck, 1971 *a,b,* 1975). On the radiograph, a line is drawn along the top of the sacrum to measure the degree of pelvic inclination (for all practical purposes the sacrum moves with the pelvis; its independent motion is no more than 4 degrees). A second line is drawn along the shaft of the femur. The angle formed by the intersection of these two lines is called the *sacrofemoral angle.* In normal persons this angle measures between 50 and 65 degrees (Fig. 6–14A and B).

In patients with a hip flexion deformity and flexed knees, the sacrofemoral angle measured less than 50 degrees, and the femora were horizontally parallel with the sacrum (Fig. 6–15A and B).

When the patient had a spastic quadriceps and extended knees, or after a hamstring lengthening procedure, the sacrofemoral angle was less than 50 degrees, and the femora were vertically parallel with the sacrum (Fig. 6–16A and B).

With acceptable compensation for the hip flexion deformity, the sacrofemoral angle, although less than normal, was approximately 35 to 45 degrees (Fig. 6–17A and B).

Practically all *lordosis* was confined to the lumbosacral joint. When lordosis between the second and fifth lumbar vertebrae was measured by the Cobb method,

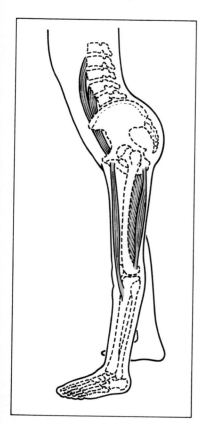

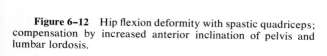

Figure 6-11 Hamstrings severely weakened with persistent hip flexion deformity; compensation by increased anterior inclination of pelvis and forward trunk lean.

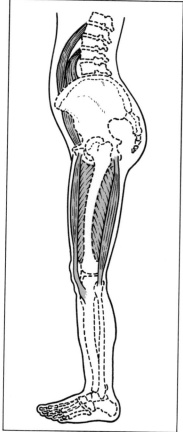

Figure 6-12 Hip flexion deformity with spastic quadriceps; compensation by increased anterior inclination of pelvis and lumbar lordosis.

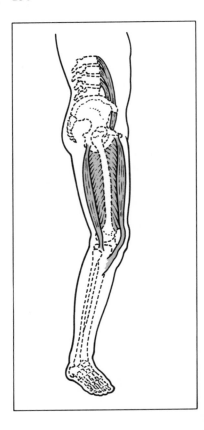

Figure 6–13 Posture is balanced after iliopsoas is lengthened, or recessed, when hamstrings have been transferred or lengthened.

Figure 6–14 A. Normal posture for 13-year-old. B. Standing lateral radiograph of lumbar spine, pelvis, and proximal femur in normal subject. Sacrofemoral angle is normal (52 degrees).

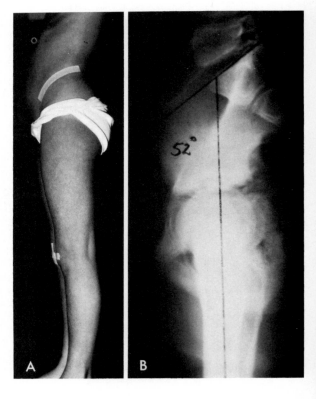

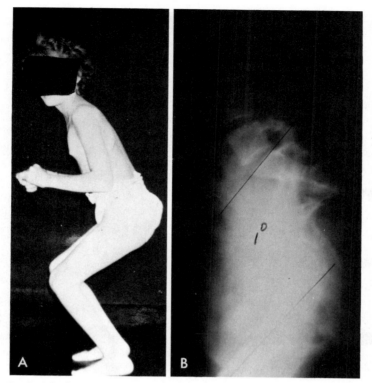

Figure 6–15 A. Hip flexion deformity (50 degrees) and flexed knees (3 years after Yount-Ober fasciotomy). B. Standing lateral radiograph of lumbar spine, pelvis, and proximal femur. Sacrofemoral angle is 1 degree. Femur is horizontally parallel with top of sacrum.

the angles were found to be within the limits of normal in a range of 45 to 65 degrees and did not vary either with the degree of the hip flexion deformity or with the sacrofemoral angle (Bleck, 1975b).

Excessive *anterior bowing of the femoral shaft* does not seem to occur in response to the hip flexion deformity. In 27 patients who had spastic hip flexion deformities and sacrofemoral angles that ranged from 15 to 48 degrees, the anterior bow of the femur, when measured on lateral radiographs, had a mean angle of 8 degrees (range 1 to 20 degrees). The normal femoral anterior bow is considered to be as high as 7 degrees.

The *clinical measurement* of the hip flexion deformity has been described in Chapter 2. Both the Thomas and Staheli methods of measurement are advised.

Pelvic-femoral fixation is another factor that adds to the spastic gait abnormality. It can be demonstrated by asking the child to stand on one limb and hold onto a table with one hand, and then swing the other limb back and forth. The femur moves as a unit with the pelvis. This partial pelvic-femoral fixation is due to spasticity and contracture of the hip musculature. The flexion deformity limits the hip extension that is so essential during gait; the lumbar spine absorbs this limited extension. These patients walk with a pelvic roll (and transverse rotation of the pelvis is also increased

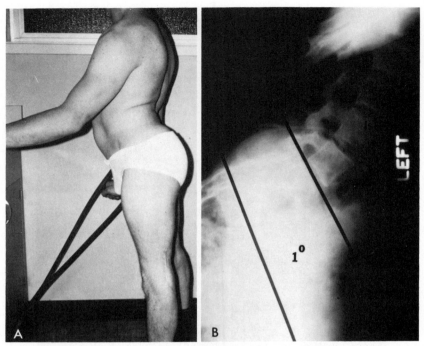

Figure 6–16   A. Hip flexion deformity (60 degrees) and extended knees (15 years after hamstring transfer). B. Standing lateral radiograph of lumbar spine, pelvis, and proximal femur. Sacrofemoral angle is 1 degree. Femur is vertically parallel with top of sacrum.

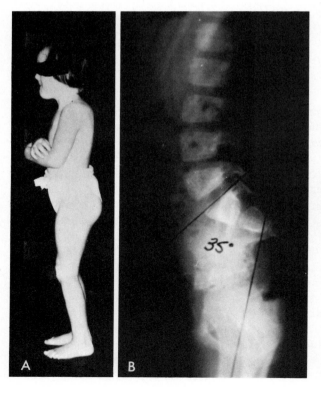

Figure 6–17   A. Spastic diplegia. Acceptable compensatory posture for the hip flexion deformity (15 degrees). B. Standing lateral radiograph of lumbar spine, pelvis, and proximal femur. Sacrofemoral angle (35 degrees) denotes mild hip flexion deformity.

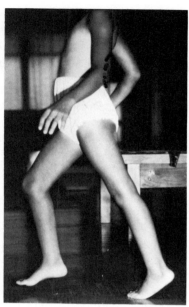

Figure 6–18 Spastic hip flexion deformity gait. During the stance phase of the gait the hip extensor limitation is compensated for by anterior pelvic inclination and lordosis.

[Bleck, 1975b]). Their gait is similar to that of patients who have had arthrodesis of the hips (Fig. 6–18).

Three spastic gait patterns can be discerned, based on the following abnormal features (Bleck, 1971a, b) (Fig. 6–19):

1. Flexed internally rotated hips and flexed knees — spastic hamstrings.
2. Flexed internally rotated hips and hyperextended knees — spastic quadriceps.

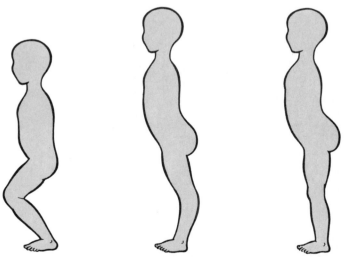

Figure 6–19 Three patterns of gait in spastic diplegia: (1) Flexed hips and flexed knees. (2) Flexed hips and hyperextended knees. (3) Flexed hips and phasic knee muscle function. (All have hip internal rotation.)

3. Flexed internally rotated hips and balanced knees — neither hamstring nor quadriceps spasticity predominates. (These children walk with an in-toeing gait that is almost identical to that of normal children without paralysis, but they have excessive femoral anteversion [Crane, 1959].)

Indications for Surgery of the Hip Flexion Deformity.   If measurements of the hip flexion deformity are taken repeatedly in a spastic cerebral palsied child, it is extremely rare to document an actual decrease in the hip flexion deformity brought about by physical therapeutic methods or by orthotics. Compensation with increased pelvic inclination is more commonly observed. If the compensation appears to be satisfactory, there is no need to apply direct surgical treatment (Fig. 6–17). In general, if the hip flexion deformity is more than 15 to 20 degrees, surgical correction is indicated (Fig. 6–20A and B).

Surgical Procedures.   Orthopaedic surgeons have applied the same procedures used with poliomyelitis to spastic paralysis, with disappointing results.

The *Ober-Yount fasciotomy* of the iliotibial band and fascia of the hip muscles has consistently failed to correct the deformity (Fig. 6–15).

The *Soutter* or *Campbell muscle slide* operation, in which the origins of the sartorius, rectus femoris, and tensor fascia femoris muscles are detached, has not been successful often enough to recommend it. Lamb and Pollock (1962) reported a 66 percent recurrence rate with this operation.

Rectus femoris tenotomy in particular has been most disappointing in correction of the hip flexion deformity. Furthermore, tenotomy of its tendinous origin allows

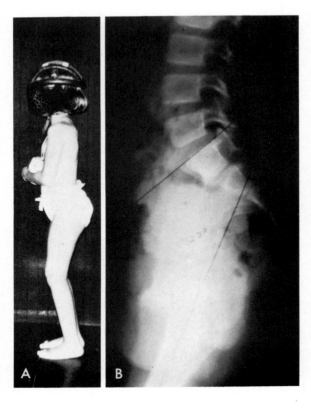

Figure 6–20   A. Hip flexion deformity (30 degrees), flexed knees (25 degrees), and lordosis. Surgical correction is indicated. B. Standing lateral radiograph of lumbar spine, pelvis, and proximal femur. Sacrofemoral angle is 29 degrees.

the muscle to retract distally, thus effectively weakening it. Quadriceps spasticity is diminished to such an extent that hamstring spasticity predominates, resulting in a crouch gait within 6 months to 1 year postoperatively.

Myotomy of the anterior fibers of the gluteus medius as an addition to the release of the sartorius and tensor fascia femoris origins has been reported by Roosth (1971). Certainly this procedure diminishes the hip internal rotation during gait because the major internal rotators of the hip are eliminated. Few electromyographic studies of the gluteus medius muscle in patients with spastic paralysis have been done. Perry and Hoffer (1977) have done such studies in patients with cerebral palsy and adult stroke. In all these patients electrical activity of the gluteus medius was normal and occurred only as it should in stance phase (Fig. 6–8).

The gluteus medius is essential for pelvic stabilization in weight shifting during walking. I have had no experience with the Roosth procedure and have been reluctant to perform it because of the great importance of the stance phase musculature in energy conservation during gait. These abductor muscles prevent excessive lateral and vertical displacement of the body during gait.

Iliopsoas tenotomy, lengthening, or recession is done because the iliopsoas is the major flexor of the hip, and it seems logical that this muscle might be the primary cause of hip flexion deformity. The iliopsoas also has a function in gait (Fig. 6–8), and for this reason it appears desirable to decrease the contracture and spasm of the muscle but at the same time to preserve its strength. Consequently, tenotomy of the iliopsoas tendon does not seem advisable in the ambulatory patient. In the non-ambulatory patient or in one whose prognosis for walking is poor (see Chapter 3), iliopsoas tenotomy is satisfactory. Furthermore, it is a simpler operation than lengthening or recession of the iliopsoas.

Bleck and Holstein (1963) performed iliopsoas tenotomy on 17 patients with spastic paralysis. All had a permanent loss of hip flexion power that has not returned in 13 years of follow-up observation. Fortunately, the patients selected for the procedure were dependent on crutches, and this masked the non-functional result. Hoffer (1969) and I tagged the end of the iliopsoas tendon at the time of tenotomy with metallic sutures. Postoperative radiographs showed retraction of the tendon to various unpredictable levels superiorly. Some tendons retracted to the level of the femoral head and others to the midilium (Fig. 6–21).

In normal non-spastic children in whom tenotomy of the iliopsoas is performed for congenital dislocation of the hip, no functional loss of hip flexion has been noted as a result of the operation. However, the iliopsoas muscle in cerebral palsied children is spastic and thus can retract too far superiorly, so that in effect the muscle is overlengthened by tenotomy.

Therefore, in the ambulatory patient, either lengthening or recession of the iliopsoas muscle is preferred. Lengthening by the Z method was reported by Anthonsen (1966) and Baumann (1970) with apparent good results. The postoperative regimen, according to Anthonsen, entailed a prolonged hospital stay in which the patient was kept in the prone position and the hips were maintained in extension.

Lengthening of the iliopsoas tendon appears disadvantageous to me for three reasons:

1. When we performed iliopsoas tenotomy, we could passively externally rotate the extended hip approximately an additional 10 degrees (Fig. 6–22A, B, and

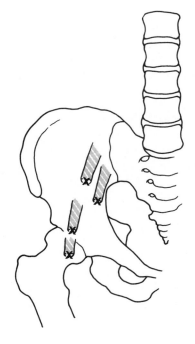

Figure 6-21 Results of tagging cut end of iliopsoas tendon in spastic paralysis. Note various levels to which the tendon is retracted.

C). The iliopsoas tendon tightly compresses the medial capsule of the hip, and tenotomy probably releases the tenodesis effect of the tendon. For this reason, I prefer to remove the tendon from its medial capsular position rather than to increase the risk of additional compression and the tenodesis effect that would be anticipated in the ensuing healing with scar formation.

2. Because we observed in cases of cup arthroplasty of the hip that transfer of the iliopsoas tendon to the anterior remnant of the capsule at the base of the neck of the femur did preserve hip flexion, we applied the same operative procedure to the spastic hip flexion deformity.

3. After Z-lengthening of the tendon, healing must occur by scar formation. As with all cicatrix formation, contracture of the scar occurs. Hence, early recurrence of the flexion deformity is a risk with iliopsoas lengthening. Indeed, in one patient in whom we did a lengthening procedure on one side and a recession on the other, contracture recurred within 3 weeks postoperatively. Fortunately, intensive physical stretching overcame this complication within 6 weeks.

ILIOPSOAS RECESSION. Iliopsoas recession is indicated in patients with flexion deformities of the hip of more than 15 to 20 degrees and either a flexed knee gait pattern due to spastic hamstrings or a hyperextended knee gait pattern due to a spastic quadriceps. It is particularly important to reduce the hip flexion deformity surgically if the crouch gait is to be corrected by lengthening, transfer, or tenotomy of spastic hamstrings. If the hamstrings alone are weakened in such patients, increased pelvic inclination and lumbar lordosis can be anticipated as a compensation (Fig. 6-11). This postural adaptation to the spastic hip flexion deformity does not decrease over a period of time, and low back pain due to lumbar lordosis occurs as the patient gets older. I recommend that a preoperative lateral radiograph of the lumbar spine be taken in all patients with a crouch gait in whom hamstring

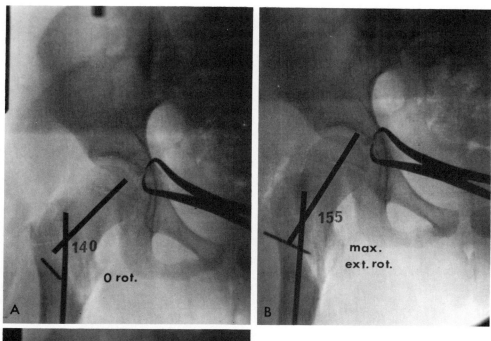

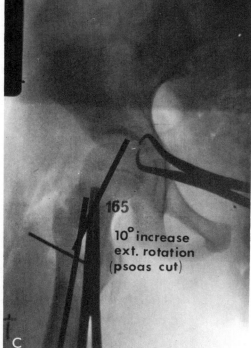

Figure 6–22 Anteroposterior radiographs of hip at time of operation. A. Spastic hip flexion deformity: patient relaxed under general anesthesia. Metal pin in greater trochanter marks rotation. Hip is in neutral rotation. B. Hip is in maximum external rotation. Note 15 degree change in femoral neck angle. C. Hips after iliopsoas tendon is cut. External rotation of the hip is increased 10 degrees.

surgery is anticipated because spondylolisthesis may already exist and may become greatly exaggerated after surgery if the hip flexion deformity is not also at least partially corrected.

The best results of iliopsoas recession have been achieved in children between the ages of 5 and 7 years. Iliopsoas recession can be combined with other surgical procedures on the lower limbs at the same time if other deformities exist — e.g., adduction spasticity and contracture (adductor myotomy and anterior branch obturator neurectomy or origin transfer are indicated in this case), flexed knees due to spastic contracted hamstrings (semitendinosis tenotomy, lengthening, or transfer and semimembranosus lengthening are indicated), or hyperextended knees due to spastic quadriceps (rectus femoris release is indicated).

Operative Technique (Fig. 6–23 A and B).   The patient is supine. An incision is made beginning about 1.5 cm distal and lateral to the anterior superior iliac spine and continuing distally and obliquely parallel with the groin crease. The incision terminates approximately at the junction of the medial one third and the lateral two thirds of the anterior surface of the thigh.

The medial border of the sartorius is identified and retracted laterally with the lateral femoral cutaneous nerve. The origin of the rectus femoris tendon is identified; medial to this is the iliacus muscle. The femoral nerve on the superior surface of the iliacus muscle under the deep fascia is dissected free from the iliacus muscle and retracted gently medially. The iliacus muscle is dissected free from the anterior capsule of the hip. A blunt instrument such as a muscle dissector is placed between the iliacus muscle and the joint capsule and pushed medially so that it underlies the psoas tendon. The psoas tendon is approximately 1 to 1.5 cm wide over the anterior capsule of the hip, and it is partly covered by the iliacus muscle fibers. After the tendon has been identified, the hip is externally rotated and flexed, and the iliacus muscle fibers are sectioned down to the tendon. The iliopsoas tendon is then cut off as close to the lesser trochanter as possible and is brought up into the wound; after exposure of the anterior capsule of the hip with blunt dissection, the tendon is sutured near the base of the neck of the femur on the anterolateral surface of the joint capsule. Two heavy non-absorbable (or absorbable synthetic) sutures are used. The iliacus fibers are then tacked down over the psoas tendon in this location with a suture or two.

If the patient walks with a hyperextended knee gait pattern, the rectus tendon origin is sectioned and the tendon allowed to retract. Otherwise, the tendon is not disturbed.

In most wounds, we use closed suction drainage, and the wound is closed as usual with absorbable synthetic sutures subcutaneously reinforced with ¼-inch sterile adhesive strips.

Postoperative Care.   We do not use spica casts. Additional plaster immobilization is used only if the hamstrings have been lengthened or transferred.

The patient is kept in bed, and sitting is not allowed for 3 weeks except in a position of 30 to 40 degrees of trunk elevation during meals. During the 3-week period, bed exercises are instituted, namely, hip extension, abduction, and external rotation. At the end of 3 weeks, gait training is instituted, first in parallel bars and then, as balance improves, the patient may walk outside of the parallel bars or, if he was a crutch-walking patient, crutches are used. It is usual for the patient to be out of the parallel bars and walking independently 6 weeks postoperatively.

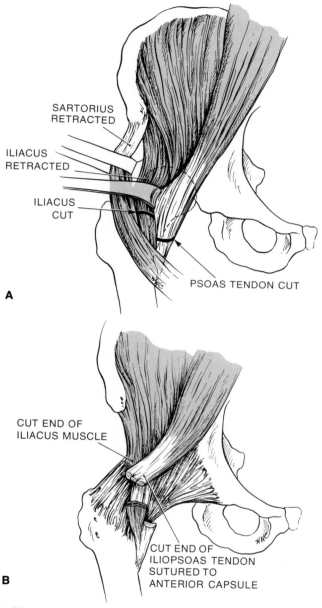

SARTORIUS
RETRACTED

ILIACUS
RETRACTED

ILIACUS
CUT

PSOAS TENDON CUT

A

CUT END OF
ILIACUS MUSCLE

CUT END OF
ILIOPSOAS TENDON
SUTURED TO
ANTERIOR CAPSULE

B

Figure 6–23 A. Dissection exposes the iliacus and psoas tendon for iliopsoas recession. B. Iliopsoas tendon cut and sutured to the anterior capsule of the hip.

Supervised exercise and balance training have been continued for approximately 6 months after surgery.

Results. The longest follow-up has been 11 years, and 23 patients have been followed for a mean of 9 years. The flexion contracture of the hip has been corrected by an average of 62 percent. The younger the patient, the greater the chance for correction of the flexion contracture. In patients who had iliopsoas recession at the age of 7 years or under, the mean amount of correction of the hip flexion contracture was 67 percent; in those over the age of 7 years the mean correction was 56 percent (Table 6–2). Postoperative standing lateral radiographs of the lumbar spine, pelvis, and proximal femur and measurements of the sacrofemoral angle confirmed the 32 percent mean decrease in the flexion contracture of the hip (Tables 6–2 and 6–3). Some hip flexion power has been lost in all patients, but it has not seriously compromised hip function. Within the limits of manual muscle testing in spastic patients, the majority of hip flexors were graded good to fair postoperatively, with a maximum range of active hip flexion of 115 degrees (normal, 100 to 125 degrees). In patients in whom hamstring lengthening or transfer was performed for a crouch gait, iliopsoas recession prevented excessive lumbar lordosis and forward leaning of the trunk postoperatively. Patients were able to climb stairs, ride bicycles, and engage in sports that were consistent with the amount of spasticity remaining and the adequacy of their equilibrium reactions.

Of the first 25 patients who had iliopsoas recession, hip flexion was weak in three patients throughout the 9-year follow-up period. In one patient this was due to almost total lack of voluntary control of the musculature of the lower limb. In the other two patients, it is probable that the absorbable sutures initially used to fix the

Table 6–2   CORRECTION OF HIP FLEXION CONTRACTURE BY
ILIOPSOAS RECESSION

Patient Number	Age at Surgery (years)	Follow-up (years)	Preoperative Flexion Contracture (degrees)	Postoperative Flexion Contracture (degrees)	Percent Correction
1	11	11	60	30	50
2	12	*	60	60	0
3	6	11	45	10	88
4	4	11	40	20	50
5	8	11	45	15	66
6	7	11	60	10	84
7	14	11	30	10	66
8	9	10	60	10	84
9	5	9	40	5	88
10	4.5	9	45	20	56
11	7.5	*	45	10	82
12	2.5	9	60	20	66
13	6	9	50	20	40
14	9	9	30	10	66
15	9	11	30	15	50
16	8	11	40	20	50
17	6	11	60	15	75
18	8	10	30	15	50
19	9	10	30	10	66
20	6	10	20	10	50
21	11	9	45	20	56
22	9	10	30	15	50
23	6	*	30	10	66
24	7	9	40	15	62
25	4.5	9	40	5	88

*Lost to follow-up after 4 years.

Table 6–3   CORRECTION OF SACROFEMORAL ANGLES
BY ILIOPSOAS RECESSION

| Patient Number | Sacrofemoral Angles (degrees) | | Percent Improvement |
	PREOPERATIVE	POSTOPERATIVE	
1	17	10	−58
2	35	20	−57
3	20	45	56
4	*	62	
5	25	50	50
6	28	30	7
7	30	45	34
8	20	30	34
9	25	45	45
10	30	40	25
11	25	22	−1
12	*	26	
13	*	40	
14	32	50	36
15	24	35	32
16	50	57	13
17	*	55	
18	20	45	56
19	27	45	40
20	27	42	36
21	56	55	−1
22	40	50	20
23	45	55	19
24	30	50	40
25	15	30	50

*Unable to obtain preoperative standing lateral radiograph.

iliopsoas tendon to the capsule of the hip pulled out in the postoperative period. Since we have been using heavy non-absorbable or synthetic absorbable sutures, I have not observed postoperative weakness of hip flexion of more than one grade lower than the preoperative manual muscle tests.

Temporary postoperative quadriceps paralysis was reported to me by another surgeon. This can be avoided by gentle and minimal retraction of the femoral nerve during the procedure.

The rectus femoris tendon *should not be released even though it appears tight* in an attempt to correct the flexion deformity at the time of iliopsoas recession unless there is a hyperextended knee gait pattern. If the knee is well-balanced during walking, there is no need to upset the balance by weakening the quadriceps and allowing the hamstring spasticity to take over. If the rectus femoris is released in such a patient, one can anticipate an increasing crouch gait within 6 months after the operation.

Correction of the hip flexion deformity fails in some patients over the age of 11 years. Anterior incision of the joint capsule, while seemingly logical in theory, has not in practice resulted in additional correction. In patients in whom this was done initially, I observed a limited passive flexion of the hip to 90 degrees, possibly due to increased anterior scarring of the hip as the capsular incision healed.

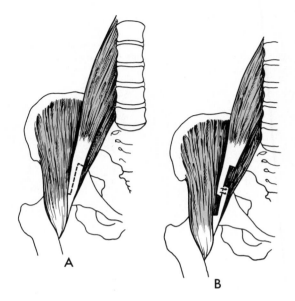

Figure 6–24 Technique of iliopsoas lengthening.

OPERATIVE TECHNIQUE FOR ILIOPSOAS LENGTHENING (BAUMANN, 1970). The same incision used for iliopsoas recession is used in this procedure; it exposes the tendon, which is then Z-lengthened (Fig. 6–24), and the ends of the lengthened tendon are sutured.

The postoperative care must be carefully supervised so that the patient lies prone most of the time, and the hips are frequently extended the maximum amount. This supervised postoperative period should probably be continued for 6 weeks to prevent recontracture.

I have used iliopsoas lengthening in a small number of patients who have a mild hip flexion contracture (less than 20 degrees) as an important additional procedure accompanying a derotation femoral osteotomy. The reason for including iliopsoas lengthening or recession in the correction of femoral anteversion by osteotomy is discussed in the following section.

HIP INTERNAL ROTATION DEFORMITY

Anatomy, Physiology, and Mechanisms. The following muscles are considered to be the internal rotators of the hip: the gluteus medius and minimus, the semitendinosus, the adductors, and the tensor fascia femoris (Duchenne, 1959; Brunnstrom, 1962).

Studies have established that the anterior portion of the gluteus medius is the main internal rotator of the hip (Hollinshead, 1951; Grant, 1952; Duchenne, 1959; Brunnstrom, 1962). Clinical experience confirms this theory — if the tendon of the gluteus medius is cut or transferred (Steel, 1977*b*), the hip will no longer rotate internally. Direct measurements of transverse rotations of the segments of the lower limb during level gait show that all segments rotate internally during swing phase and continue to do so until midstance, when there is an abrupt shift to external rotation that continues until toe-off at the beginning of the swing phase (see Figure 2–4). The gluteus medius contracts at the beginning of stance and continues to contract until about midstance (Fig. 6–8). This stance phase electrical activity coexists with the internal rotation of the entire limb.

Electromyograms of the gluteus medius in spastic patients show that the phasic activity of this muscle is no different in the child with spastic paralysis than it is in the normal child (Perry and Hoffer, 1977).

I have seen only four patients who had abductor spasticity. In these patients, almost no flexion contracture was found, and all had a normal or limited range of hip internal rotation (Fig. 6–25 A, B, and C).

These clinical and electromyographic data indicate that it is doubtful that gluteus medius spasticity is the cause of excessive hip internal rotation in spastic gait patterns.

The *semitendinosus muscle* is capable of internally rotating the hip. Electromyographic studies demonstrate activity of this muscle at the beginning of stance and the end of swing phase (Fig. 2–49). Duchenne (1959) noted that the semitendinosus rotated the thigh medially when the knee was extended but this rotation diminished as knee flexion increased. The medial rotation was less pronounced than the lateral rotation produced by the biceps femoris. Duchenne found no evidence of rotation function in the semimembranosus. Sutherland et al. (1969) reported that

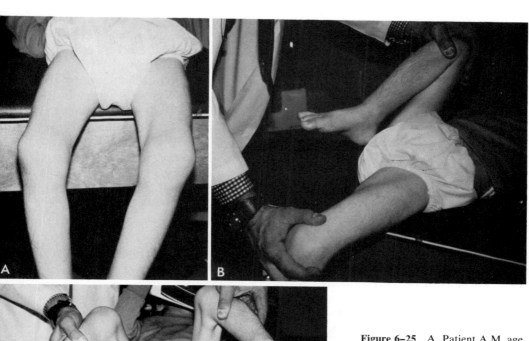

Figure 6–25 A. Patient A.M. age 6 years, spastic quadriplegia with hip abductor spasticity. B. Thomas test shows mild hip flexion contracture (5 degrees). C. Hip internal rotation is within normal limits.

there was prolonged contraction of the semitendinosus throughout stance phase in seven children who had spastic paralysis and a gait characterized by hip internal rotation. Our own studies (Bleck et al., 1975a) of spastic gait patterns show that practically all children demonstrate dysphasic and prolonged activity of the semitendinosus. These data do not contradict the suggestion that the semitendinosus may contribute to hip internal rotation, but they do indicate that other factors may account for the internal rotation gait.

The *adductors,* according to Duchenne (1959), are lateral rotators. The lower portion of the adductor magnus has been described as a powerful internal rotator. Electromyographic studies of the adductors have shown that they contract in late stance (Mann et al., 1973); an additional burst of activity has been reported in early stance (Brunnstrom, 1962). Most electrical activity occurs after heel contact. These authors consider the adductors to be weak internal rotators.

If hip flexion is combined with adduction on internal rotation, contraction of the adductor longus can be observed. Clinical observations do not support the view that the adductor muscles are primary internal rotators in spastic paralysis.

In patients with *only* hip adductor spasticity and mild hip flexion deformity little internal rotation of the hip during gait can be discerned. I have observed patients who toed in without clinically demonstrable adductor spasticity or limited hip abduction. All of these patients had excessive femoral anteversion, an increased range of passive internal rotation of the hip (over 60 degrees), and a hip flexion contracture.

The *tensor fascia femoris* is a weak internal rotator (Duchenne, 1959). This fact is confirmed by the disappointing results of transfer of its origin posteriorly (Majestro and Frost, 1971).

The rotary function of the *iliopsoas* has been controversial. Electromyographic studies of the iliacus muscle during gait seem to discount any rotary function of this muscle (Basmajian, 1962; Close, 1964), but Keagy's (1966) electromyographic study of the psoas major during level gait confirmed activity of the psoas beginning with heel rise and continuing through the first 40 percent of the swing phase. These data can be correlated nicely with Strange's concept (1965) that the psoas contracts to counteract the lateral rotation of the pelvis. When weight is placed on the hip as the body is propelled forward, a force is generated that leaves the pelvis behind. The iliopsoas muscle probably prevents excessive lateral pelvic rotation and even rotates the pelvis medially to a small degree.

A spastic and contracted iliopsoas results in excessive medial pelvic rotation due to pelvic-femoral fixation. An increase in transverse rotation of the pelvis has been found in patients who have spastic gait patterns (Bleck, 1975b).

In view of the lack of convincing evidence of spastic muscles as the cause of excessive hip internal rotation gait in spastic paralysis, some other mechanism must be responsible. This mechanism, which has been studied and verified by several investigators, is excessive femoral anteversion.

FEMORAL ANTEVERSION.   Clinical and anatomical analysis supports the concept that the one consistent deformity associated with hip internal rotation gait in patients with cerebral palsy and spastic paralysis is excessive femoral anteversion (or torsion). This means that the head, neck, and trochanteric region of the femur are twisted forward with respect to the transcondylar axis of the knee beyond the range anticipated and measured for normal humans at a given age.

Radiographic measurements using the Magilligan (1956) or the Ryder-Crane

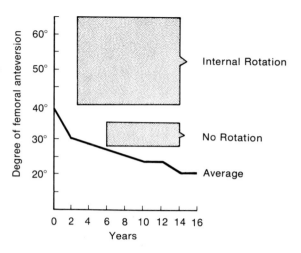

Figure 6–26 Comparison of degrees of femoral anteversion in 50 patients with cerebral palsy and hip internal rotation gait patterns with those of 10 cerebral palsy patients who did not internally rotate, and with normal averages, according to age in years. Increased femoral anteversion is a consistent finding in those who internally rotate during gait.

(1953, 1972) technique for measuring femoral anteversion in ambulatory cerebral palsied children who had hip internal rotation gaits demonstrated femoral anteversion beyond the range of normal for their age (Fig. 6–26). A study of 29 cerebral palsied patients who did not have excessive hip internal rotation showed that they also lacked excessive femoral anteversion. Lewis et al. (1964), Fabry et al. (1973), and Beals (1969) have all documented excessive femoral anteversion in cerebral palsied patients.

In anteroposterior radiographs femoral anteversion has been frequently mistaken for coxa valga (i.e., a femoral neck-shaft angle of greater than 145 degrees). This radiographic misinterpretation is not surprising, as radiographs are merely shadows of the bone projected in one dimension. When the true angles of femoral neck inclination were measured in 60 hips of cerebral palsied children who had excessive femoral anteversion, only three were above the normal ranges for age as reported by Shands (1958). These measurements were made using the Magilligan technique and ranged from 118 to 148 degrees. Coxa valga, then, must be a rare deformity in cerebral palsy.

Natural History. At birth, most infants are born with an angle of femoral anteversion in the range of 10 to 60 degrees (mean, 31 degrees [Michele, 1962]; 38 degrees [Shands and Steele, 1958]) (Fig. 6–27). During skeletal maturation, this angle gradually decreases to the adult value of 19 degrees (Shands and Steele, 1958; Crane, 1959; Fabry et al., 1973) (Fig. 6–28). This spontaneous decrease probably has a biomechanical basis.

At birth, the proximal end of the femur (head, neck, and greater trochanter) is entirely cartilaginous and pliable; this proximal segment is fixed to a rigid osseous diaphysis that terminates at the subtrochanteric level. When fresh stillborn specimens are manipulated, the proximal end of the femur can be made to rotate on the fixed diaphysis. Mechanically and mathematically, the point of torsion has been located in the subtrochanteric region of the femur (Michele, 1962). With progressive ossification of the femoral head, neck, and trochanter, the elasticity of cartilage is lost, and consequently no further derotation can occur. Fabry et al. (1973) have documented that after the age of 8 years, no further correction of femoral anteversion occurs.

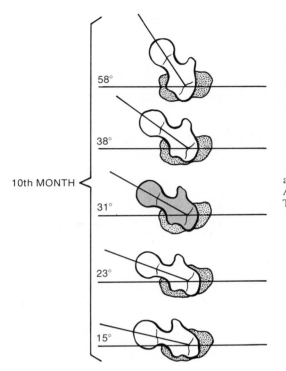

Figure 6–27 Mean and range of femoral anteversion at birth. (Redrawn from Michele, A. A. (1962) *Iliopsoas*, Springfield, Charles C Thomas.)

Lee (1977*a*) studied the cause of derotation of the proximal femur in the hips of fresh stillborn specimens. He found that 2 to 4 degrees of external torque strain was needed to derotate the proximal end of the femur at the growth plate. This strain had to be applied while the femoral head was relatively fixed by the capsule of the joint. The torque strains in external rotation were diminished when the hip was flexed 90 degrees. Wilkinson (1962) demonstrated in skeletally immature rabbits that femoral anteversion could be created when their hips were held for several weeks in internal rotation; retroversion resulted when the hips were held in external rotation. These data strongly suggest that in humans the mechanisms necessary for the diminution of

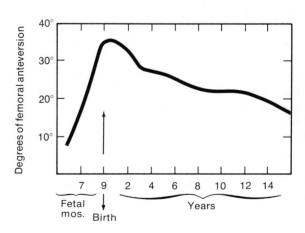

Figure 6–28 Normal mean values of femoral anteversion from the sixth fetal month to age 16 years.

newborn femoral anteversion are (1) external rotation of the hip, and (2) hip extension to produce optimal derotation.

Pressure Effects on Epiphyseal Growth.   The experiments of Arkin et al. (1956) demonstrated that epiphyseal growth responds to stress on the physis. Torque causes torsional growth. All changes in bone shape are due to new bone laid down with the cartilage cells aligned in the strained pattern.

All *newborn* children have a *flexion contracture of the hip* of 28 degrees (mean value [Haas et al., 1973]). At 6 weeks, the flexion contracture decreases to a mean value of 19 degrees, and at 3 to 6 months it decreases to 7 degrees (Coons et al., 1975). As the hip extends, the range of internal rotation decreases (p = 0.005 [Coon et al., 1975]).

With these experimental and clinical data, a *hypothesis* can be constructed to explain the persistence of newborn femoral anteversion in children who have spastic diplegia. These children are born with spastic paralysis that causes persistent spasticity of the iliopsoas muscle and continuation of the newborn hip flexion contracture beyond the normal time. The persistent pull of the iliopsoas does not permit the normal stretching of the anterior capsule. (In normal newborns all of the hip flexion contracture was in the capsule of the joint and not in the muscle; this was demonstrated by dissection of stillborn term infants [Lee, 1977a]). In addition, this lack of hip extension in spastic paralysis decreases the torque strains on the proximal end of the femur in external rotation. It may be further postulated that spasm and contracture of the iliopsoas limit hip external rotation in extension. In *summary,* we may deduce that persistent flexion contracture of the hip from birth causes persistence of the fetal femoral anteversion.

In-Toed Gait and Femoral Anteversion.   Why does excessive femoral anteversion result in the in-toed gait seen in some normal children and in cerebral palsied children? The best explanation is that offered by Merchant (1965) in his mechanical model study of the function of the gluteus medius. This hip abductor muscle is known to be the major stabilizer of the pelvis; it allows the lateral shift of the trunk and its center of gravity over the head of the femur on the stance limb during gait. Merchant's model showed that the hip abductors exert optimum force when the insertion of the abductors on the greater trochanter is in a neutral relationship to the origin. If the greater trochanter is in a posterior position, as it is in excessive femoral anteversion, we may surmise that the child automatically rotates his hip internally throughout the stance phase of gait in order to gain the maximum output of the hip abductors, since only in this way can the lateral trunk shift occur with optimal efficiency and minimal expenditure of energy to keep the center of gravity as level as possible during forward progression. Clinical observations seem to confirm this premise. Normal children with in-toeing due to excessive femoral anteversion usually toe-in more toward the end of the day when they are fatigued; if the normal child with excessive femoral anteversion is asked to stand and balance on one foot with his hip maximally externally rotated, he is not as steady, and lateral bend of the trunk occurs, shifting the center of gravity over the head of the femur.

Radiographic Examinations.   The degree of femoral anteversion can be measured utilizing biplane radiographs. Two techniques have been used — the Magilligan (1956) and the Ryder-Crane (1953) techniques. In the Magilligan technique, an anteroposterior radiograph of the hips is made with the hips in neutral rotation; the angle of femoral neck inclination is measured on the film. Next, a true lateral radiograph is taken with the hip in neutral rotation; the film cassette is placed parallel with the neck of the femur according to the measurement of the femoral angle of inclination taken from the anteroposterior radiograph. The projected angle of anteversion is obtained from this lateral film by drawing one line along the shaft and a second along the center of the neck of the femur. Based upon a trigonometric calculation, the angle of rotation of the neck of the femur can be calculated from these two lines. Magilligan has constructed a chart so that from the two angles of femoral inclination obtained, the true angle of femoral anteversion and the angle of femoral neck inclination can be found directly. In the Ryder-Crane technique, an anteroposterior radiograph of the hips in neutral rotation is taken, and the angle of femoral neck inclination is measured. The second radiograph is an anteroposterior projection with the hips abducted exactly 30 degrees and flexed to 90 degrees. A special frame is utilized (MacEwen, 1972), and from the radiograph obtained, the projected angle of femoral neck anteversion is measured. Trigonometry is used to figure the true angle of anteversion. Ryder (1972) has produced computer calculations from which one can read off the true angle of anteversion from the measurements obtained with the two radiographs. The disadvantage of the Magilligan technique is that it demands a true lateral radiograph of the hip. The disadvantage of the Ryder-Crane technique is that the hip must have a range of abduction of 30 degrees. In children with spastic and contracted adductors, it may not be possible to obtain 30 degrees of abduction with the hip flexed 90 degrees.

Surgical Procedures to Correct Hip Internal Rotation. *Posterior transposition of the origin of the tensor fascia femoris* was originally described by Durham (Edmunson, 1963). In my experience and that of others, it has failed to correct the deformity (Majestro and Frost, 1971).

Adductor myotomy with anterior branch obturator neurectomy or *transfer* of the adductor origins to the ischium has not been uniformly successful in overcoming hip internal rotation (Majestro and Frost, 1971; Baumann, 1972).

Neurectomy of the superior gluteal nerve was tried by Majestro and Frost (1971) and was a failure.

Gluteus medius and minimus tendon transfer has been done by Steel (1977b) in 81 hips. In 2- to 11-year follow-up studies of 43 hips in 32 patients, 80 percent walked with their hips in neutral or external rotation. Failure to correct the deformity occurred in 19 percent; these patients had a more severe Trendelenburg gait. Femoral anteversion (measured clinically) decreased more than 25 percent in those children who had surgery before the age of 7 years. No increase in the valgus inclination of the femoral neck occurred.

The operation consists of removing the tendinous insertion of the gluteus medius and minimus muscles by removing a thin sliver of bone from the apophyseal insertion of the tendon. The insertion is then transferred to the origin of the vastus intermedius muscle on the anterior aspect of the femur. Fixation of the osteoperiosteal insertion is done with two crossed pins. The hips are held in external rotation and abduction (10 degrees less than the maximal range) in a double hip spica for 6 weeks.

Although motion picture films of the preoperative and postoperative gait show impressive corrections, I have been reluctant to perform the procedure. My reluctance is based upon the following reasons:

1. Limited electromyographic studies show that the gluteus medius muscle is not spastic in cerebral palsy. Thus, a normal muscle is transferred.

2. This normal muscle has a most important function in stabilizing the pelvis

during the stance phase of gait. Will this important function be compromised if the insertion is transferred anteriorly (19 percent of patients had a severe Trendelenburg gait postoperatively)? Perry et al. (1975) noted that the hip abductors are not often part of the primitive locomotor pattern in spastic paralysis. These patients will have a Trendelenburg drop of the pelvis due to lack of proprioceptive "awareness" and selective motor control. If such a patient is asked to stand on one limb, he falls *wholly* to the unsupported limb and fails to catch himself.

If the patient merely has weak abductors and stands on one limb, his pelvis drops on the unsupported limb side; his trunk leans to that side but his whole body does not, and he is aware of his instability and tries to catch himself. It may be that those patients who respond to the Trendelenburg test in this way without falling respond best to the transfer described by Steel.

3. If the gluteus medius and minimus muscles pass more anterior to the hip after transfer, it is possible that the hip flexion contracture will be aggravated, hip extension will be more limited, and gait thus compromised.

Semitendinosus transfer to the anterior-lateral femur (Baker and Hill, 1964; Sutherland et al., 1969) has had unpredictable results in my experience. Often the transfer is not sufficient to overcome the hip internal rotation during the stance phase of gait. Furthermore, patients who have a predominantly spastic quadriceps will have increased spasticity of the quadriceps after the counterbalancing effect of the semitendinosus is removed. An extended knee gait is less functional and more energy-consuming than a gait depending upon slightly flexed knees with hip internal rotation. After a 12-year trial with this procedure, I've given it up. My intent is to avoid repetitive surgical procedures in children.

Iliopsoas recession performed before the age of 7 years has resulted in a gradual decrease of the hip internal rotation gait and a decrease in the passive range of internal rotation of the hip over a period of 3 to 5 years (Bleck, 1971). In a 9- to 11-year follow-up of 23 patients who had iliopsoas recession, five required subtrochanteric femoral rotation osteotomies to correct noticeable in-toeing. Two were bilateral osteotomies and three were unilateral. Although the case load is too small to permit statistically valid conclusions, the median age of the patients who did not require femoral osteotomy was 7 years and their ages ranged from 1½ to 14 years. Given the data on the failure of spontaneous correction of femoral anteversion in otherwise normal children after the age of 8 years, it seems logical to suggest that surgery to decrease hip flexion contracture and thus increase hip extension is best done before the age of 8 years.

In the past year we have attempted to force hip external rotation during gait by using an auditory biofeedback orthosis. Preliminary data indicate success with this orthosis after iliopsoas recession.

Derotation subtrochanteric femoral osteotomy of the femur has produced definite and permanent results (Majestro and Frost, 1971; Bost and Bleck, 1975). This operation is indicated in the child 8 years of age or older in whom a marked in-toed gait persists, if the passive range of hip internal rotation remains 80 to 90 degrees and external rotation is limited to less than 30 degrees with the hip extended. In our study of 29 hips in 22 patients who were followed an average of 6 years, the mean age at the time of surgery was 11.7 years. Improvement was obtained in 90 percent of hips.

OPERATIVE TECHNIQUE OF FEMORAL DEROTATION OSTEOTOMY. Because a hip flexion deformity is always present in these patients and is aggravated by the derotation osteotomy, I first perform an iliopsoas recession at the time of the osteotomy. Therefore, two separate incisions are required. The incision for the derotation femoral osteotomy begins at the tip of the greater trochanter and extends distally for 10 to 15 cm, depending upon the size of the child and the accommodation that will be necessary for the femoral fixation plate. The fascia lata is incised in the same line of the skin incision, and the origin of the vastus lateralis is detached at the base of the greater trochanter.

We prefer to perform this operation under radiographic control, using the image intensifier. With the hip in internal rotation, one guide pin is introduced through the greater trochanter transversely across the base of the neck of the femur so that it will lie parallel to the intended subtrochanteric osteotomy, which is marked with a second guide pin. The first guide pin in the base of the neck of the femur should be slightly higher than the intended position for the 90-degree angle compression nail (ASIF).

The size of the nail (whether for child, adolescent, or adult) is dependent upon the age and size of the patient's bone. With a special chisel, a channel for the nail portion is made across the base of the neck of the femur parallel to the previously placed guide pin. A radiograph is taken, and, if the position is satisfactory, the nail is driven in to the point where the plate portion of the nail rests against the femoral shaft. A third pin is placed in the greater trochanter and into the neck of the femur parallel with the floor, and a fourth pin is placed in the distal shaft of the femur so that it creates an angle of the desired amount of derotation. For example, if there are 90 degrees of passive internal rotation of the hip, and 30 to 40 degrees of internal rotation are desired at the conclusion of the operation, then the two pins are set at an angle of 60 to 50 degrees. The osteotomy at the subtrochanteric level is performed with a reciprocating power saw, and when it is completed, the distal fragment is rotated externally so that the pin in the distal shaft is parallel with the pin in the proximal end of the femur. The shaft of the femur is then clamped with a bone plate clamp against the plate portion of the nail. The compression device is applied, and the plate is fixed to the shaft of the femur with screws (Fig. 6–29). At the conclusion of the procedure, it should be possible to rotate the hip internally 30 to 40 degrees with the hip extended and flexed. Closed suction drainage is used in all cases. The wound is closed as usual.

Postoperative care after femoral derotation osteotomy consists of keeping the patient from bearing weight for 8 weeks in the average case. For the first 3 weeks the patient is not allowed to sit up but must remain supine or prone or on the side in bed. Bed exercises, particularly quadriceps exercises, hip external rotation, isometric abduction, and foot dorsiflexion exercises, are carried out by the patient three times a day. At the end of the 8 weeks, union is usually secure, and the patient may walk in parallel bars or with a walker, progressing to crutches. At the end of 12 weeks, it is usually possible to discard the crutches entirely. Ordinarily, we do not use plaster casts except for a long leg cylinder or a long leg plaster if hamstring lengthening or foot surgery has been done at the same time. Because internal fixation is secure, hip spicas have not been necessary.

Errors of Derotation Femoral Osteotomy.   In analyzing our own failures and those of other surgeons, we have recognized five complications and have suggested how these may be minimized.

1. Increased postoperative hip flexion deformity. If the patient has hamstring spasticity, compensation for the hip flexion deformity occurs by knee flexion, and a crouch gait results within 6 months. If quadriceps spasticity is the predominant

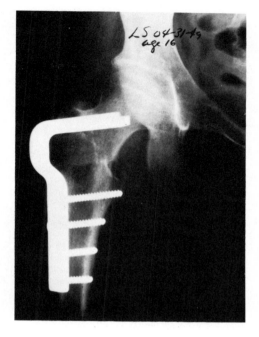

Figure 6–29 Anteroposterior radiograph of the hip postoperative derotation subtrochanteric femoral osteotomy with 90 degree compression nail-plate.

pattern, severe compensatory lumbar lordosis is the result (Fig. 6–30). The mechanism responsible for the increased hip flexion deformity after rotation osteotomy appears to be increased tension on the psoas muscle, regardless of whether the osteotomy was above or below the lesser trochanter. If above the trochanter, internal rotation of the proximal femur pulls on the psoas tendon; if below, external rotation of the distal femur pulls on the tendon (Fig. 6–31). For this reason, we recommend iliopsoas lengthening or recession through a separate incision as the initial procedure at the time of osteotomy.

2. Undercorrection of the deformity. This can be avoided by preoperative measurements of the range of hip internal rotation and the use of two pins set at the appropriate angle as described in the preceding section.

3. Overcorrection is far more common than undercorrection. Overcorrection to the point where only 0 to 10 degrees of internal rotation remain compromises a smooth gait because external pelvic rotation cannot occur. In unilateral osteotomies, overcorrection causes a persistent anterior rotation of the pelvis on the side of the osteotomy.

To avoid overcorrection, we recommend that 30 to 40 degrees of hip external rotation be preserved. The use of two pins to determine the correct amount of derotation has been described in the section on operative technique.

4. Failure to recognize and correct excessive compensatory external tibial-fibular torsion (Fig. 6–32). If the preoperative examination documents external tibial-fibular torsion of greater than 35 degrees, internal rotation osteotomy of the proximal tibia and fibula may be necessary in addition to femoral external rotation osteotomy (Fig. 6–33). If not recognized and corrected, the patient will have a distinct ungainly duck-like gait after femoral osteotomy.

5. Inadequate internal fixation. Small bone plates do not always hold the sub-

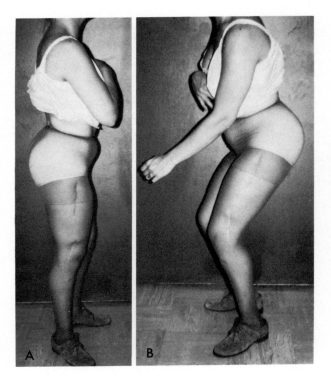

Figure 6–30 A. Patient N.C., spastic diplegia, age 26 years, 14 years post–bilateral derotation subtrochanteric femoral osteotomy. The hip flexion deformity was worse postoperatively. (Of interest is that she is 16 years post–Ober-Yount fasciotomy with no correction of the hip flexion contracture.) B. The lumbar lordosis is fixed, Even with knee flexion lumbar lordosis remains fixed. The iliopsoas was *not* lengthened or recessed at the time of rotation osteotomy.

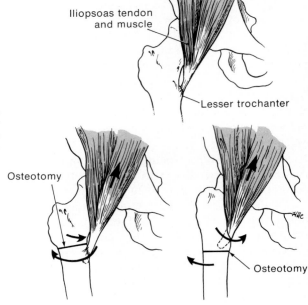

Figure 6–31 Explanation for the increased hip flexion deformity after rotation osteotomy. No matter where the osteotomy is located, rotation increases the tension on the iliopsoas.

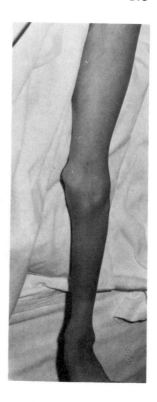

Figure 6–32 Spastic diplegia, lower limb, with severe internal femoral torsion (note position of patella). Despite internal rotation of the femur, the foot is externally rotated owing to excessive external tibial-fibular torsion.

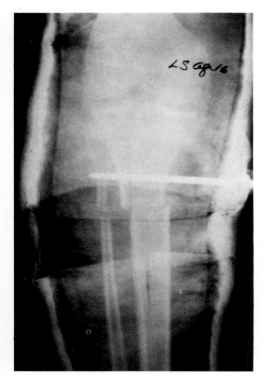

Figure 6–33 If there is a concomitant excess external tibial-fibular torsion, it should be corrected by internal rotation osteotomy of the tibia and fibula either at the time of femoral osteotomy or at a later date.

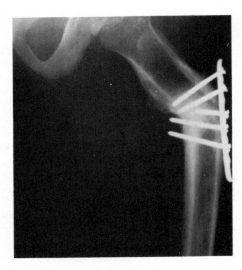

Figure 6–34 Inadequate internal fixation of a femoral rotation osteotomy.

trochanteric osteotomy securely even with plaster spica immobilization (Fig. 6–34). We avoid plaster immobilization and the attendant prolonged recovery of joint function by the use of rigid internal fixation with the 90-degree hip compression nail (Fig. 6–29).

We do not perform supracondylar femoral osteotomy instead of subtrochanteric osteotomy for the following reasons. Almost always these patients have spastic knee muscles that can cause displacement of the osteotomy. Supracondylar osteotomies need plaster immobilization if done without internal fixation, and immobilization delays recovery. If internal fixation is used in the supracondylar region, more dissection of the important knee musculature is required, and this presents the risk of postoperative limitation of knee motion. In gait, the knee is perhaps the most important joint in compensating for structural limitations in the lower limb; hence, optimum mobility of the knee is desirable (see the discussion of the major determinants of gait in Chapter 2).

SUBLUXATION AND ACETABULAR DYSPLASIA

Mechanism. Subluxation of the hip and acetabular dysplasia in spastic diplegia or paraplegia are usually acquired. Initially, acquired hip subluxation has no acetabular dysplasia, whereas in the congenital type, acetabular dysplasia is evident from the beginning. As in acquired paralytic subluxation of the hip, acetabular dysplasia is secondary to the lateral displacement of the femoral head from the acetabulum. Animal experiments have demonstrated that when the femoral head loses complete contact with the acetabulum, it does not develop and becomes shallow.

In spastic paralytic subluxation of the hip, the major muscle groups causing the deformity are the adductors and the iliopsoas. As the infantile flexion contracture of the hip persists owing to spasticity of the iliopsoas, the fetal femoral anteversion also persists, according to our data. When ambulation is delayed and weight-bearing is limited owing to the necessary use of crutches or walkers, the abductor muscles do not function maximally to stabilize the pelvis because crutches or walkers reduce the weight-bearing load on the head of the femur; there is no need to balance the head, trunk, and upper limbs over the head of the femur during the stance phase of gait. Spastic hip adduction contributes to the lateral uncovering of the femoral head. Flexion without weight-bearing in the presence of femoral anteversion allows the hip to rotate externally; the femoral head exerts pressure anteriorly and laterally on the joint capsule, and subluxation ensues.

The effects on the hip of persistent flexion contracture and concomitant persistent newborn femoral anteversion depend upon the ambulatory status of the patient: (1) If the patient is non-ambulatory, the effect is dislocation of the hip; (2) if the patient is partly weight-bearing with crutches, subluxation ensues; (3) if the patient is independently ambulatory, internal rotation results.

Indications for Correction.   Correction of this deformity is always advisable when it is first discovered. It is only many years later that the symptoms of degenerative arthritis of the hip will become evident. If the patient is an independent crutch-walking adult, degenerative arthritis of the hip may change his status from that of a community walker to a household walker or even a non-walker. Physiological reconstructive surgery of the hip is much more difficult in the adult than in a child.

In the child under 8 years of age, subluxation of the hip can be treated with release of the spastic muscles alone (Fig. 6–35 A, B, C, D). Although it is almost always

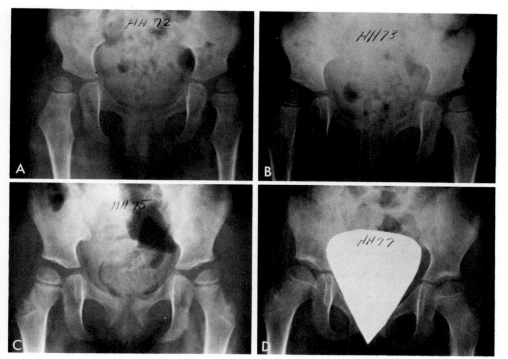

Figure 6–35   A. Patient H. H., a 3-year-old, non-ambulatory spastic diplegic with a good prognosis for bilateral subluxation of hips. Hip flexion contracture is 30 degrees: abduction for each hip, 35 degrees; internal rotation, 90 degrees;   external rotation, 15 degrees. B. One year post-iliopsoas recession. C. Three years postoperative. Now walks independently. D. Five years post-iliopsoas recession. No bone surgery required to locate hips.

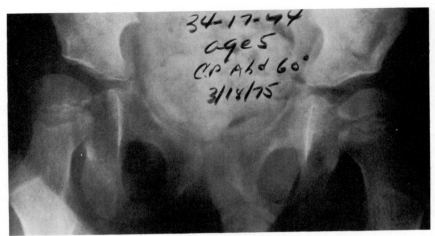

Figure 6–36   Anteroposterior radiograph of hips. Patient is a 5-year-old spastic diplegic. Each hip abducts to 60 degrees. *Without hip adduction contracture,* subluxation of the right hip is seen. Iliopsoas recession was performed to correct 30 degree hip flexion contracture. Adductor myotomy, anterior branch obturator neurectomy, or adductor transfer was not indicated.

necessary to perform an adductor myotomy and anterior branch obturator neurectomy, there are patients with subluxation of the hip who do not have any demonstrable adduction deformity. In these patients, only an iliopsoas recession is required to relieve the deforming spastic hip flexion contracture (Fig. 6–36).

The surgeon can wait for a year after such surgery to determine whether or not the deformity persists and whether or not additional bone surgery will be required. In general, in patients over the age of 8 years, in addition to iliopsoas recession, adductor myotomy, and anterior branch obturator neurectomy, bony deformities should be corrected with a subtrochanteric derotation varus osteotomy and an iliac osteotomy (Salter, 1961).

The Salter osteotomy is best done before the patient is 10 or 11 years old. In the adolescent years, I have found that the Salter osteotomy is more difficult and have used the Chiari osteotomy instead (described in Chapter 7). Sutherland et al. (1977) resolved the difficulty of performing a Salter osteotomy in older children and adolescents by adding to the procedure an osteotomy of the pubis 1 cm medial to the pubic symphysis (Fig. 6–37). Prior to this innovation, Steel (1977*a*) described a triple innominate osteotomy that facilitated anterior and lateral rotation of the acetabular portion of the hip. I have not used either procedure.

Operative Techniques.   The principle of surgery in the management of spastic paralytic subluxation of the hip is always to relieve the deforming force by muscle surgery in addition to correcting the structural abnormality of the bones. All the procedures can be done at the same time in the following order: (1) adductor myotomy and anterior branch obturator neurectomy and/or iliopsoas recession in the ambulatory patient (iliopsoas tenotomy can be done in the non-ambulatory patient): (2) varus derotation subtrochanteric femoral osteotomy; and (3) iliac osteotomy.

The iliopsoas recession can be done through the same incision as that used for the Salter iliac osteotomy. I use an oblique incision paralleling the groin, beginning 1 cm distal to the anterior superior iliac spine. This incision can be extended laterally and the proximal flap reflected to expose the anterior half of the inner and outer walls of the ilium for the osteotomy that is done after the femoral osteotomy.

A derotation and varus osteotomy can be performed through a separate lateral thigh incision as described previously in the technique for the subtrochanteric derotation osteotomy. Since the major femoral bone deformity is excessive femoral anteversion, a derotation osteotomy alone will usually result in centralization of the head of the femur in the acetabulum. The degree of varus angulation obtained during the osteotomy should be kept to a minimum because reducing the femoral neck angle to less than 135 degrees by removal of too large a wedge of bone at the osteotomy site will result in weakening of the abductor mechanism and a gluteus medius limp. I prefer to use 90-degree osteotomy compression nail plates for fixation.

If a compression nail plate is used and derotation and varus osteotomies are to be combined, the nail portion of the device should be inserted into the femoral neck at an angle that will correspond with the degree of varus inclination to be accomplished by the osteotomy. If, for example, a varus angle of 15 degrees is desired at the osteotomy, the nail is inserted at a 15-degree angle to what would be the horizontal subtrochanteric osteotomy. (The same angle can be obtained by inserting the nail in the neck of the femur at an angle of 105 degrees to the shaft.) As in the technique used for derotation osteotomy, radiographic control using guide pins prior to nail insertion is essential. The track for the nail is cut in the neck of the femur with a special chisel, and the nail is then inserted into the neck of the femur just to the point where the plate portion abuts against the lateral femoral shaft. Using a reciprocating power saw, a transverse subtrochanteric osteotomy is performed. The first cut is straight across and perpendicular to the femoral shaft. In the proximal fragment, an oblique cut is made parallel to the nail in the neck of the femur so that a wedge of bone with the base medial can be removed. The nail is then driven completely into the femoral head and neck. When the two surfaces are brought together and the derotation of the distal fragment is completed, the nail in the neck of the femur should lie almost parallel to the osteotomy site so that compression of the cut bone surfaces is obtained (Fig. 6–38 A and B).

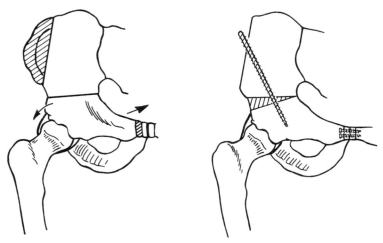

Figure 6–37 Modification of Salter's innominate osteotomy for older children (Sutherland, 1977). The superior ramus of the pubis is cut 1 cm lateral to the symphysis. This permits anterior and lateral rotation of the distal portion of the innominate bone. The pubic osteotomy is fixed with threaded wires.

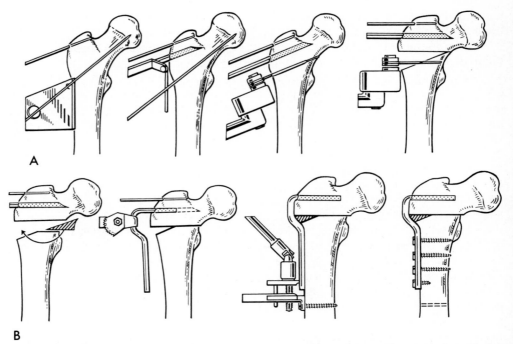

Figure 6–38 Technique for varus derotation subtrochanteric osteotomy with compression nail-plate fixation. For rotation osteotomy alone, no wedge is removed. (Redrawn from ASIF technique manual, Synthes Corporation.)

I no longer use or recommend a two-pin external fixation for a femoral osteotomy (Bleck, 1966), since it requires plaster spica immobilization beyond the 6 weeks necessary for the iliac osteotomy to heal sufficiently. With the excellent fixation afforded by hip compression nails, such prolonged and difficult immobilization is now unnecessary.

Iliac osteostomy, performed exactly as described by Salter (1961), completes the procedure. The operative technique is so well known and described in standard orthopaedic texts that repetition here is unwarranted (Tachdjian, 1972).

POSTOPERATIVE CARE OF ILIAC AND FEMORAL OSTEOTOMIES. Mobilization can begin within 6 to 8 weeks following the surgery and removal of the plaster spica cast. The iliac fixation pins, which should be palpable under the skin over the crest of the ilium, can be removed under local or brief general anesthesia. It may take 1 to 2 weeks before the joints in a child with cerebral palsy are sufficiently mobilized for ambulation with crutches. Usually it is safe to begin weight-bearing with crutches 8 weeks postoperatively. Since practically all of these patients are crutch-walkers, crutches present little problem to the patient.

Results of Surgery. In 90 percent of the patients, the results of surgery have been quite satisfactory on follow-up continued beyond skeletal maturity (25- and 30-year follow-up studies are not available) (Fig. 6–39 A, B). Failures have occurred. Usually resubluxation occurs because the muscles responsible for the deformity have not been removed (Fig. 6–40 A, B, C). Patients who have hyperelasticity of all connective tissue and ligamentous structures, in addition to spastic paralysis, may be more prone to recurrence of subluxation of the hip.

HIP ABDUCTION DEFORMITY

In clinical observations of four cases of spastic hip abduction deformity, the main spastic muscle was a hypertrophied tensor fascia femoris. These patients had mild hip flexion deformities, a normal or limited range of internal rotation, and a greater range than normal of external rotation. Curiously, two of these patients had internal tibial torsion.

Surgical Treatment. If the abducted position of the hip is such that the standing base from heel to heel is greater than 20 cm when the patient attempts to stand, the iliotibial band can be sectioned just distal to the tensor fascia femoris muscle. If a

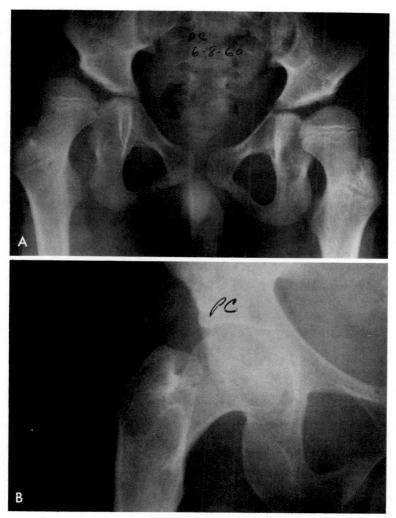

Figure 6–39 A. Patient P. C., a 9-year-old spastic diplegic with bilateral hip subluxation and 45 degree flexion contracture of hip preoperatively. B. Ten years post-bilateral iliopsoas recession, adductor myotomy, anterior branch obturator neurectomy, and varus-derotation subtrochanteric osteotomy. Acetabular dysplasia is minimal; iliac osteotomy is not necessary.

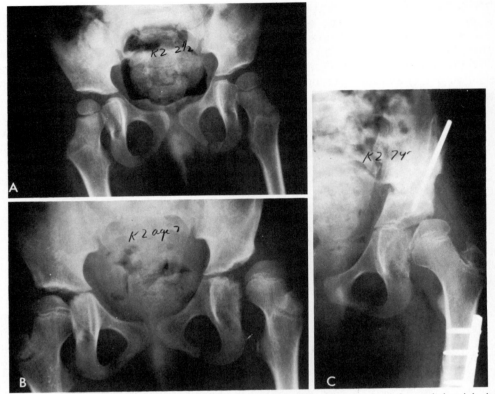

Figure 6–40   A. Patient K.Z., age 2½ years, has marked dysequilibrium and left spastic hemiplegia, only partially weight bearing in walker. B. Age 9 years. Note subluxation of left hip. C. Ten months post-Salter iliac osteotomy and derotation femoral osteotomy (I do not recommend shaft osteotomy as was done in this case). Subluxation persists. Note persistent pre- and postoperative widening of medial joint space due, possibly, to the iliopsoas and capsular invagination.

contracture of the iliotibial band is not yet present and abductor spasticity is the main cause of the deformity, lidocaine or 45 percent alcohol myoneural blocks of the tensor fascia femoris muscle can be done to assess the probable effects of surgery.

Knee

There are only two significant deformities of the knee, one the opposite of the other — knee flexion and knee hyperextension.

KNEE FLEXION DEFORMITY

The *mechanism* of the knee flexion deformity may be primary, due to a spastic and contracted hamstring muscle, or it may be secondary to a hip flexion deformity. Usually it is a combination of both. If the knee flexion deformity due to the spastic hamstrings is allowed to persist, the capsule of the knee joint contracts, and the knee flexion contracture is superimposed upon the initiating contracture of the hamstring muscles. Secondary shortening of the sciatic nerve occurs in cases of long-standing knee flexion contracture.

The literature is replete with reports on the management of knee flexion deformities (Keats and Kambin, 1962; Hein, 1969; Porter, 1970; Hayashi, 1970; Frost, 1971; Banks, 1972; Reimers, 1974; Feldkamp and Katthagen, 1975). More references will be found in the text that follows.

Assessment. *Clinical assessment* of gait and of hamstring spasticity and contracture has been described in Chapter 2.

Electromyography of the hamstring muscles in the spastic patient during gait will demonstrate a prolongation of the contraction of the hamstrings throughout the stance phase and in some patients even through the entire swing phase. The electromyograph itself does not show whether or not the hamstrings are responsible for the knee flexion deformity. Our studies (Bleck et al., 1975) have shown that most patients with spastic diplegia have both dysphasic hamstring contraction and quadriceps contraction. The two defects frequently balance each other, so no flexion deformity may be evident. Consequently, electromyography must be combined with clinical observations and, when available, with electrogoniometry or photographic measurements of knee flexion and extension during gait.

Preoperative assessment also includes an estimation of the *strength of the quadriceps* and its voluntary control. With the patient lying supine with his knees flexed over the edge of the table, he is asked to extend his knees. If knee extension is possible to the full range of extension permitted by the underlying contracture of the hamstrings and/or the joint capsule contracture, the muscle power is at least fair and should be sufficient to sustain the erect posture during standing and level walking. If the extension of the knee is less than the range of motion passively permitted, the quadriceps is weak and may need reinforcement.

Underlying *spasticity of the quadriceps* can be assessed as described in Chapter 2. The knowledge that spasticity of the quadriceps is present is most important in deciding the extent of hamstring weakening; in most cases quadriceps spasticity will maintain the surgical result and will preclude orthotics that keep the knee extended postoperatively.

A *lateral radiograph* with the knee flexed 30 degrees will determine whether or not the patella is high-riding (patella alta). We use the Insall-Salvati method of measurement in which measurements are made on the lateral radiograph of the length of the patella and the distance between the inferior pole of the patella and the tibial tubercle. Normally, the ratio of these two lengths should not exceed 1 to 1.25. If it does, then the patella is high-riding. It is not usually necessary to make such refined measurements, since it will be obvious in most cases that the patella is superior to the normal position in the patellar-femoral articulation.

Indications for Hamstring Weakening. Surgical lengthening of the hamstring muscles is indicated if the knee flexion deformity is greater than 15 degrees during the stance phase of gait. This recommendation is based not only on clinical observations but on experimental studies as well. Patients who tolerate the 15 degrees of knee flexion are those who have good hip extension that locks the hip and brings the trunk forward anterior to the knee. In addition, the ankle plantar flexors serve to overcome the flexed knee at midstance and beyond (Perry et al., 1975).

In a study of knee flexion contracture in gait, Perry et al. (1975) measured the quadriceps force needed to stabilize the knee: in 15 degrees of flexion, 75 percent of the load on the femoral head was taken up by the knee; at 30 degrees of flexion, 210 percent; and at 60 degrees of flexion, 400 percent. The quadriceps muscle force exerted at 15 degrees of flexion was equivalent to 20 percent of the maximal quadriceps strength; at 30 degrees of flexion, this force was equivalent to 30 percent of the quadriceps strength.

The quadriceps force needed when the knee is flexed beyond 15 degrees is greatly increased because the weight-bearing surfaces of the femoral condyles are relatively flat up to 15 degrees of flexion, but beyond this point the condyles are rounder, and thus more muscle strength is required for weight-bearing.

Biomechanical calculations have shown that if a 70-kilogram person stands with the knees flexed 50 degrees, not only is the force of the quadriceps increased to 752.4 kilograms, but also joint pressure is enormously increased to 1038.4 kilograms (Kottke, 1966). It is not surprising, therefore, that patients who have knee flexion deformities will eventually have more disability and pain caused by degenerative joint disease.

Surgical Procedures. Because flexed knees are so obvious, the surgeon may be tempted to treat this deformity without consideration of the associated hip flexion and equinus deformities. Foster and Munger (1977) attempted to determine which joint deformity was responsible for the crouched gait by using cylinder plaster casts to evaluate the effect of knee extension and short leg plasters to evaluate the effect of equinus of knee flexion. If the patient could stand erect with a cylinder plaster, only the hamstrings were lengthened; if he could stand erect with a short leg walking plaster, only the Achilles' tendon was lengthened; if there was forward trunk lean with either cast, iliopsoas recession was recommended.

If there are structural deformities at hip and ankle, these deformities should be corrected at the same time as the knee flexion deformity. If the hamstrings are weakened and a hip flexion deformity of over 15 degrees is present, unacceptable lumbar lordosis and trunk lean can be anticipated (Figs. 6–42 and 6–43). Studies of the sacrofemoral angle measured on standing radiographs after hamstring lengthening have consistently shown a decrease in the angle measurements, indicating pelvic and lumbar spine adaptation to the hip flexion deformity (Bleck, 1966).

INDICATIONS FOR HAMSTRING TENOTOMY, LENGTHENING, TRANSFER, AND PROXIMAL RELEASE. *Tenotomy.* Except for the gracilis and semitendinosus hamstrings, there is a risk with tenotomy of the hamstrings of permanent overcorrection in knee extension and loss of knee flexion function that is so essential in gait. Diamond (1978) had good results from semitendinosus tenotomy. I have been unable to discern any difference between tenotomy and lengthening of this muscle. Because of its great excursion and straight fibers, the cut tendon of the semitendinosus retracts to the middle third of the femur (Evans, 1975).

Lengthening. I prefer lengthening to all other methods. Lengthening can be selective and controlled. The results of lengthening have been indistinguishable from those of hamstring transfer (Evans, 1975). Green and McDermott (1942) recommended fractional lengthening of the hamstrings a quarter of a century ago. Flexion power is preserved with this method.

Transfer. The promise that transfer of the hamstring tendon insertions to the femoral condyle would assist in extension of the hip has, unfortunately, not been fulfilled (Eggers, 1952). I have given up this procedure because the additional surgery did not seem worthwhile when the end-results were compared with those of hamstring lengthening.

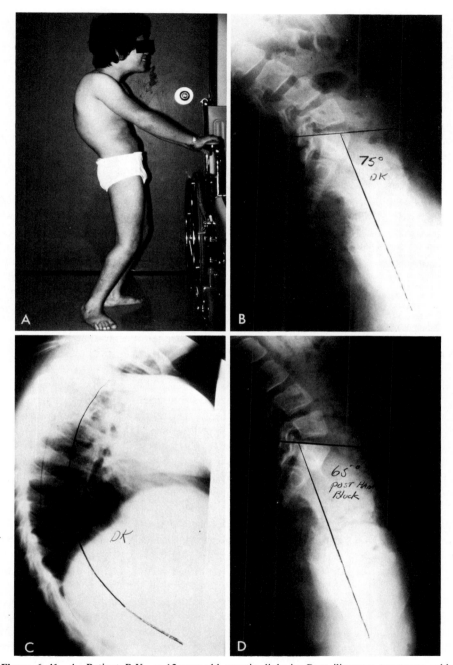

Figure 6–41   A. Patient P.K., a 12-year-old spastic diplegic. Post–iliopsoas tenotomy, adductor myotomy and anterior branch obturator neurectomy. Quadriceps and hamstrings are very spastic. Note severe thoracolumbar kyphosis (C). B. Standing lateral radiograph. Pelvis is inclined posteriorly, with a 75 degree sacrofemoral angle. Note flattening of lumbar spine and compensatory kyphosis. D. Standing lateral radiograph after 0.5 per cent lidocaine infiltration of hamstring muscles. The posterior pelvic inclination has decreased. Sacrofemoral angle is 65 degrees. This result indicates that proximal hamstring release will be beneficial in decreasing both the severe posterior inclination of the pelvis and the compensatory kyphosis.

Proximal Release. Proximal release of the hamstring origins was proposed by Seymour and Sharrard (1968) and by Drummond et al. (1974); it was recommended by Dunn (1974) if the patient had a "tight hamstring gait" manifested by a short stride length and if "swing-through" was accomplished by the pelvis. Of 14 patients who had this procedure, Dunn reported that 3 were much improved and 11 were improved. None were unchanged or worse.

Sharrard (1975) recommended that the origins of the hamstrings be divided if the quadriceps muscle was very strong so that hip flexion was limited and the stride length was short. In the study of gait, it seems that hip extension is more important in determining the length of stride than hip flexion. Hoffer (1972) had two patients whose knee flexion contracture was not corrected after proximal release of the hamstrings.

Occasionally there may be a rare patient who might benefit from proximal release of the hamstrings. This is the patient who does not have hip flexion deformity but does have spastic quadriceps and hamstrings, causing the pelvis to incline posteriorly and resulting in severe kyphosis of the thoracolumbar spine. A myoneural block of the hamstring muscles with 0.5 percent lidocaine may help in evaluating the potential effects of proximal release. If the pelvis inclines anteriorly after paralysis of the hamstrings with local anesthetic, proximal release may help in redistributing pelvic balance to allow lumbar lordosis and a decrease in the compensatory kyphosis (Fig. 6–41 A, B, C, D).

Other surgeons (Frost, 1971) seem to be discouraged with hamstring surgery and have accepted the crouch but advise surgery if there are structural changes, presumably contracture of the knee joint capsule and the hamstrings.

POSTERIOR CAPSULOTOMY OF THE KNEE JOINT. This is necessary if there is a knee flexion contracture. Capsulotomy is recommended in addition to hamstring lengthening. Preoperatively, knee joint capsular contracture can be ascertained if the knee will not extend completely when the extended limb is resting on the examining table and the patient in the supine position.

OPERATIVE TECHNIQUE OF HAMSTRING LENGTHENING. In children, generally only the medial hamstrings need lengthening. Medial *and* lateral hamstring lengthening may be required if (1) the contracture is of long duration in the adolescent or adult, and (2) if there is no underlying quadriceps spasticity.

In the usual spastic diplegic child, I prefer to use the following method. An incision approximately 7 to 8 cm long is made longitudinally over the semitendinosus tendon and extended to the popliteal crease. A tenotomy of the gracilis tendon can then be performed. The semitendinosus tendon is larger, more lateral, and more subcutaneous than that of the gracilis. The semitendinosus tendon is Z-lengthened and then retracted to expose all sides of the broad bandlike semimembranosus tendon. A long serpentine S incision (or a broad V) is made just through its tendinous portion to expose the muscle beneath. Straight leg raising to 70 to 75 degrees should be possible. The ends of the semitendinosus tendon can be resutured; if the proximal end retracts inadvertently into the proximal thigh out of the wound, it can be left alone as a tenotomy. At the time of this writing, I am not certain that the postoperative result of lengthening of this muscle can be distinguished from that of tenotomy.

In more severe cases of hamstring contracture when biceps femoris contracture is suspected, and in adults and adolescents, the method used by Westin (1973) is preferred. With the patient supine, an assistant flexes the hip 90 degrees and extends the knee to its limit. A straight incision is made in the midline of the distal one third of the thigh. The medial and lateral hamstring muscles are exposed at their musculotendinous junctions and dissected distally to their tendons. The epimysium of the muscles is incised circumferentially in a proximal to distal direction as the knee is progressively extended to a point where it lacks approximately 15 degrees of complete extension. The muscular portions, although remaining intact, do stretch and some fibers may tear.

In more severe contractures, it may be necessary to lengthen the semimembranosus and biceps tendons, but I have rarely done so.

In patients with long-standing contractures, the *sciatic nerve* will be shortened. Sciatic nerve stretch paralysis can be minimized if this structural change is appreciated, the nerve is palpated, and efforts to forcibly stretch the knee into extension under anesthesia are avoided. In this type of problem, gradual extension of the knee must be accomplished postoperatively with wedging plasters.

Postoperative Care. If no foot or ankle surgery has been performed, a long leg cylinder plaster provides sufficient immobilization. I allow the patient to walk as soon as possible, providing no additional procedures on the foot, ankle, or hip that preclude weight-bearing were done at the same time. Three weeks of immobilization are sufficient. After the plasters have been removed, the antagonistic quadriceps spasticity is usually sufficiently effective to eliminate orthoses to keep the knee extended.

Results and Complications. Recurrence of the knee flexion deformity has been the dominant concern of surgeons. Lutman (1976) examined 152 patients 3 years after hamstring surgery and found a 32 percent recurrence rate of the deformity. He related this to the presence of patella alta in 72 percent of the patients (Blumensaat's method of radiographic measurement was used). It was thought that patella alta decreased the power of the quadriceps in terminal extension because a shorter moment arm would be the result of the abnormal proximal position of the patella. If this were the true explanation of recurrence, then the deformity should have recurred in 72 percent of patients; however, only 32 percent were affected. Recurrence of the knee flexion deformity has not been the major problem in surgery of the flexed knee in patients with spastic diplegia. Other problems have been more prominent, among them:

1. Increased postoperative lumbar lordosis (Bleck, 1975b) (Fig. 6–42). This can be partially avoided by surgical treatment of the hip flexion deformity, particularly if the hip flexion contracture is greater than 20 degrees.

2. Hyperextended knee gait. Quadriceps spasticity that becomes evident after hamstring weakening can assist in maintaining the correction of the flexion deformity. It can be discerned preoperatively. However, too much quadriceps spasticity leading to postoperative limited knee flexion and genu recurvatum is a greater functional disability than knee flexion of up to 15 degrees (Fig. 6–43). The zeal of the surgeon has been conditioned by the fear of recurrence of flexion. Consequently, surgeons usually err on the side of overlengthening too many hamstrings or transferring all hamstrings to the femoral condyles. In children with spastic diplegia, semitendinosus gracilis tenotomy, and aponeurotic semimembranosus lengthening are sufficient most of the time.

3. Failure to correct the deformity and a persistence of the crouch gait. This discouraging result is more common when the deformity has been untreated beyond the age of 8 years. Two reasons account for failure: (a) inability to achieve complete extension of the knee due to secondary contracture of the posterior capsule of the joint; (b) quadriceps weakness, lack of terminal extension associated with patella alta,

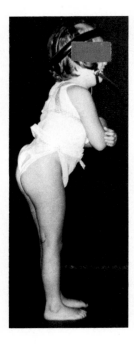

Figure 6–42 Eight-year-old spastic diplegic following semitendinosus transfer, gracilis tenotomy, and semimembranosus lengthening. Untreated hip flexion contracture causes lordosis and forward trunk lean.

and little if any quadriceps spasticity. To obtain complete knee extension, posterior capsulotomy of the joint followed, if necessary, by wedging casts is required. Quadriceps augmentation is discussed in the following section.

4. Crouch position caused by overlengthening of the gastrocnemius-soleus muscles. If the function of the gastrocnemius-soleus to resist forward acceleration of the tibia during stance is lost, knee flexion occurs. When this possibility is suspected in a crouched patient who has a range of ankle dorsiflexion of more than 5 degrees,

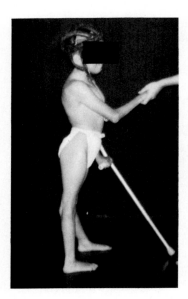

Figure 6–43 Nine-year-old spastic diplegic one year after medial and lateral hamstring lengthening (had a 40 degree flexed knee posture preoperatively). Patient now has severe quadriceps spasticity, genu recurvatum, and lumbar lordosis.

bilateral short leg walking plasters to block ankle dorsiflexion can be applied as a test of gastrocnemius-soleus function. If they are successful, rigid plastic ankle-foot orthoses may be used to correct this unfortunate result.

5. Sciatic postoperative neuropathy. This may occur in patients with severe (over 30 degrees) long-standing knee flexion contractures if the knee is forcibly extended at the time of surgery. Shortening of the sciatic nerve does occur; in such patients, gradual knee extension in wedging casts after the operation will usually allow stretching of the nerve without compromising its function.

The symptoms and signs of sciatic neuropathy include pain on the plantar aspect of the foot and hypesthesia on the plantar aspect of the toes and foot.

QUADRICEPS AUGMENTATION. As previously stated, recurrence of the knee flexion deformity occasionally occurs; it is caused, not by recurrent hamstring contracture, but usually by a lag in quadriceps function. Preoperatively, such patients have a high-riding patella and are unable to completely extend the knee against gravity in the range of motion permitted by the contracture. These patients will not have quadriceps spasticity of any significant amount.

The problem is difficult to resolve. Two solutions are suggested: (1) patellar tendon advancement in the patient whose epiphyses have closed; (2) transfer of the spastic semitendinosus to the patella.

Patellar Tendon Advancement (Chandler, 1933; Roberts and Adams, 1953; Baker, 1956; Keats and Kamblin, 1962). This procedure must be accompanied by hamstring lengthening. In children with open epiphyses, there is a definite risk of premature arrest of the proximal anterior tibial physis when the patellar tendon is detached from its insertion. This has occurred even with the Baker modification (1956), in which the tendon is skived off its insertion rather than removed with a block of bone. For this reason, I do not perform the procedure in children.

Through a lateral parapatellar incision that extends 3 cm distal to the tibial tubercle, the patellar tendon is dissected free medially and laterally. The dissection is continued proximally to include the joint capsule. Together with a 1.0 to 1.5 cm block of bone, the patellar tendon insertion is removed and pulled distally with sufficient tension so that the knee can be flexed 45 degrees. A block of bone is removed at this location on the anterior medial aspect of the tibial shaft, and the patellar tendon insertion bone is placed in this well. An alternative method is to detach only the patellar tendon from its insertion with thin slivers of bone, anchoring this distally with a 3- or 4-pronged staple or a screw. Additional sutures are used to anchor the patellar tendon to the adjacent soft tissues.

Plaster immobilization is continued for 6 weeks. Knee flexion and extension exercises will be required. Frequently, a knee-ankle-foot orthosis with a knee lock will be necessary until full quadriceps strength is regained.

A possible risk with this procedure is the development of knee pain due to chondromalacia patella. When the patella has been high-riding and its articular cartilage has been out of contact with the normal opposing femoral articular cartilage, degeneration of the patellar articular surface can be anticipated. Plain radiographs may show spurring of the poles of the patella when chondromalacia is far advanced. Gross radiographic changes of the patella consisting of fragmentation of the lower pole and elongation of the patella in patients who have knee flexion deformities in cerebral palsy have been described (Kaye and Freiberger, 1971; Rosenthal and Levine, 1977). A preoperative arthroscopic examination can determine the status of the patellar articular cartilage.

Transfer of the Semitendinosus to the Patella. Other surgeons (McCullough,

1972) and I have tried this procedure. The number of cases has been small and the results have not been analyzed. It appears to be a logical procedure in view of the beneficial effects of retaining some quadriceps spasticity in maintaining knee extension. It has done no harm.

In transferring the semitendinosus to the patella at the time of hamstring lengthening, the patient should be supine; an assistant flexes the hip 90 degrees and extends the knee. Hamstring lengthening proceeds in the usual way through the longitudinal incision over the semitendinosus tendon. The tendon is followed distally to the pes anserinus insertion, where it is cut. A 3-cm transverse incision over the semitendinosus muscle at the level of the distal and middle thirds of the thigh exposes the muscle and tendon; the tendon is pulled out through this wound.

A third 3- to 4-cm transverse incision is made over the junction of the proximal and middle thirds of the patella. A long forceps (uterine packing) is used to create a subcutaneous tunnel from the patella to the incision in the thigh. With the knee extended, the tendon is held under maximum tension and is woven through the quadriceps tendon and through an osteoperiosteal tunnel in the anterior aspect of the proximal patella, where it is firmly sutured.

Postoperative care is similar to that described for patellar tendon advancement.

The only risk with this procedure is a postoperative saphenous neuropathy. The saphenous nerve lies along the posterior border of the sartorius and is in the region of dissection of the semitendinosus tendon. Inadvertent cutting or entrapment of this nerve is understandable.

HYPEREXTENSION DEFORMITY

Mechanisms.   Two explanations for the hyperextended knee gait have been offered: (1) a spastic quadriceps (Bleck et al., 1975*a*) and (2) poor regulation of ankle plantar flexion power (Simon et al., 1977).

Although the spastic rectus femoris muscle was once thought to be an isolated entity (Duncan 1955; Sutherland, 1975), it seems clear now that all segments of the quadriceps muscle are spastic. In normal subjects, all four portions of the quadriceps contribute to knee extension; the vastus intermedius is a particularly strong extensor (Perry and Lieb, 1967).

The sophisticated electrical and computer-plotted study of Simon et al. (1977) of genu recurvatum in patients with cerebral palsy and spastic paralysis indicates that a number of factors are responsible. The most prominent defect found in this study was poor ankle plantar flexion, which caused an abrupt halt in tibial motion in early stance if the calf muscles were weak or in late stance if the calf muscles were strong. Simon and his co-workers concluded that the rigid plastic ankle-foot orthosis was effective in overcoming genu recurvatum because of its locking effect on the ankle.

Indications for Surgery.   If the patient has hyperextension of the knee during the stance phase of gait and if the knee does not flex sufficiently in swing phase so the foot can clear the floor, the gait is functionally disabling.

Confirmation of the spasticity of the quadriceps is obtained by the tests described in Chapter 2. Electromyography will show almost continuous activity of the rectus femoris and the vastus muscles throughout both phases of gait.

OPERATIVE   TECHNIQUE   OF   RECTUS   FEMORIS   TENOTOMY   (DUNCAN,

1955).   This simple operation is performed through an oblique incision 1.5 cm below the anterior superior iliac spine parallel with the groin crease. The sartorius is retracted laterally. The rectus femoris tendon is hidden by a veil of fatty tissue. When this is removed, the white shining tendon is easily seen. A reflection of fascia from the iliacus muscle to the tendon is sectioned. The direct head of the tendon is dissected free and cut near its origin. It then retracts distally (Fig. 6–44).

I perform this procedure in association with iliopsoas recession if the patient has a hyperextended knee gait pattern (Bleck 1971*a*, *b*, *c*).

The *results of rectus femoris release,* although not extraordinary, have produced gait improvement. Sutherland et al. (1975) reported that of eight patients, six improved; the major improvement was initial knee flexion at the beginning of the swing phase in gait.

QUADRICEPS TENDON LENGTHENING. *Quadriceps tendon lengthening* has been performed in three patients who had no knee flexion during gait due to severe quadriceps spasticity after total hamstring release for a flexed knee gait.

The operative technique is quite direct. Through a transverse incision, the quadriceps tendon is Z-lengthened and resutured with the knee flexed 45 degrees. Plaster immobilization for 6 weeks with the knee flexed 30 degrees has been sufficient.

The results have been satisfactory. The knees could flex 75 to 90 degrees when the patient was seated (preoperatively knee flexion was only 30 to 40 degrees), and the gait, while not normal, was improved.

Foot and Ankle

EQUINUS DEFORMITY

The management of equinus deformity has been covered in Chapter 4. In spastic diplegia, this deformity is usually bilateral. Overlengthening should be avoided (Fig.

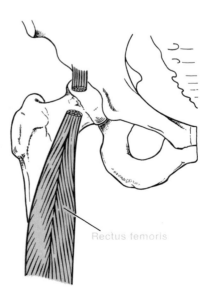

Figure 6–44   Rectus femoris release. The straight head of its tendinous insertion is cut, causing the distal portion to retract.

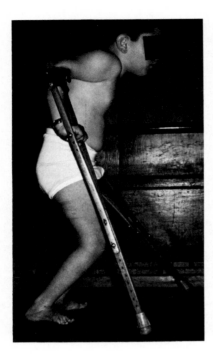

Figure 6–45 Postoperative crouch due to an overlengthened Achilles tendon.

6–45). Increased ankle dorsiflexion aggravates the flexed knee posture. Recurrence or a slight residual equinus inclination is preferred to irreparable calcaneus.

PES VALGUS

Anatomy. Pes valgus in patients with spastic diplegia consists of eversion and equinus inclination of the calcaneus and abduction of the midfoot, resulting in prominence of the head of the talus medially. It is a flexible deformity; the foot can be passively manipulated into the corrected position by plantar flexion of the ankle and inversion of the foot.

Standing lateral radiographs show greater than normal plantar flexion of the talus and varying degrees of loss of dorsiflexion of the calcaneus (Fig. 6–46). The normal angle of plantar flexion of the talus is 26.5 degrees (S.D. 5.3 degrees) (Bleck and Berzins, 1977) (Fig. 6–47). In children under 5 years of age, the plantar flexion of the talus normally may be as much as 35 degrees, so that a line through the talus falls just inferior to the first metatarsal shaft rather than through it. The normal calcaneal dorsiflexion angle is 16.8 degrees (S.D. 5.6 degrees) (Fig. 6–47).

On anteroposterior radiographs made with the patient bearing weight, the normal angle between the axes of the talus and calcaneus is a mean of 18 degree (S.D. 5 degrees). If this angle is greater than 25 degrees, a valgus angle is present; if less than 15 degrees, the heel is in varus (Fig. 6–48).

Mechanisms. The *axis of rotation of the subtalar joint* is probably more horizontal than oblique, and accounts more for eversion of this joint than inversion. When measured on anatomical specimens, the mean angle of inclination as projected on the sagittal plane was 42 degrees, with a very great range of 20.5 to 68.5 degrees (Inman,

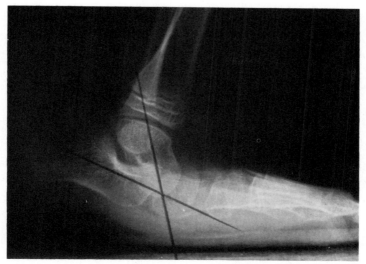

Figure 6–46 Lateral radiograph made with weight–bearing from a patient with severe spastic pes valgus, 80 degree talus plantar flexion, and calcaneus in equinus position.

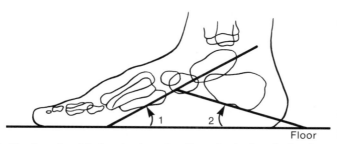

Figure 6–47 Tracing of weight-bearing lateral radiograph. Angle 1 is the plantar flexion angle of talus; angle 2 is the dorsiflexion angle of calcaneus. Normal means: talus, 26.5 degrees (S.D. 5.3 degrees); calcaneus, 16.8 degrees (S.D. 5.6 degrees).

Figure 6–48 Tracings of weight-bearing anteroposterior radiographs showing talar–calcaneal divergent angle in normal, varus, and valgus feet. Normal mean: 18 degrees (S.D. 5 degrees); varus: less than 15 degrees; valgus: more then 25 degrees.

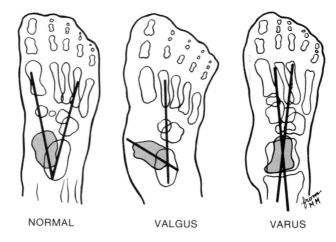

NORMAL   VALGUS   VARUS

1976). If this is true, then a more horizontally inclined axis should result in greater eversion.

It is possible that *spasticity of the peroneal muscles* deforms the subtalar joint, bringing its axis of rotation into a more horizontal alignment. In addition, however, it seems evident that the spastic peroneals abduct the mid- and forefoot so much that the talus loses the support of the navicular bone and its plantar ligament. The result of this lost support is talar plantar flexion.

Calcaneal plantar flexion due to gastrocnemius-soleus contracture contributes to the deformity but unfortunately is not the sole cause. If it were, Achilles tendon lengthening would prevent and correct pes valgus. This we know does not occur. Equinus deformity is seen without valgus and even with varus deformities.

Persistent fetal medial deviation of the neck of the talus may account for a portion of the deformity. The fact that the newborn talus has a greater degree of medial deviation of its neck at birth than in the adult form has been documented (Lisowski, 1967), and the persistence of the newborn talar neck angle as a cause of in-toeing in children has been reported (Bleck, 1976). I have observed normal children who originally toed-in develop pes valgus with a prominent head of the talus on the medial aspect of the foot. Standing anteroposterior radiographs of the ankle have permitted a measurement of the projected talar neck angle (Fig. 6–49A) and appear to confirm the increased talar neck angle in some cases of pes valgus. In the discussion of the risks of subtalar arthrodesis, this possible mechanism of medial deviation of the talar neck is important. Thus, if the navicular is brought into alignment with the talar head and it is medially deviated, a toed-in posture results.

Assessment.   In addition to the clincial examination of the deformity, the surgeon will want to confirm the flexibility and correctibility of the foot by passive manipulation; the foot will have to be brought into varying degrees of equinus before it can be put into a corrected position. If in doubt about the mobility of the talus, a lateral radiograph with the foot in equinus inclination and inversion resolves the question and differentiates a fixed from a flexible deformity.

Anteroposterior and lateral radiographs of the foot when standing, and an anteroposterior radiograph of the ankles during weight-bearing are essential. The anteroposterior radiographs of the ankle are most important in defining the tilt (if any) of the ankle mortise (Fig. 6–50).

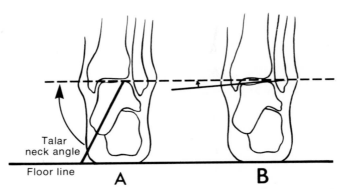

Figure 6–49   Tracings of weight-bearing anteroposterior radiographs of ankle. A. Measurement of talar neck deviation. B. Measurement of valgus tilt of the ankle joint.

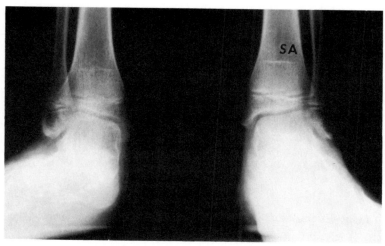

Figure 6–50 Weight-bearing anteroposterior radiograph of ankles in a 14-year-old male spastic diplegic with severe pes valgus. Is the ankle joint change secondary to the neglected correction of the pes valgus?

Indications and Timing of Surgery. Surgical correction is advised for an obvious and severe deformity. It should be performed before the occurence of secondary changes such as hallux valgus and callus formation on the medial border of the great toe. However, based upon our own study, surgery should not be done too early. The best results of corrective surgery have been obtained in patients who are more than 7 years old but have not yet reached skeletal maturity. Lee (1977*b*) found that when surgery was performed in patients under age 7 years, 11 out of 13 feet in my series were failures. If surgery is delayed until adolescence, triple arthrodesis is usually required. Because triple arthrodesis entails bone removal, the height of the foot is decreased, and the malleoli impinge uncomfortably on the shoe (Banks, 1976).

If surgery is done in young children (before age 5 years), the corrections may be inadequate owing to the smallness and cartilaginous bulk of the bones.

Surgical Procedures. Six procedures are possible. For early correction only two are recommended, and for late correction, only one.

1. PERONEAL TENDON TRANSFER OR LENGTHENING. Attractive as transfer or lengthening of the spastic peroneal muscle appears, the results are usually very poor; varus deformity is the frequent result. Keats (1974) issued a stern warning about re-routing the peroneus longus and brevis tendons. In my own experience, good results were obtained in only two of seven feet that had peroneal tendon lengthening using the Grice procedure (Lee, 1977*b*).

2. SUBTALAR EXTRA-ARTICULAR ARTHRODESIS (Grice, 1952). This has been the most widely used procedure (Baker and Dodelin, 1958). Despite its popularity, numerous problems have been encountered with it. Ross et al. (1977) reported a 64 percent failure rate, and 28 percent had complications. Moreland and Westin (1977) analyzed their results in 302 feet; 73 percent were satisfactory and 26 percent were unsatisfactory. Banks (1977) reported a success rate of 86 percent, of which 63 percent were excellent.

My own results were studied by Lee (1977*b*). Of 44 Grice procedures performed in patients with cerebral palsy, the rate of good corrections was only 50 percent with

Table 6–4   METHODS OF CORRECTION OF POSTOPERATIVE VARUS
AND VALGUS IN GRICE PROCEDURES*

VARUS
    (1) posterior tibial tendon transfer
    (3) posterior tibial tendon lengthening
    (1) anterior tibial tendon transfer
    (2) closed wedged lateral calcaneal osteotomy
VALGUS
    (2) peroneus brevis tendon lengthening

*Lee, C. (1977) The Grice subtalar extra-articular arthrodesis in cerebral palsy. Unpublished thesis —fellowship from United Cerebral Palsy Research and Education Foundation and Children's Hospital at Stanford.

the first surgery. Eventually, with secondary procedures, the results were satisfactory in 85 percent (for details of correction of postoperative varus or valgus deformities see Table 6–4).

These data are not encouraging, but neither do they indicate abandonment of the operation. It seems clear that the technique is demanding (the results are better in Boston). It should be performed on children who are 7 years old or older; on children under age 7 years, my failure rate was 85 percent! This operation apparently is not needed for every valgus deformity. Of 300 of my patients who required surgery for cerebral palsy, only 24 needed a Grice procedure (44 feet).

3. POSTERIOR CALCANEAL FACET OPEN WEDGE OSTEOTOMY (Baker and Hill, 1964).   Because of the fear that this procedure would be insufficient to correct the deformity and would not preserve subtalar joint motion as originally intended due to arthrofibrosis, I have not performed it as the sole procedure. When Baker's procedure was combined with the Grice procedure, the results improved dramatically: with the Grice procedure alone, 83 percent failed, but with the Grice and Baker procedures combined only 25 percent failed.

The rationale for adding Baker's calcaneal facet osteotomy to the Grice proce-

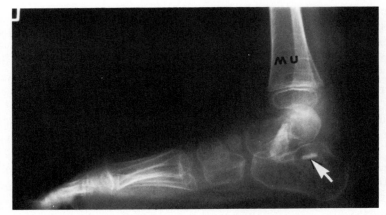

Figure 6–51   Weight-bearing lateral radiograph of ankle following Grice procedure and horizontal calcaneal osteotomy (Baker). The white horizontal density below the posterior calcaneal facet (arrow) is the bone graft used for the open wedge horizontal osteotomy.

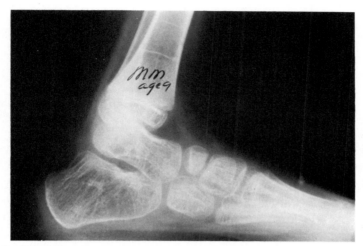

Figure 6–52 Weight-bearing lateral radiograph of ankle one year after Grice procedure and horizontal calcaneal osteotomy. Even though the tibial bone graft in the sinus tarsi resorbed, the correction was maintained.

dure was that if the tibial bone graft used in the sinus tarsi in the Grice procedure resorbed or did not unite, the calcaneal facet osteotomy would hold the corrections (Figs. 6–51 and 6–52).

4. SUBTALAR EXTRA-ARTICULAR ARTHRODESIS, MODIFIED. Brown (1968) and Seymour and Evans (1968) used a fibular bone graft (modified by Batchelor) that was driven through a hole in the neck of the talus and into the calcaneus to create the arthrodesis. Graft fracture has been a complication with this procedure. It is no wonder — because the graft is inserted almost exactly parallel (if not in exact alignment) with the axis of rotation of the subtalar joint. This alignment is not conducive to immobilization of the joint. Ideally, the graft should be placed perpendicular to the subtalar joint axis; it will then be under compression, and rotation will be minimal.

To simplify the correction of spastic pes valgus using the principle of extra-articular subtalar arthrodesis Cahuzac (1977) and the orthopaedic surgeons of Montpellier have used the technique of Cavalier and Judet (cited by Trouillas, 1978). The foot was manipulated into the corrected position, and a screw was inserted obliquely posteriorly through the superior surface of the talar neck into the calcaneus (Fig. 6–53). The screw maintained the correction. Bad results occurred in only 10 percent of the 50 feet reported by the Montpellier group.

Dennyson and Fulford (1976) combined the screw fixation technique with the insertion of a cancellous bone graft from the ilium into the sinus tarsi. The reported results were good (93.7 percent fusion rate). The bone graft appears to be a wise measure because with the screw alone loosening is likely to occur; the screw is in the same axis of rotation as that of the subtalar joint. The screw holds the correction while rapid extra-articular arthrodesis occurs. The advantage of this procedure is that it allows early weight bearing in short leg plasters for 6 to 8 weeks postoperatively. At the Newington Children's Hospital the surgeons (Cary, 1978) seem pleased with the results.

5. CALCANEAL OSTEOTOMY, OPEN WEDGE (Silver et al., 1967, 1974, 1977). Calcaneal osteotomy has been proposed to preserve the mobility of the

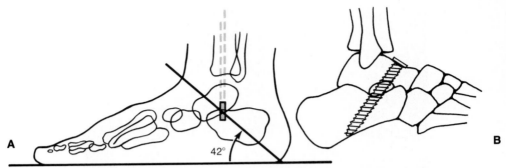

Figure 6–53   A. Correct alignment of the tibial bone graft in the Grice procedure. The axis of rotation of the subtalar joint has a mean of 42 degrees. The graft should cross this axis and not be aligned with it. B. The foot is manipulated into the corrected position and a single screw is inserted through the superior neck of the talus into the os calcis in order to hold the correction. To assure early fusion, iliac bone grafts are placed in the sinus tarsi. When the screw is inserted, only a small incision need be made over the neck of the talus and a drill guide can be used to protect the soft tissues from the threads of the screw as it is being inserted. Radiographic control is indicated.

subtalar joint and correct the valgus deformity by shifting the weight-bearing area of the calcaneus. Silver has had success with this procedure, but others have reported failure or recurrence of the original problem. From a study of Silver's publications, it appears that calcaneal osteotomy will realign the valgus foot if it has moderate plantar flexion of the talus of 45 to 55 degrees. If plantar flexion of the talus is greater than this (60 to 80 degrees), calcaneal osteotomy may not offer enough correction (Sage, 1977; Samilson, 1972) (Fig. 6–46).

6. TRIPLE ARTHRODESIS.   This standard orthopaedic operation is reserved for adolescent and adult patients with severe pes valgus who have reached skeletal maturity. Although triple arthrodesis offers good correction of varus deformities, the results have not been as satisfactory in patients with valgus deformities (Horstmann and Eilert, 1977; Duckworth, 1977). All too often after triple arthrodesis, the foot still appears to have a valgus inclination. I have added the tibial bone graft prop in the sinus tarsi (Grice procedure) to improve the difficult correction of valgus feet by triple arthrodesis.

OPERATIVE TECHNIQUES

Subtalar Extra-Articular Arthrodesis (Grice, 1952).   If there is hindfoot equinus deformity, a Hoke Achilles tendon lengthening is performed first so that the tendon will slide as the surgeon manipulates the foot into the correct position.

A posteriorly inclined incision is made in the sinus tarsi beginning at the talar head and extending to the peroneal tendon sheath. The deep fascia and fat are incised in the sinus tarsi to expose the inferior aspect of the talus and the calcaneal floor of the sinus tarsi distal to the subtalar joint. It is best to preserve some of the fat and connective tissue in the sinus tarsi in order to facilitate wound closure.

The inferior aspect of the talar neck and the superior aspect of the calcaneus are denuded of all soft tissue. The foot is manipulated into the correct position. An osteotome wide enough to span the space between the talar neck and the calcaneus is inserted *parallel* with the tibia. With the osteotome in place, eversion should be blocked and correction maintained with the foot in neutral dorsiflexion.

A bone graft 3 to 4 mm wider than the osteotome is cut from the anterior proximal

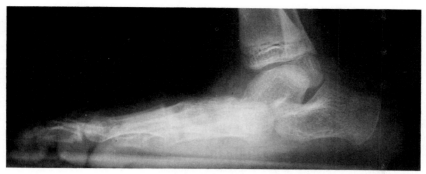

Figure 6–54 Weight-bearing lateral radiograph showing 60 to 70 degree plantar flexion of talus. There may be more deformity than can be corrected with calcaneal osteotomy.

cortex of the tibia. Originally, two grafts were used, but I have found that one is sufficient, as has Banks (1977). With a curette, a shallow channel is prepared to receive the graft on the cortex of the talar neck and calcaneus. It is most important *not to penetrate the cortex* so that the graft sinks into the soft cancellous bone. The graft can be trimmed to fit snugly in the sinus tarsi. It must be placed parallel to the tibia so that it crosses the axis of rotation of the subtalar joint (Figs. 6–53 to 6–55). The graft is tapped to secure a tight fit. The foot is placed in the corrected position of neutral dorsiflexion and the heel is placed in neutral position. The heel position can be checked with a simulated weight-bearing anteroposterior radiograph in the operating room. The divergent angle between the talus and the calcaneus should be between 15 and 20 degrees for a neutral heel. Angles of less than 15 degrees will cause a varus deformity.

I have added the horizontal osteotomy, described by Baker and Hill (1964) to the Grice procedure. It is an insurance measure in case the graft in the sinus tarsi is absorbed or displaced. After the Grice procedure is completed, the lateral aspect of the calcaneus just inferior to its articular surface is easily exposed. No additional incisions are required. A straight osteotome the width of the posterior calcaneal articular surface is driven horizontally through the subchondral bone, parallel with the joint. The articular surface is raised with the osteotome, and the wedge is held open with small bone grafts from the tibia.

If the graft in the sinus tarsi seems unstable, a Kirschner wire or a small

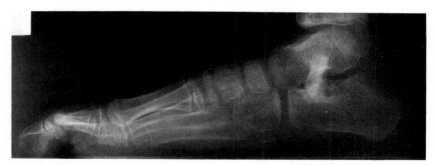

Figure 6–55 Weight-bearing lateral radiograph of ankle following Grice procedure. A single tibial graft is sufficient, and it is in the correct position.

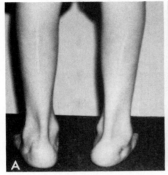 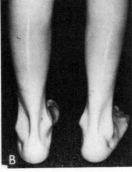

Figure 6-56 A. Patient P.L., a spastic diplegic who, following Grice procedure, has unacceptable fixed varus deformity of the left heel. B. Post-closed wedge calcaneal osteotomy performed after Grice procedure to correct fixed varus deformity.

Steinmann pin can be inserted through the heel pad into the talus. The pin will hold the correction while a padded plaster is applied from the toes to the mid-thigh.

The tourniquet is always released before wound closure, and bleeding vessels are coagulated. If the bone bleeds excessively, closed suction drainage of the wound is used for 24 to 48 hours.

Postoperative care entails plaster immobilization for 8 weeks with no weight-bearing, and 4 weeks in a short leg walking plaster. In children who are over 9 years old or are large for their size, the foot should be protected with a molded plastic ankle-foot orthosis (Fig. 6-2) for 6 months.

Risks of the Grice procedure are:

1. Overcorrection and a postoperative varus deformity. When the subtalar joint has fused in varus (Fig. 6-56A), the problem can be corrected by closed wedge lateral osteotomy of the calcaneus (Fig. 6-56B).

2. Loss of correction due to graft absorption or displacement. Both of these complications can be minimized by making certain that the graft is aligned parallel with the tibia (Fig. 6-53).

3. Recurrence of valgus deformity of the forefoot due to spastic peroneal muscles. If the peroneals are very spastic, I lengthen only the peroneus brevis. In 44 feet, only two required peroneal lengthening because of persistent postoperative peroneal spasticity. Lengthening of both peroneals should not be done, nor should they be transferred. Electromyography during gait may help in deciding which peroneal is spastic (Hoffer, 1976).

4. Varus deformity of the mid- and forefoot usually occurs if the peroneal tendons have been lengthened. In this situation, the midfoot is flexible and passively correctible. The posterior tibial muscle is spastic and should be lengthened. If the heel is in neutral position and arthrodesis of the subtalar joint has been successful, osteotomy of the os calcis is unnecessary.

5. Valgus deformity of the ankle. Valgus tilt of the ankle mortise may have been present preoperatively. Standing anteroposterior radiographs of the ankle will alert the surgeon to this additional deformity (Fig. 6-50).

Valgus deformity of the ankle may develop if a segment of the fibula has been removed for the graft and fails to reossify. This complication has been reported by Wiltse (1972) and Hsu et al. (1974). For this reason, I do not use a fibular bone graft. Why increase the risk?

6. Postoperative in-toed gait. This unwelcome result can be confused with varus inclination of the hindfoot (overcorrection of pes valgus or posterior tibial muscle

spasticity). The gait problem may be due to internal rotation of the entire foot. In some cases, both varus deformity and internal rotation may be combined.

Internal rotation of the foot may be due to either internal tibial-fibular torsion or persistent fetal medial deviation of the talar neck or both. Internal rotation of the foot becomes evident only after surgery when the navicular bone is aligned in its normal position on the head of the talus (Figs. 6–57 and 6–58). In some valgus deformities, the forefoot with the navicular bone is abducted at the talonavicular joint.

This end result can be avoided by anticipating it in the preoperative examination and passively maneuvering the foot into the correct position. Then the internal rotation will be evident. If it is, derotation osteotomy of the proximal tibia and fibula should be planned, either at the time of subtalar extra-articular arthrodesis or as a second stage procedure. Because the bone graft for the Grice procedure is taken at the osteotomy site, rotation osteotomy would not be wise until several weeks have elapsed. For this reason and to avoid prolonged immobilization, I have performed the rotation osteotomies without difficulty at the time of the Grice procedure in three patients.

Operative Technique of Calcaneal Osteotomy, Open Wedge (Silver) (Fig. 6–59). An oblique incision is made on the lateral side of the heel; it begins anteriorly and extends to the Achilles tendon insertion to the plantar aspect of the calcaneus, almost parallel to the peroneal tendons. A limited width of the lateral aspect of the calcaneus is exposed subperiosteally so that an osteotome can be driven across the calcaneus just posterior to its articular facet. The osteotomy is opened so that the weight-bearing area of the heel is inverted and shifted medially. The osteotomy is held open with an allograft cortical bone graft obtained from the tibial bone of an autoclaved cadaver (freeze-dried bone grafts can be used). The entire amount of correction must be obtained at surgery, and no further correction can be expected from manipulation or growth. Consequently, it depends upon the surgeon's visual and

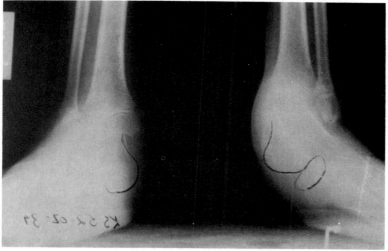

Figure 6–57 Weight-bearing anteroposterior radiograph of ankle of patient with spastic pes valgus. As a result of correction the navicular moves medially, and if the talar neck is deviated more medially than normal (18 to 20 degrees), internal axial rotation of the foot may occur.

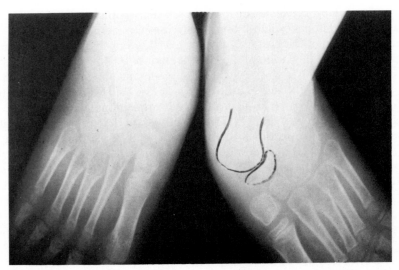

Figure 6–58 Weight-bearing anteroposterior radiograph of foot of patient with spastic pes valgus. Navicular is displaced laterally. If correction is obtained, navicular should rest on the center of the talar head. This may result in an in-toed gait if the talar neck has persistent fetal medial deviation.

perceptual skills to ensure that the valgus deformity is corrected but not overcorrected.

A non–weight-bearing long leg plaster is used for 8 weeks postoperatively. After plaster removal no special shoes or orthotics are necessary.

Operative Technique for Triple Arthrodesis for Valgus.   Because of the many failures of correction with triple arthrodesis (only 2 of 17 feet were satisfactorily corrected in Horstman and Eilert's series [1977]), I have combined the procedure with the tibial bone graft in the sinus tarsi (Grice procedure).

Williams and Menelaus (1977) have also been disenchanted with the ordinary triple arthrodesis in valgus feet. Their technique involves a tibial bone graft that is embedded in a rectangular trough cut into the sinus tarsi and across both the

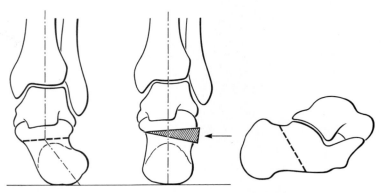

Figure 6–59   Diagram of Silver technique for open wedge calcaneal osteotomy to correct pes valgus. An autogenous bone graft (autoclaved tibial shaft) is shaped to keep the osteotomy open.

Figure 6–60 Diagram of the Williams and Menelaus technique for triple arthrodesis in the valgus foot. A trough is excised from the sinus tarsi to include the talonavicular and calcaneo-cuboid joints. Into this a tibial bone graft, slightly oversized, is hammered to fit snugly. Subtalar joint cartilage is removed with a gouge and the cavity is packed with bone chips. (Redrawn from Williams, P. F., and Menelaus, M. B. (1977). Triple arthrodesis by inlay grafting—a method suitable for undeformed or valgus foot. *Journal of Bone and Joint Surgery* 59B:333–336.)

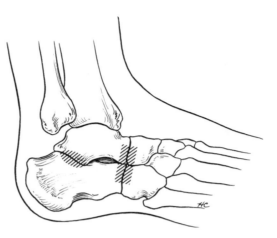

talonavicular and the calcaneocuboid joints. An area of subtalar joint cartilage is removed with a gouge and packed with the bone obtained from the trough (Fig. 6–60). Plaster immobilization lasts for 3 months.

If there is an equinus deformity, a Hoke Achilles tendon lengthening is performed so that the foot can be dorsiflexed to a neutral position and manipulated into the correct position after the arthrodesis.

The arthrodesis is performed through an oblique incision that begins at the talar head and stops at the peroneal tendons. It bisects the sinus tarsi, which is denuded of its fat. Care should be taken to preserve a thick layer of subcutaneous tissue so that the skin can be closed without tension after the correction.

With a half-inch osteotome, an osteoperiosteal flap that contains the extensor digitorum brevis muscle is raised across the calcaneocuboid joint. A right angle retractor under this flap exposes the calcaneocuboid joint, which is denuded of its cartilage.

The capsule of the talonavicular joint is opened, and a large Cobb elevator or sharp spoon is inserted into the joint and swept around the talar head to reflect the capsule. With the Cobb elevator in place medially against the talar head, the articular cartilage of the talar head is removed, preserving its spherical shape. The articular cartilage of the navicular bone is then removed with a large curette.

Then the articular surfaces of the subtalar joint are removed with an osteotome and a curette. A curved narrow elevator or similar instrument held on the medial side of the joint protects the neurovascular bundle.

Although usually not necessary to any great extent, appropriate medially based wedges of bone may be removed to correct the valgus.

The foot is manipulated into the correct position and held in varus and plantar flexion to bring the talus into alignment with the calcaneus. An osteotome of appropriate width is placed in the sinus tarsi parallel with the tibia to support the neck of the talus. From the width of the osteotome, it is easy to determine the size of the bone graft removed from the proximal anterior tibial shaft. The graft is tapped into place in the sinus tarsi.

With the foot corrected and dorsiflexed to the neutral postion, two Steinmann pins are used for fixation: one is driven through the plantar aspect of the heel into the talus, and the other is introduced on the distal and dorsal aspect of the foot and driven proximally across the talonavicular joint.

Closed suction drainage of the wound is used for 24 to 48 hours. A bulky postoperative dressing applied as a sandwich of dorsal and plantar ABD pads secured with several layers of rolled cast padding ensures against constriction by the plaster. The plaster should extend from the toes to the midthigh with the knee flexed 30 degrees.

Postoperative care. At the end of 4 weeks, the pins and plaster are removed, and a short leg plaster is applied. In 8 weeks, weight-bearing in plaster is begun and is continued for 4 more weeks.

After plaster removal, edema is controlled with elastic bandages or stockings. Regular shoes can be worn.

Because union will not be evident radiographically until 6 months to 1 year postoperatively, both patient and surgeon can be relieved of anxiety if solid union is not seen at 12 weeks when the final plaster is removed.

TIBIAL-FIBULAR TORSION, INTERNAL OR EXTERNAL

Excessive external tibial-fibular torsion is commonly associated with excessive femoral torsion. It appears to be compensatory. It also may be due to the overpowering external rotation force of the biceps femoris after the medial hamstrings have been lengthened, although I have seen no documentation of this mechanism.

Internal tibial-fibular torsion is probably congenital and is occasionally seen in patients with spastic diplegia. Spontaneous correction after the age of 6 years is most unlikely.

Derotation Osteotomy.   The problem can be corrected by derotation osteotomy of the proximal tibia and fibula. I prefer a transverse osteotomy of the proximal tibia just below the tibial tubercle and a fibular osteotomy 1 to 2 cm distal to the tibial site. To control the proximal tibial fragment so that the cast can be wedged to correct malalignment postoperatively, a Steinmann pin is inserted medially to engage both cortices of the tibia (Fig. 6–33). It is unnecessary to penetrate the lateral muscular compartment or the skin.

With the hip in neutral position and the knee extended, the correct degree of rotation can be determined by employing 10 degrees of external axial rotation of the foot.

COMPLICATIONS.   Like so many apparently simple and direct operations, proximal tibial osteotomy is fraught with complications, such as the following:

1. Anterior Compartment Syndrome.   After 20 years without this complication, we had three cases in one year. In children, this is a difficult phenomenon to recognize in the first two or three postoperative days. The only important symptom is unusual pain, which is difficult to assess in children. In our patients it was only after the osteotomy had healed and the plaster had been removed that weakness of the extensor hallucis longus muscle was noted. In two patients, this weakness disappeared in 90 and 120 days. In the third patient, 4 years have passed with no recovery of great toe extension.

To prevent this complication, we now routinely perform a fasciotomy of the anterior compartment throught the same incision used for the tibial osteotomy. Only a single linear cut with a blunt scissors proximally and distally for 5 to 7 cm in the fascia is necessary.

It is possible that insertion of the Steinmann pin from the lateral side could impale a branch of the nerve to the extensor hallucis longus. For this reason, all pins are inserted medially and do not cross the anterior lateral muscular compartment.

2. *Severance of the Posterior Tibial Artery.* This large vessel lies directly posterior to the proximal tibial osteotomy. Without protection from the osteotome or saw, it could be easily cut (I have seen this happen only once). Prevention is accomplished by total subperiosteal exposure of the tibia at the osteotomy site and envelopment of the posterior aspect of the tibia with ribbon or spade retractors (Chandler or similar type).

REFERENCES

Anthonsen, W. (1966) Treatment of hip flexion contracture in cerebral palsy patients. *Acta Orthopaedia Scandinavica* 37(4):387–393.

Arkin, A. M., and Katz, J. F. (1956) The effects of pressure on epiphyseal growth. *Journal of Bone and Joint Surgery* 38A:1056–1076.

Baker, L. D. (1956) A rational approach to the surgical needs of the cerebral palsy patient. *Journal of Bone and Joint Surgery* 38A:313–323.

Baker, L. D., and Dodelin, R. A. (1958) Extra-articular arthrodesis of the subtalar joint (Grice procedure). *Journal of the American Medical Association* 168:1005–1008.

Baker, L. D., and Hill, L. M. (1964) Foot alignment in the cerebral palsy patient. *Journal of Bone and Joint Surgery* 46A:1–15.

Banks, H. H., and Green, W. T. (1960). Adductor myotomy and obturator neurectomy for correction of the hip in cerebral palsy. *Journal of Bone and Joint Surgery* 42A:111–126.

Banks, H. H. (1972) The knee and cerebral palsy. *Orthopaedic Clinics of North America* 3(1):113–129.

Banks, H. H. (1975) The foot and ankle in cerebral palsy. *Orthopaedic Aspects of Cerebral Palsy* (Ed. Samilson, R. L.), Philadelphia, J. B. Lippincott Co.

Banks, H. H. (1972) Management of spastic deformities of the foot and ankle. *Clinical Orthopaedics and Related Research* 122:70–76.

Basmajian, J. V. (1972) *Muscles Alive,* Baltimore, The Williams & Wilkins Co.

Baumann, J. V. (1970) *Operative Behandlung der infantilen Zerebralparesen,* Stuttgart, Georg Thieme.

Baumann, J. V. (1972) Hip operations in children with cerebral palsy. *Reconstructive Surgery and Traumatology* 13:68–82.

Beals, R. K. (1969) Developmental changes in the femur and acetabulum in spastic paraplegia and diplegia. *Developmental Medicine and Child Neurology* 11:303–313.

Bleck, E. E., and Holstein, A. (1963) Iliopsoas tenotomy for spastic hip flexion deformities in cerebral palsy. Paper presented at the annual meeting of the American Academy of Orthopaedic Surgeons, Chicago.

Bleck, E. E. (1966) Management of hip deformities in cerebral palsy. *Current Practice in Orthopaedic Surgery* (Ed. Adams, J. P.), St. Louis, C. V. Mosby Co.

Bleck, E. E. (1971a) The shoeing of children: sham or science? *Developmental Medicine and Child Neurology* 13:188–195, 1971.

Bleck, E. E. (1971b) Surgical management of spastic flexion deformities of the hip with special reference to iliopsoas recession. *Journal of Bone and Joint Surgery* 53A:1468–1488.

Bleck, E. E. (1971c) The hip in cerebral palsy. *Instructional Course Lectures,* American Academy of Orthopaedic Surgeons, St. Louis, C. V. Mosby Co.

Bleck, E. E., Ford, F., Stevik, A. C., and Csongradi, J. (1975a) Electromyography telemetry study of spastic gait patterns in cerebral palsied children. *Developmental Medicine and Child Neurology* 17:307.

Bleck, E. E. (1975b) Spinal and pelvic deformities in cerebral palsy. *Orthopaedic Aspects of Cerebral Palsy* (Ed. Samilson, R. L.), Philadelphia, J. B. Lippincott Co.

Bleck, E. E. (1976) Persistent fetal medial deviation of the neck of the talus: a common cause of in-toeing in children. Paper presented at the annual meeting of the American Academy of Orthopaedic Surgeons, New Orleans.

Bleck, E. E., and Berzins, U. J. (1977) Conservative management of pes valgus with plantar flexed talus flexible. *Clinical Orthopaedics and Related Research* 122:85–94.

Bost, F. W., and Bleck, E. E. (1975) Rotation osteotomies for spastic paralytic internal rotation deformities of the femur. Paper presented at the annual meeting of the American Academy for Cerebral Palsy, Denver.

Brown, A. (1968) A simple method of fusion of the subtalar joint in children. *Journal of Bone and Joint Surgery* 50B:369–371.

Brunnstrom, S. (1962) *Clinical Kinesiology,* Philadelphia, F. A. Davis Co.

Cahuzac, M. (1977) *L'Enfant Infirme Moteur d'Origine Cérébrale,* Paris, Masson.

Carey, J. (1978) Personal communication.

Chandler, F. A. (1933) Re-establishment of normal leverage of patella in knee flexion deformity in spastic paralysis. *Surgery, Gynecology and Obstetrics* 57:523–527.

Close, J. R. (1964) *Motor Function in the Lower Extremity,* Springfield, Illinois, Charles C Thomas.

Coon, V., Donato, G., Houser, C., and Bleck, E. E. (1975) Normal ranges of hip motion in infants six weeks, three months and six months of age. *Clinical Orthopaedics and Related Research* 110:256–260.

Couch, W. H., DeRosa, G. P., and Throop, F. B. (1977) Thigh adductor transfer for spastic cerebral palsy. *Developmental Medicine and Child Neurology* 19:343–349.

Crane, A. (1959) Femoral torsion and its relation to toeing-in and toeing-out. *Journal of Bone and Joint Surgery* 41A:421–428.

Dennyson, W. G., and Fulford, R. (1976) Subtalar arthrodesis by cancellous grafts and metallic fixation. *Journal of Bone and Joint Surgery* 58B:507–510.

Diamond, L. (1978) Personal communication.

Drummond, D. S., Rogala, E., Templeton, J., and Cruess, R. (1974) Proximal hamstring release for knee flexion and crouched posture in cerebral palsy. *Journal of Bone and Joint Surgery* 56A:1598–1602.

Duchenne, G. B. (1959) *Physiology of Motion* (Transl. Kaplan, E. B.), Philadelphia, W. B. Saunders Co.

Duckworth, T. (1977) The surgical management of cerebral palsy. *Prosthetics and Orthotics International* 1:96–104.

Duncan, W. R. (1955) Release of rectus femoris in spastic children. *Journal of Bone and Joint Surgery* 37A:634.

Dunn, H. K. (1974) A clinical rationale for surgery to improve crouch gait in spastic cerebral palsy. *Instructional Course Syllabus,* 28th annual meeting of the American Academy for Cerebral Palsy.

Edmunson, A. S. (1963) *Campbell's Operative Orthopaedics,* St. Louis, C. V. Mosby Co.

Eggers, G. W. N. (1952) Transplantation of hamstring tendons to femoral condyles in order to improve hip extension and to decrease knee flexion in cerebral spastic paralysis. *Journal of Bone and Joint Surgery* 34A:827–830.

Evans, E. B. (1975) The knee in cerebral palsy. *Orthopaedic Aspects of Cerebral Palsy* (Ed. Samilson, R. L.), Philadelphia, J. B. Lippincott Co.

Evans, E. B. (1977) Personal communication.

Fabry, G., MacEwen, G. P., and Shands, A. R. (1973) Torsion of the femur. *Journal of Bone and Joint Surgery* 55A:1726–1738.

Feldkamp, M., and Katthagen, E. W. (1975) Results of surgical correction of flexion contractures of the knee joint in cerebral palsy children. *Zeitschrift für Orthopaedie and ihre Grenzgebiete* (Stuttgart) 113(2):181–188.

Foster, R. S., and Munger, D. H. (1977) Evaluation of crouch gait due to spastic cerebral palsy. Paper submitted for scientific program of the American Academy for Cerebral Palsy and Developmental Medicine.

Frost, H. M. (1971) Cerebral palsy, the spastic crouch. *Clinical Orthopaedics and Related Research* 80:2–8.

Garrett, A. L. (1976) Discussion of papers by Couch et al. and Griffin et al. on adductor transfer at the annual meeting of the American Academy for Cerebral Palsy, Los Angeles.

Garrett, A. L., Lister, M., and Drenan, J. (1966) New concept in bracing for cerebral palsy. *Journal of American Physical Therapy Association* 46:728.

Grant, J. C. B. (1952) *A Method of Anatomy,* 5th Ed., Baltimore, The Williams & Wilkins Co.

Green, W. T., and McDermott, L. J. (1942) Operative treatment of cerebral palsy of the spastic type. *Journal of the American Medical Association* 118:434–440.

Grice, D. S. (1952) Extra-articular arthrodesis of the subtalar joint for correction of paralytic flat feet in children. *Journal of Bone and Joint Surgery* 34A:927–940.

Griffin, P. P., Wheelhouse, W. W., and Shievi, R. (1977) The adductor transfer for adductor spasticity: a clinical and electromyographical gait analysis. *Orthopaedic Transactions* 1:76.

Haas, S. S., Epps, C. H., and Adams, J. P. (1973) Normal ranges of hip motion in newborn. *Clinical Orthopaedics and Related Research* 91:114–118.

Hagy, J. L., Mann, R. A., and Keller, C. (1973) Normal gait electromyograms and lower limb ranges of motion. Shriner's Hospital for Crippled Children, San Francisco.

Hayashi, Y. (1970) The surgery of hamstring tendons for knee flexion contracture in cerebral palsy. *Journal of the Kumamoto Medical Society* 44:144–149.

Hein, W. (1969) Surgical therapy of the knee contracture in cerebral pareses. *Zeitschrift für Orthopaedie and ihre Grenzgebiete* (Stuttgart) 106:755–759.

Hoffer, M. M. (1969) Personal communication.

Hoffer, M. M. (1972) Personal communication. *Annual Review of Cerebral Palsy Surgery,* Rancho Los Amigos Hospital, Downey, California.

Hoffer, M. M. (1976) Basic considerations and classification of cerebral palsy. *Instructional Course Lectures,* American Academy of Orthopaedic Surgeons, St. Louis, C. V. Mosby Co.

Hoffer, M. M. (1977) Personal communication.

Hollinshead, W. H. (1951) *Functional Anatomy of the Limbs and Back,* Philadelphia, W. B. Saunders Co.

Horstmann, H. M., and Eilert, R. E. (1977) Triple arthrodesis in cerebral palsy. Paper presented at the annual meeting of the American Academy of Orthopaedic Surgeons, Las Vegas.

Hsu, L. C. S., O'Brien, J. D., Yau, A. C. M. C., and Hodgson, A. R. (1974). Valgus deformities of the ankle in children with fibular pseudoarthrosis. *Journal of Bone and Joint Surgery* 56A:503–510.

Inman, V. T. (1947) The functional aspects of the abductor muscles of the hip. *Journal of Bone and Joint Surgery* 29A:607–619.

Inman, V. T. (1976) *The Joints of the Ankle,* Baltimore, The Williams & Wilkins Co.

Kaye, J. J., and Freiberger, R. H. (1971) Fragmentation of the lower pole of the patella in spastic lower extremities. *Radiology* 101:97–100.

Keagy, R. D., Brumlik, J., and Bergin, J. J. (1966) Direct electromyography of the psoas major muscle in man. *Journal of Bone and Joint Surgery* 48A:1377–1382.

Keats, S. (1974) Warning: serious complications caused by the routine re-routing of the peroneus longus and brevis tendons in performing the Grice procedure in cerebral palsy (abstract). *Journal of Bone and Joint Surgery* 56A:1304.

Keats, S., and Kambin, P. (1962) An evaluation of surgery for the correction of knee-flexion contracture in children with cerebral spastic paralysis. *Journal of Bone and Joint Surgery* 44A:1146–1154.

Keats, S., and Kouten, J. (1968) Early surgical correction of the planovalgus foot in cerebral palsy. *Clinical Orthopaedics and Related Research* 61:223–233.

Kottke, F. J. (1966) The effects of limitation of activity upon the human body. *Journal of the American Medical Association* 196:825–830.

Krom, W. (1969) An evaluation of the posterior transfer of the adductor muscles of the hip in the ambulatory patient with cerebral palsy. Resident conference paper, Rancho los Amigos Hospital, Downey, California.

Lamb, D. W., and Pollock, G. A. (1962) Hip deformities in cerebral palsy and their treatment. *Developmental Medicine and Child Neurology* 4:488–497.

Lee, C. (1977*a*) Forces acting to derotate exaggerated femoral anteversion of the newborn hip. Unpublished thesis — fellowship from United Cerebral Palsy Research and Education Foundation, and Children's Hospital at Stanford, Palo Alto.

Lee, C. (1977*b*) The Grice subtalar extra-articular arthrodesis in cerebral palsy. Unpublished thesis — fellowship from United Cerebral Palsy Research and Education Foundation, and Children's Hospital at Stanford, Palo Alto.

Lewis, F. R., Samilson, R. L., and Lucas, D. B. (1964) Femoral torsion and coxa valga in cerebral palsy — a preliminary report. *Developmental Medicine and Child Neurology* 6:591–597.

Lisowski, F. P. (1967) Angular growth changes and comparisons in the primate talus. *Folia Primat* 7:81–97.

Lotman, D. B. (1976) Knee flexion deformity and patella alta in spastic cerebral palsy. *Developmental Medicine and Child Neurology* 18:315–319.

Magilligan, D. J. (1956) Calculations of the angle of anteversion by means of horizontal lateral roentgenography. *Journal of Bone and Joint Surgery* 38A:1231–1246.

MacEwen, G. D. (1972) Adjustable frame for the lower limb for femoral anteversion radiographs by the Ryder-Crane technique. Personal communication.

McCullough, N. (1972) Personal communication.

Majestro, T. C., and Frost, H. M. (1971) Cerebral palsy: spastic internal femoral torsion. *Clinical Orthopaedics and Related Research* 79:44–56.

Majestro, T. C., and Frost, H. M. (1971) Posterior transposition of the origins of the anatomical internal rotators of the hip. *Clinical Orthopaedics and Related Research* 79:57–58.

Mann, R., and Hagg, J. (1973) Normal electromyographic data. Shriner's Hospital for Crippled Children. San Francisco.

Merchant, A. C. (1965) Hip abductor force muscle. *Journal of Bone and Joint Surgery* 47A:462–475.

Michele, A. A. (1962) *Iliopsoas,* Springfield, Illinois, Charles C Thomas.

Moreland, J. R., and Westin, G. W. (1977) Further experience with Grice subtalar arthrodesis. *Orthopaedic Transactions* 1:109.

Morinaga, H. (1973) An electromyographic study on the function of the psoas major muscle. *Journal of Japanese Orthopaedic Association,* 47:47, (reprints in English).

Murray, M. P., and Sepic, S. B. (1968) Maximum isometric torque of hip abductor and adductor muscles. *Physical Therapy* 43:1327–1335.

Perry, J., and Lieb, F. J. (1967) A study of the quadriceps extension mechanism at the knee. *Final Project Report.* Rancho los Amigos Hospital, Downey, California.

Perry, J., Antonelli, D., and Ford, W. (1975) Analysis of knee joint forces during stance phase. *Journal of Bone and Joint Surgery* 57A:961–967.

Perry, J., Hoffer, M. M., Antonelli, D., Plut, J., Lewis, G., and Greenberg, R. (1976) Electromyography before and after surgery for hip deformity. *Journal of Bone and Joint Surgery* 58A:201–208.

Perry, J., and Hoffer, M. (1977) Electromyographic studies of the gluteus medius during gait of cerebral palsy and adult stroke patients. Personal communication.

Porter, R. E. (1970) Hamstring transfers in cerebral palsy. *New York State Journal of Medicine* 70:1866–1867.

Reimers, J. (1974) Contracture of the hamstrings in spastic cerebral palsy. A study of three methods of operative correction. *Journal of Bone and Joint Surgery* 56B:102–109.

Roberts, W. M., and Adams, J. P. (1953) The patellar-advancement operation in cerebral palsy. *Journal of Bone and Joint Surgery* 35A:958–966.

Roosth, H. P. (1971) Flexion deformity of the hip and knee in spastic cerebral palsy: treatment by early release of spastic hip-flexor muscles. *Journal of Bone and Joint Surgery* 53A:1489–1510.

Rosenthal, R. K. (1975) A fixed-ankle below-the-knee orthosis for the management of genu recurvatum in spastic cerebral palsy. *Journal of Bone and Joint Surgery* 57A:545–549.

Rosenthal, R. K., and Levine, D. B. (1977) Fragmentation of the distal pole of the patella in spastic cerebral palsy. *Journal of Bone and Joint Surgery* 59A:934–939.

Ross, P. M., Lyne, E. D., and Eilert, R. E. (1977) The long term evaluation of the Grice procedure. *Orthopaedic Transactions* 1:10.

Ryder, C. T. (1972) Computerized calculations for femoral anteversion with the Ryder-Crane technique. Personal communication.

Ryder, C. T., and Crane, L. (1953) Measuring femoral anteversion: the problem and a method. *Journal of Bone and Joint Surgery* 35A:321–328.

Sage, F. (1977) Personal communication.

Salter, R. B. (1961) Innominate osteotomy in the treatment of congenital dislocation and subluxation of the hip. *Journal of Bone and Joint Surgery* 43B:518–539.

Samilson, R. L., Carson, J., James, P., and Raney, F. (1967) Results and complications of adductor tenotomy and obturator neurectomy in cerebral palsy. *Clinical Orthopaedics and Related Research* 54:61–73.

Samilson, R. L. (1972) Personal communication.

Saunders, J. B., Dec, M., Inman, V. T., and Eberhart, H. D. (1953) The major determinants in normal and pathological gait. *Journal of Bone and Joint Surgery* 35A:543–586.

Scrutton, D. R. (1969) Foot sequences of normal children under five years old. *Developmental Medicine and Child Neurology* 11:44–53.

Seymour, N., and Evans, D. K. (1968) A modification of the Grice subtalar arthrodesis. *Journal of Bone and Joint Surgery* 50B:372–375.

Seymour, N., and Sharrard, W. J. W. (1968) Bilateral proximal release of the hamstrings in cerebral palsy. *Journal of Bone and Joint Surgery* 58B:274–277.

Shands, A. R., and Stelle, M. K. (1958) Torsion of the femur. *Journal of Bone and Joint Surgery* 40A:803–816.

Sharrard, W. J. W. (1975) The hip in cerebral palsy. *Orthopaedic Aspects of Cerebral Palsy* (Ed. Samilson, R. L.), Philadelphia, J. B. Lippincott Co.

Silver, C. M., Simon, S. D., and Lichtman, H. M. (1966) The use and abuse of the obturator neurectomy. *Developmental Medicine and Child Neurology* 8:203–205.

Silver, C. M., Simon, S. D., Spindell, E., Eichtman, H. M., and Scala, M. (1967) Calcaneal osteotomy for valgus and varus deformities of the foot in cerebral palsy. *Journal of Bone and Joint Surgery* 49A:232–246.

Silver, C. M., Simon, S. D., and Lichtman, H. M. (1974) Long term followup observations on calcaneal osteotomy. *Clinical Orthopaedics and Related Research* 99:181–187.

Silver, C. M., (1977) Calcaneal osteotomy results of 100 operations and 64 feet followed longer than 5 years. *Instructional Course Lectures,* American Academy of Orthopaedic Surgeons, St. Louis, C.V. Mosby Co.

Simon, S. R., Deutsch, S. D., and Rosenthal, R. K. (1977) Genu recurvatum in spastic cerebral palsy: preliminary report. *Orthopaedic Transactions* 1:75.

Steel, H. (1977a) Triple osteotomy of the innominate bone. A procedure to accomplish coverage of the dislocated or subluxated femoral head in the older patient. *Clinical Orthopedics and Related Research* 122:116–127.

Steel, H. (1977b) Gluteus medius and minimus advancement for correction of internal rotation gait in spastic cerebral palsy. Paper presented at the annual meeting of the American Orthopaedic Association, Boca Raton.

Stephenson, C. T., and Donavan, M. M. (1971) Transfer of hip adductor origins to the ischium in spastic cerebral palsy. *Developmental Medicine and Child Neurology* 13:247.

Strange, F. G. St. Clair (1965) *The Hip,* Baltimore, The Williams & Wilkins Co.

Sutherland, D. H., Schottstaedt, E. R., and Larsen, L. I. (1969) Clinical and electromyographic study of seven spastic children with internal rotation gait. *Journal of Bone and Joint Surgery* 51A:1070–1082.

Sutherland, D. H., Larsen, L. I., and Mann, R. (1975) Rectus femoris release in selected patients with cerebral palsy: a preliminary report. *Developmental Medicine and Child Neurology* 17:26–34.

Sutherland, D. H., Miller, K. E., Cooper, L., and Matthews, J. V. (1977) Surgical treatment of hip subluxation and dislocation in the older child with spastic cerebral palsy. Scientific exhibit at the annual meeting of the American Academy of Orthopaedic Surgeons, Las Vegas.

Tachdjian, M. O. (1972) *Pediatric Orthopaedics,* Philadelphia, W. B. Saunders Co.

Trouillas, J. (1978) *La Chirurgie des Membres Inferieurs chez l'Infirme Moteur Cérébrale Spastique.* Thesis for Faculty of Medicine, Montpellier.

Westin, G. W. (1973) Technique of hamstring lengthening. Personal communication.

Wilkinson, J. A. (1962) Femoral anteversion in the rabbit. *Journal of Bone and Joint Surgery* 44B:386–397.

Williams, I. (1977) The consequences of orthopaedic surgery to the adolescent cerebral palsied; medical, educational and parental attitudes. Paper presented at the Study Group on Integrating the Care of Multiply Handicapped Children, St. Mary's College, Durham, England. London, The Spastics Medical Education and Information Unit.

Williams, P. F., and Menelaus, M. B. (1977) Triple arthrodesis by inlay grafting — a method suitable for undeformed or valgus foot. *Journal of Bone and Joint Surgery* 59B:333–336.

Wiltse, L. L. (1972) Valgus deformity of the ankle. A sequel to acquired or congenital abnormalities of the fibula. *Journal of Bone and Joint Surgery* 54A:595–606.

Chapter Seven

TOTAL BODY
INVOLVEMENT

CHARACTERISTICS

Quadriplegia, trunk and head dysfunction, and sensory deficits are typical of individuals with total body involvement (Fig. 7–1). The most serious defect in many of them is an inability to communicate needs, thoughts, and feelings. The overall incidence of communication disorders in patients with cerebral palsy was estimated as 40 percent who could not write, 10 percent who were non-verbal, and 20 percent who were non-vocal (BEH Conference, 1976). (Non-verbal refers to an inability to think and talk; non-vocal indicates an ability to think but not talk.)

Deafness is common in those whose central nervous system malfunction is due to maternal rubella or erythroblastosis fetalis. Blindness due to retrolental fibroplasia associated with the respiratory distress syndrome of prematurity has fortunately decreased since the discovery of the ill effects of hyperoxygenation. Convulsive disorders, like all static encephalopathies, add to the turmoil of existence.

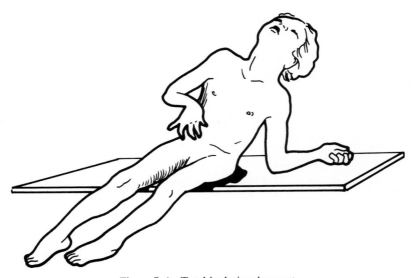

Figure 7–1 Total body involvement.

Mental retardation is not invariably present. Some non-verbal individuals were found to have normal intelligence after they were taught to communicate by non-verbal methods (McNaughton, 1975). Root (1977a) found that 55 percent of this group had I.Q.s of over 80; 36 percent of those with spastic paralysis and 68 percent of those with athetosis had normal intelligence.

Head and trunk control are usually deficient; standing equilibrium reactions are usually nil. Some patients have total extensor patterns, while others have total flexion. The upper limbs may be more involved in athetosis, and there are patients who have better foot and toe control than control of hands and fingers. Often one upper limb is not quite as involved as the other and can be controlled better. Some patients with total body involvement may be able to exercise control over only the eyes or head.

The most common orthopaedic problems in these patients are contractures and dislocations of the hip, scoliosis, knee flexion contractures, and equinus deformity. If the skeletal changes in the hip and spine persist without correction, degenerative changes occur in the joints, causing added pain and disability. As patients with athetosis age, they are particularly prone to pain in the spine and limb joints as the result of continuous contorted motion (Bleck, 1975). A particularly distressing structural change in athetosis is recurrent dislocation of the shoulder (Grove, 1972).

PROGNOSIS

Walking is usually not possible. It depends upon the presence of infantile automatisms, the absence of normal postural reflexes, and equilibrium reactions (see Chapters 2 and 3).

The level of mobility can be categorized as follows: (1) community walkers; (2) household walkers; (3) physiological walkers; (4) non-walkers in wheelchairs who can transfer themselves, need assistance, or are entirely dependent (see Chapter 4). Root (1977a) reported that 78 percent of the cerebral palsy population with total body involvement were confined to a wheelchair.

ASSESSMENT AND GOAL SETTING

Assessment of these patients entails all the methods discussed in Chapter 2. In addition, language, hearing, visual, and intellectual assessments are essential. Because these individuals present an almost overwhelming number of problems, efforts toward rehabilitation are apt to be truncated and their maximum potential as persons may be neglected. An approach to the patient based upon his functional loss will be more effective.

Goal setting and problem solving for and with the individual patient should be done according to the priorities established by adults with cerebral palsy: (1) communication, (2) activities of daily living, (3) mobility, (4) walking (see Chapter 3).

PHYSICAL AND OCCUPATIONAL THERAPY

In the *infant,* physical and occupational therapy is directed toward assessment of the patient's motor ability, physical development, and ranges of joint motion, as well as education of the parent. The therapist should find the optimum position of the trunk and limbs for hand use, feeding, and control of mobility equipment. Adaptive equipment for feeding may be necessary.

For children of *school age,* the therapist should concentrate on teaching activities of daily living with the use of adaptive equipment, seating, and mobility devices. Non-verbal communication methods can be introduced and taught. As the child matures and develops, social games and recreational activities that are and will be important should be taught. Finally, in this brief general description of the thrust of the physical and occupational program, it is worth noting that I have not mentioned stretching, which is so frequently prescribed and is entirely useless.

ORTHOTICS AND REHABILITATION ENGINEERING

With the rapid advances of technology in plastics, electronics, and electric power storage systems, the formerly routine use of braces has given way to the broader concept of rehabilitation engineering. The routine application of bilateral metal upright braces with a pelvic band ("full control brace") has been discarded in favor of selective orthotic application to control a deformity; if orthoses are not able to control it, surgical treatment can be used. Restrictive bracing around the hip has not prevented dislocation (Chapter 4).

Orthotics will not correct a contracture or a fixed deformity. The principle of treatment is to correct the deformity first by surgery and then utilize the orthosis to prevent recurrence and provide stability. The following devices are the most commonly used orthoses in the total body involved patient:

Head Control Helmet or Sling

A constant flexed position of the head precludes visual contact and learning. A helmet with a chin strap can be suspended from an overhead spring attached to a chair or walker (Fig. 7–2).

A biofeedback head position trainer has shown more promise as a therapeutic device to keep the head erect than any other method. This device consists of sensors in the helmet that respond to unwanted head positions with an auditory signal (Motloch, 1975). Russell et al. (1976) gave a preliminary report on the results obtained with this biofeedback system in 12 patients; all responded during training with the device, and three maintained the erect head position. As visual positive biofeedback the helmet sensors have been linked via telemetry to a television screen; head flexion turns off the TV program while an upright head position turns it on.

Spinal Orthosis

I have used the Milwaukee brace to control a slump and listed posture in preschool children with cerebral palsy. The cervical portion of the orthosis was modified with a padded ring around the neck attached to the head piece. The use of this device is limited, and we prefer a plastic molded thoracolumbar spinal orthosis

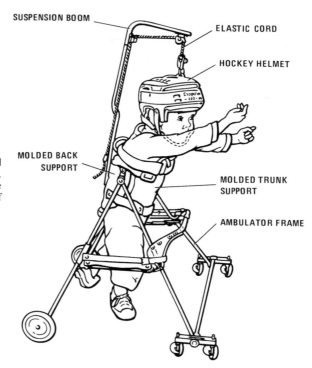

SUSPENSION BOOM

ELASTIC CORD

HOCKEY HELMET

MOLDED BACK
SUPPORT

MOLDED TRUNK
SUPPORT

AMBULATOR FRAME

Figure 7–2 Head control achieved by suspension of helmet with chin strap. The same system can be attached to the wheelchair. (For improved model of Stanford walker see Fig. 7–17.)

(TLSO) for control of scoliosis. If truncal dysequilibrium is the problem, custom molded seating has been much more successful in correcting it than the spinal orthosis.

Bunnell and MacEwen (1977) have had enough success with a plastic molded jacket (TLSO) in the early non-operative treatment of scoliosis in 48 patients with cerebral palsy to merit its use. The orthosis was worn 23 hours per day. In a 26-month follow-up, the spinal curves in 35 patients were held within 5 degrees of the original curve. Three patients' curves became worse and three did not improve. In this series 42 of 48 patients had quadriplegia, and 30 were mentally retarded. James (1977) also used the plastic spinal orthosis in 80 children with the intent of preventing scoliosis in the "collapsing spine." After a 5-year follow-up, none had developed a fixed spinal deformity; however, none had spastic paralysis.

We have also used the spinal jacket. As emphasized by Bunnell and MacEwen, the orthosis must be made from a positive plaster mold of the trunk with the spine in the corrected position. To accomplish this, the negative plaster body jacket is applied with the patient lying on a table (e.g., a Risser table) specifically designed for this purpose. Head and pelvic traction can be applied. The plaster is carefully molded so that it will apply pressure over the apices of the curves. Like James (1977) we used polypropylene lined with Plastazote for the final orthosis (Bunnell and MacEwen used Orthoplast).

Ankle-Foot Orthosis

The plastic ankle-foot orthosis (AFO) described in Chapters 3, 4, and 5 is used to control equinus deformity. If the patient is non-ambulatory or bears weight only for wheelchair transfers, this kind of orthosis after Achilles' tendon lengthening may prevent recurrence of the deformity.

Knee-Ankle-Foot Orthosis

The plastic knee-ankle-foot orthosis (KAFO) has been used after hamstring lengthening in patients who have the capability for assistive or independent wheelchair transfer.

We do not use orthotics to control hip position in non-ambulatory patients. Molded seat inserts offer better control and positioning of the thighs and hip joints.

Communication Devices

The use of devices to compensate for loss of speech is based on the theory of the existence of "inner language" in the brain. Experience with non-verbal individuals has demonstrated that this concept is correct.

The various compensatory devices can be subdivided into those used for writing, signals, and symbols and synthetic voice devices. The technology in this field is constantly changing and evolving. The devices described are examples in current use.

Writing Devices.   The simplest writing device is the electric typewriter. It can be modified with roll paper and a keyboard guard. Electric typewriters can be electronically linked for remote operation by a head stick or by switches for toe operation.

Strip printing devices such as the Porta-Printer have been made commercially. Each has its function in fulfilling the needs of the individual (Fig. 7–3).

Signals.   Hagen et al. (1973) designed and used successfully a simple yes-no auditory signal (a buzzer) for communication of the needs of non-verbal persons in an institution. The list of common needs included wants, feelings, people, and places. Example of wants were: "change position," "TV," "talk to me." Feelings included: "I am sad," "I am tired," "Why are you doing this?". Among the people represented were: "nurse," "doctor," and "family." Places categorized included: "playroom," "canteen," and "outside."

This system is a good beginning, but it does not yet have the range of human expression required by most of these people.

Symbols.   For those who have normal finger and hand dexterity, the American Sign Language is the best method. However, total body involved people do not usually have the excellent hand function required for successful communication. Also, the use of sign language demands that the receiver of the message understand signing. For preschool children, boards that depict common recognizable objects are a good way to begin communication. The objects can be identified with electrically controlled pointers and a variety of pressure-sensitive switches that do not require individual finger control (Figs. 7–4 and 7–5). Communication boards are commercially available and can be adapted to individual needs by the services of an electronic technician.

The *Bliss symbol language* devised by Bliss (1965) and introduced by the

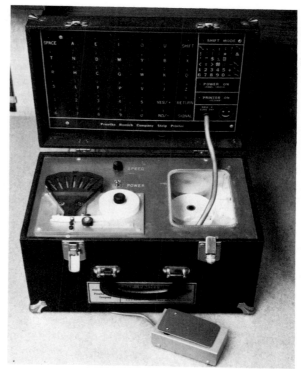
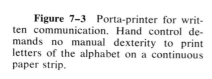

Figure 7-3 Porta-printer for written communication. Hand control demands no manual dexterity to print letters of the alphabet on a continuous paper strip.

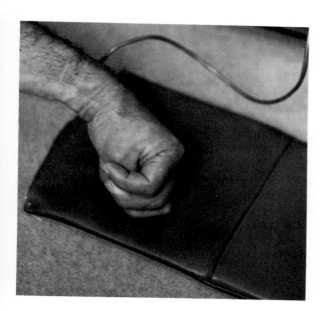

Figure 7-4 Pressure-sensitive switch that demands only gross motor control.

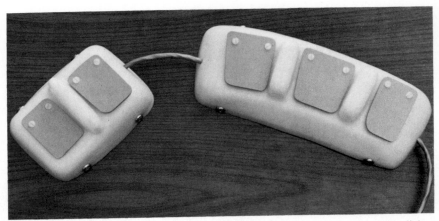

Figure 7–5 Switches for control of communication and other devices need only the slightest pressure to operate.

Ontario Crippled Children's Center has had extensive use, trial, and study (McNaughton, 1975). The symbols are ideograms that can be combined to make new words and thoughts (Fig. 7–6). Children have had no difficulty in learning 440 symbols and and in the process have learned English in Roman letters as well. They have learned rapidly to communicate with each other, their teacher, and their parents. Electronically controlled Bliss symbol communication boards have been manufactured (Figs. 7–7 and 7–8).

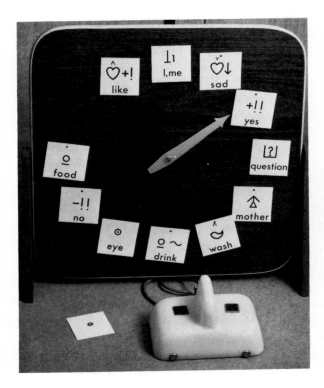

Figure 7–6 Bliss symbols for non-verbal communication. This is a simple device to teach symbol language. Only gross motor ability is required to direct the arrow via pressure-sensitive switches.

a	b	c	d	e	f	g	h	i	j
0	1	2	3	4	5	6	7	8	9
hello good-bye	question	I, me (my)	like	happy	make action	food	pen, pencil	friend	animal
please	why	you (your)	want	angry	mouth	drink	paper, page	GOD	bird
thanks	how	man	come	afraid	eye	sleep	book	house	flower
I'm sorry	who	woman	give	funny	legs	toilet	table	school	water
opposite	what thing	father	make	good	hand	pain	television	hospital	sun
much, many	which	mother	help	big	ear	clothing	news	store	weather
music	where	brother	think	young, new	nose	outing	word	show	day
	when	sister	know	difficult	head	car	light	room	week-end
	how many	teacher	wash	hot	name	wheelchair	game, toy	street	birthday

Figure 7-7   Bliss symbols.

Synthetic Voice (speech prosthesis).   Synthetic voice devices have a programmed vocabulary that can be activated by the non-verbal person so that oral communication results (Fig. 7-9). Intensive research and development need to be done before these devices are practical for use by the total body involved person with

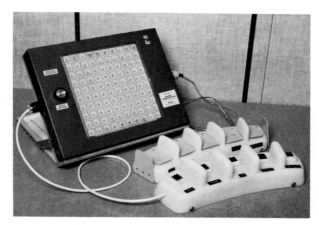

Figure 7-8 Matrix communicator for Bliss symbol language and two types of slot control switches.

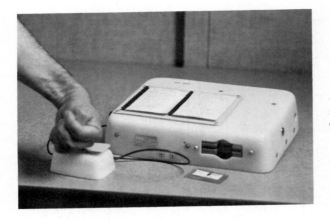

Figure 7–9 Synthetic voice device with interchangeable tape cassettes. Operated by gross upper limb control.

cerebral palsy. Commercially available speech prostheses include Speech Plus Talking Calculator, Master Specialties Talking Calculator, Master Specialties Voice Read-Out System, Handivoice, PhonicMirror/Handivoice, Computalker, and Votrax (LeBlanc, 1977). Addresses of the manufacturers of these devices are listed in Appendix B.

Activities of Daily Living

Eating. For those with moderately limited hand function, a wide variety of adaptive eating tools are available in every occupational therapy department so that testing can be done. If hand function is severely limited with no grasp at all, the Ontario Crippled Children's Centre Feeder is the best device available (Fig. 7–10). For success with this device, however, head control is essential.

Reading. Automatic electric page turners appear to be practical and are available. Projection of printed pages on a screen has also been used in special education endeavors.

Dressing. Dressing skills may be enhanced with adaptive clothing (e.g., Velcro

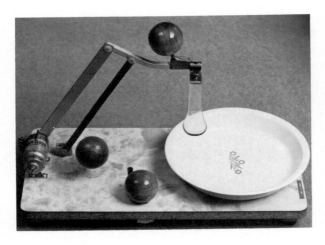

Figure 7–10 Ontario crippled children's feeder. The plate rotates, and the spoon scoops up the food, which is lifted by hydraulic mechanism. To operate, the patient needs only gross motor control to push knobs with his fisted hand. (Available from Orthopop.)

fasteners). The choice of specialized clothing must be made by the handicapped person himself. Much depends upon the level of his abilities. Complicated adaptive clothing usually is not acceptable.

Toilet and Bath. In the bath, handrails can be attached to the wall and tub. Bath seats in shower and tub are practical. A plastic water-inflatable bath seat for ease in assistive transfers is commercially available. Handrails on either side of the toilet and elevated toilet seats facilitate transfers. Commode-type toilets are particularly useful at the bedside for nighttime use. A bidet type toilet with an air dryer is available for those unable to cleanse the anus and perineum manually.

Transfers. Transers to bed, chairs, and toilet can apparently be taught with the use of a plinth (slotted wood table top) and repetition (Cotton, 1977). For those who need more assistance, adjustable poles with grab bars or rings can be wedged securely between floor and ceiling (provided the ceiling is not false).

Environmental Controls. Electronic systems that can be operated by a simple puff of breath have been manufactured. These systems will operate the telephone, radio, and other appliances for living (Fig. 7–11).

Architectural Barriers. Through the efforts of organizations of the handicapped themselves, architectural barriers in public facilities are gradually and slowly (perhaps too slowly) being eliminated. Studies of the deficiencies in public facilities and transportation have been done; the best are those that categorize handicapped persons not by disease but by functional loss (Bourgeois et al., 1977).

In the home, some barriers can be simply remedied. Doors can be made wide enough for wheelchairs, shower stall curbs can be removed, ramps can replace stairways, and light switches can be brought down low enough to manipulate when seated. If the outside entrance to the home is blocked by too many (or too steep) stair steps, elevators can be installed to lift the wheelchair person to his door.

Mobility and Seating. A series of mobility devices that change with the age and development of the patient are recommended. *Trunk stability* is of major importance. With an unstable trunk, all upper limb function is subordinate to sitting support. Consequently, seating that stabilizes the trunk and eliminates the common startle reactions is an integral part of any mobility system (Motloch, 1977).

INFANCY. A normal infant develops sitting balance (at age 4 to 8 months), which increases his visual field and experience. To compensate for delayed sitting

Figure 7–11 Environmental control system operated with puffs of breath. Telephone, stereo set, and radio can be operated without manual dexterity.

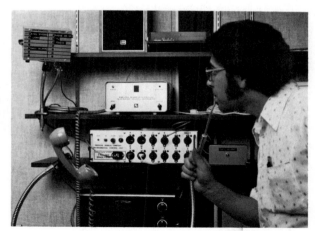

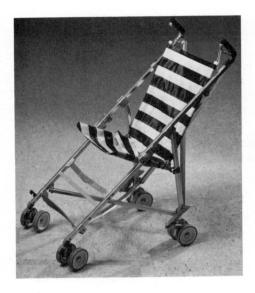

Figure 7–12 MacLaren buggy. Lightweight and collapsible. Ideal for transportation.

and lack of early visual experience, the handicapped child needs supportive seating. We have modified the infant automobile seat by lining it with plastic foam carved to fit the trunk and thighs. This seat can be set in a stroller (MacLaren-Pogom Buggy) (Fig. 7–12).

PRESCHOOL YEARS.   As the child matures in the preschool years, trunk imbalance will thwart hand function. A custom seat insert to stabilize the trunk, head and neck, and thighs can be made to place the child in a posture of optimum relaxation. The therapist and orthotist test the child in various positions and then select the best position for the insert (Fig. 7–13).

Plastic foam in the basic plywood seat is carved by hand to fit the child. We use fabric upholstery protected with Scotchguard to cover the foam. Plastic upholstery materials have been unsatisfactory because they retain body heat. The addition of a

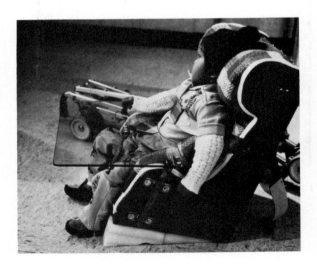

Figure 7–13 Cerebral palsy seat. Child's posture captured in the most relaxed position. Plastic lap tray aids hand function.

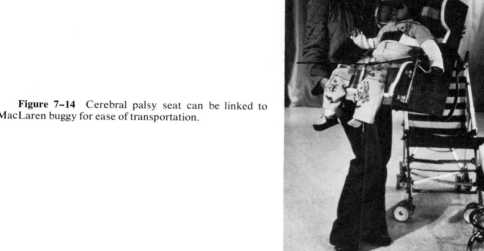

Figure 7–14 Cerebral palsy seat can be linked to MacLaren buggy for ease of transportation.

clear plastic tray facilitates early hand function. The seat can be easily lifted into the portable buggy (Figs. 7–14 and 7–15).

If the child has reciprocal use of both upper limbs, *crawling,* which allows the normal child to explore his environment, can be compensated for by a padded board mounted on swivel casters on which the child lies prone. Some children have sufficient hand grasp and movement to use a cart, which is actually a miniature wheelchair (Fig. 7–16). We have motorized the caster cart for some children who have enough hand function and sense of direction to be able to operate a switch.

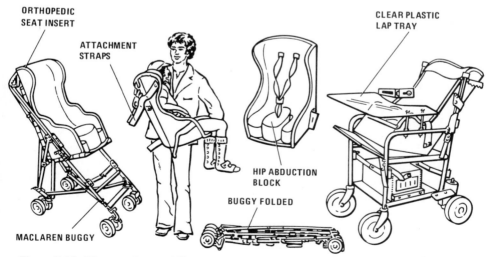

Figure 7–15 The complete mobility system and seating for the child with total body involvement from preschool to school age. (From Bleck, E. E. (1978) in Ahstrom, J. P. (Ed.). *Current Practice in Orthopaedic Surgery,* St. Louis, C. V. Mosby Company, with permission.)

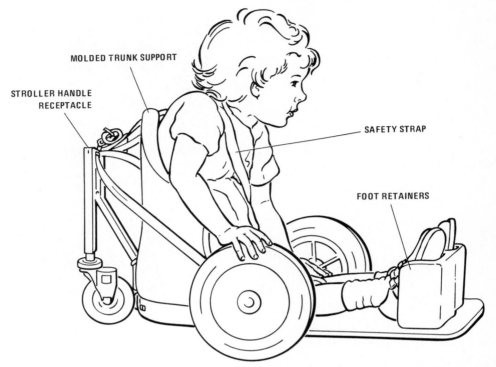

MOLDED TRUNK SUPPORT

STROLLER HANDLE
RECEPTACLE

SAFETY STRAP

FOOT RETAINERS

Figure 7–16 Caster cart, a miniature wheelchair for exploration of the environment in the preschool years. If upper limb function precludes manual operation, it can be motorized. Trunk support is built-in. (From Bleck, E. E. (1978) in Ahstrom, J. P. (Ed.). *Current Practice in Orthopaedic Surgery,* St. Louis, C. V. Mosby Company, with permission).

Because mobility is a prime developmental need, we give the total body involved child every opportunity to have this experience. Creative orthotists and therapists can devise seating and mobility aids for the individual child (Letts et al., 1976; Motloch, 1977).

Independent standing and *walking* are not usually feasible. In some children who do not have overwhelming extensor or flexor spasticity but lack mainly equilibrium reactions, the Stanford weight-relieving walker can provide mobility experience in the preschool years (Fig. 7–17). For some children, the standing A-frame can provide crutchless standing and is easier to use than the familiar standing tables or chimneys. If standing is at all possible it needs reinforcement and practice to prepare the child to undertake wheelchair transfers.

SCHOOL-AGE YEARS. In additon to seating, hand use, and communication, mobility for independence at home, in school, and for recreation is required. Up to the age of 10 to 12 years, the *steerable walker* allows participation in recreation with other children in the neighborhood. This is a highly stable, four-wheel walker with an anterior molded trunk support into which the child can lean. The steering mechanism is designed so that turns can be made merely by flexion or extension of the upper limbs (Fig. 7–18). A similar walker with a banana seat can be used for children who do not need trunk support.

Three-wheeled cycles for those who have adequate lower limb control can be

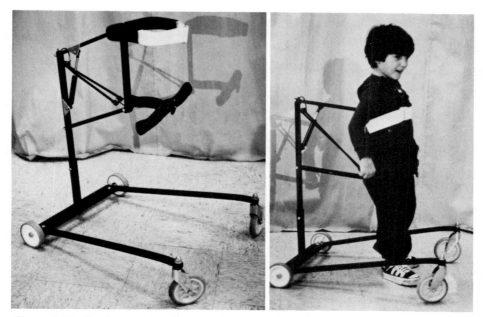

Figure 7–17 Stanford weight-relieving walker. If trunk and head balance are normal, the walker allows mobility without the need for hand pushing by reciprocal lower limb function. The walker follows the child.

tried. The Ontario Crippled Children's Centre designed a tricycle driven by pedals situated in the rear to accommodate those who have extensor patterns.

Wheelchairs. Basically, two types of wheelchair must be considered: hand-driven and power-driven. The hand-driven types are indicated in children who have sufficient function and power in both upper limbs to move the wheelchair with

Figure 7–18 Steerable walker for school age children's recreation and mobility. Lack of trunk balance is compensated for by anterior molded support. Steering mechanism requires only upper limb extension and flexion (not rotation). (Courtesy of Ontario Crippled Children's Centre.)

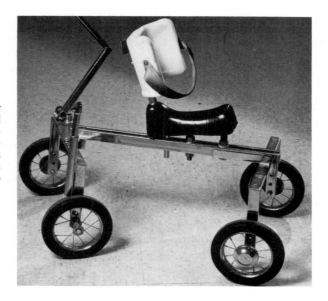

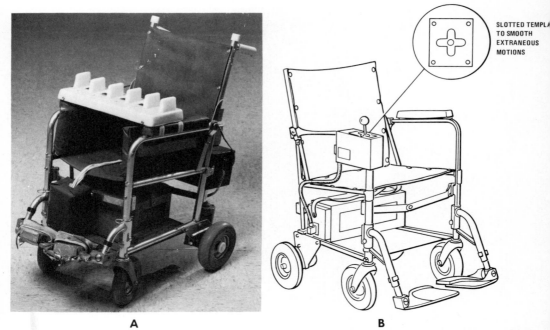

SLOTTED TEMPL/
TO SMOOTH
EXTRANEOUS
MOTIONS

A   **B**

Figure 7–19 A. Portable electric chair (available from ABEC Electric Wheelchair, Inc., 10889 Wilshire Blvd. Suite 2, Los Angeles). B. Control has been modified by a template to limit extraneous motions. Accelerator controls added to prevent sudden stops and starts (developed by Rehabilitation Engineering Center, Children's Hospital at Stanford). (From Bleck, E. E. (1978) in Ahstrom, J. P. (Ed.) *Current Practice in Orthopaedic Surgery,* St. Louis, C. V. Mosby Company, with permission.)

reasonable efficiency and speed. Voluntary alternating control of both upper limbs is required to steer the wheelchair. If the child has only one functional upper limb, I recommend a power-driven wheelchair, since the unilateral drive (so-called hemiplegic) chairs are heavy, cumbersome, and inefficient, and consume more energy than the child can afford to expend and still accomplish more important tasks, for example, learning. For young children, the ABEC-powered transportable chair* has proved to be reasonably durable and efficient. For older children and adults, the Everett-Jennings powered wheelchair is a standard item.

All powered wheelchairs must be recharged daily. A charger can be plugged into any 120-volt outlet, and usually one charger is kept at home with the patient and one is kept at the educational facility.

Powered wheelchairs can be controlled with a variety of switches that are adapted to the best functioning part of the child. Obviously, the hand joystick is the most commonly used control if the hands are functional. If the child has gross forward, backward, and side-to-side upper limb motion but does not have sufficient fine motor control, a template can be placed over the joystick so that it can be moved only in the four directions without wavering and turning the child in his chair in a complete circle (Fig. 7–19).

For patients who do not have sufficient dexterity to control the powered chair by a joystick, pressure-sensitive switches mounted in a lightweight plastic slotted control panel can be used successfully (Fig. 7–20).

---

*ABEC Electric Wheelchair, Inc., 10889 Wilshire Blvd., Suite 2, Los Angeles, CA 90024

Some children require a molded insert that can be placed in the wheelchair to stabilize the trunk and head and to break up the extensor pattern that tends to slide the child out of the wheelchair. Sliding causes pressure on the sacral area with resultant abrasions and decubiti. Clear plastic lap boards that can be attached to the wheelchair for desk work or for communication should be considered when prescribing the wheelchair (Figs. 7–13 and 7–15).

A *prescription for any type of wheelchair* should not be made by simply looking up a model in a catalog and purchasing it. The child should be carefully analyzed by an occupational or physical therapist and an orthotist or rehabilitation engineer, and his functional losses, the limbs or organs with the most normal function, the position in which they function best, and the best seating position should be identified. Measurements of his sitting height, thigh length, leg length, and foot and arm length are all included in the prescription. The need for a head rest, type of armrests (generally detachable upholstered desk arms are best), and foot support should be specified.

If a child needs a powered wheelchair for optimum mobility and independence, he should first be tested in several types of powered chairs by the occupational therapist and the rehabilitation engineer or orthotist. For this purpose, we keep on hand several different types of powered chairs and various control mechanisms.

Costs. In general, there has been a great deal of reluctance to prescribe and pay for powered chairs for children on the part of therapists, physicians, and third party fiscal intermediaries. However, once these professional people recognize and appreciate that the patient is a person and not a diagnosis to be manipulated, these attitudes will slowly change. The high cost of seating and wheelchair mobility is the usual reason given for non-approval, but if the therapist's time spent in futile attempts to make the total body involved child walk or to "de-program" the brain to

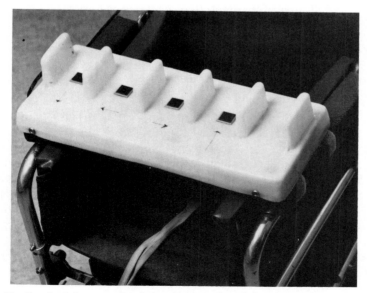

Figure 7–20 Stanford slot control switches for operation of electric wheelchair and communication devices with solenoid switches. Five slots are used: forward, backward, right, left, and rest positions. (Developed by Rehabilitation Engineering Center, Children's Hospital at Stanford.)

eliminate pathological reflexes was cost-accounted (as are all rehabilitation engineering devices), this prejudice toward powered wheelchairs would no doubt be somewhat modified. The cost of a parent who must attend the child day in and day out (including weekends and vacations when the medical team is off-duty) is also a factor that is missing in calculations. If a mobility system can free a mother or attendant of direct care for even half a day and the child can remain at home rather than in a state institution, a very large cost indeed can be calculated as a saving.

Travel and Transportation. Of all factors that limit adult independence and employment the most important is the inability to get out of the home (Bachman, 1972). Root (1977a) found that only 16 percent of total body involved patients had the capability or means for independent travel. Public transportation still presents too many barriers for the handicapped. In France, a study of the autobus and its barriers for public transportation of the handicapped concluded that these facilities were inadequate (Bourgeois et al., 1977). Airplane travel in commercial carriers in the United States, however, is a feasible means of transportation for the handicapped.

Probably independent travel by the wheelchair-dependent person is easiest in the autovans now being manufactured. Vans can be equipped with ramps or hydraulic elevators for ease of entry and exit. We are convinced of the practicality of autovan travel.

The ability to operate a motor vehicle is dependent upon eyesight, visual-motor coordination, perception reaction times, sense of direction, and hand use. Pushbutton controls are feasible. All of these factors should be accurately assessed before a person can be certified as safe to drive. Unfortunately, the issue of a certificate to learn how to drive is based upon the diagnosis of the disease and the physician's signature. To implement full integration of the handicapped in society and to give them this equal opportunity, detailed functional assessments should be performed instead of asking for a simple yes or no from the physician. Such assessment centers could be established under the direction of occupational therapy departments.

STRUCTURAL DEFORMITIES

Spine

Scoliosis occurs more often in patients with cerebral palsy than in the normal population (Robson, 1968; Balmer and MacEwen, 1970; Samilson and Bechard, 1973; Rosenthal et al., 1974). Total body involved patients have an incidence of structural scoliosis of between 25 and 38 percent.

Curve Patterns. In total body involved patients the thoracolumbar (T8–L4) curve pattern occurs most often (in 45 percent in Samilson's series). Thoracolumbar curves are particularly prone to progression (Fig. 7–21). Consequently, an early curve should be controlled if possible with the spinal orthoses discussed earlier in this chapter (Fig. 7–22).

Surgical Correction. Spinal curves of 42 to 50 degrees may not respond to an orthosis. If the curve is over 50 degrees, most experts feel surgical correction and spinal fusion are indicated.

Because scoliotic spines in cerebral palsy are often rigid, one-stage surgical correction can fail. Preoperative radiographs of the spine, with the patient lying

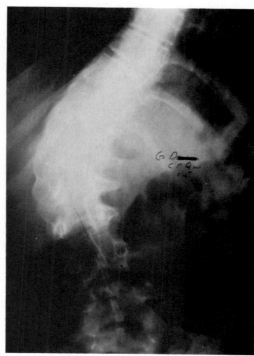

Figure 7–21 Anteroposterior sitting radiograph of the spine of a 15-year-old spastic quadriplegic, showing typical thoracolumbar scoliosis.

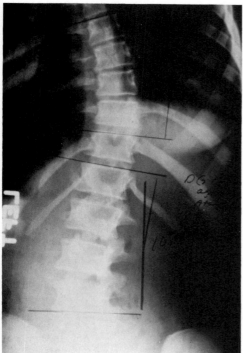

Figure 7–22 Anteroposterior radiograph of the spine in a patient with total body involvement and total lack of equilibrium reactions. This curvature is prone to progression and should be held in a corrective molded plastic orthosis.

prone and manual pressure applied over the curve apex, or bending films will determine curve flexibility.

Pelvic obliquity may be due to unbalanced adduction contractures of the hips and/or dislocation of the hip. Certainly, hip contracture and dislocation should be corrected first. Most often, however, pelvic obliquity is caused by the spinal curvature that in effect includes the pelvis as part of the vertebrae (Fig. 7–23). Surgical correction of this type of paralytic scoliosis has evolved from the Harrington procedure (MacEwen, 1968; Bleck, 1975) to the Dwyer procedure involving anterior spinal fusion (Bonnett, 1972) to a combination of both (Bonnett et al., 1976). The use of either procedure alone led to too many cases of lost correction and pseudoarthrosis.

If the curve is rigid, a four-stage procedure can be recommended:
chair (Stagnara, 1971). Femoral traction can be used but not with patients who
1.   Myotomy of the spastic and contracted spinal muscles and application of a halo.
2.   Halo traction, which seems to be best tolerated with the patient seated in his chair (Stagnara, 1971). Femoral traction can be used but not with patients who have subluxation of the hips. A pelvic halo is another method; however, a total body involved patient may be difficult to manage in this apparatus, and pelvic pin tract infection is a risk with the major procedure, Dwyer instrumentation and anterior fusion.
3.   After 7 to 10 days' traction, anterior correction with Dwyer instrumentation is performed.

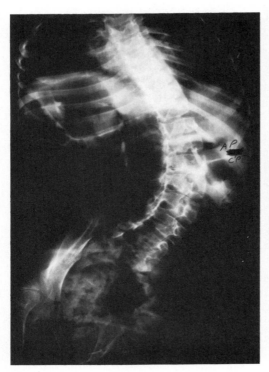

Figure 7–23 Anteroposterior radiograph of spine in a 14-year-old with total body involvement, tension athetosis, and subluxation of right hip. Milwaukee brace for four years gave unsuccessful results. Patient will require release of hip contractures and myotomy of paraspinal muscles, anterior Dwyer instrumentation and spinal fusion L5 to T9, and Harrington instrumentation and spinal fusion from sacrum to T4 or above.

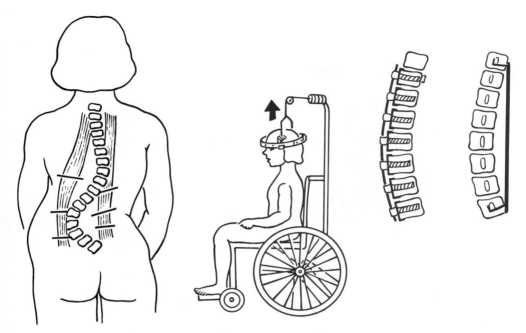

Figure 7–24 Scheme and stages of treatment for the usual rigid severe scoliosis in the patient with total body involvement. (Halo traction suspension in wheelchair [Stagnara, 1971].)

4. Three to 4 weeks after the anterior surgery, Harrington instrumentation and posterior spinal fusion are done (Fig. 7–24).

 If there is pelvic obliquity, the Harrington correction and fusion must include the sacrum. A long posterior fusion to the upper thoracic vertebra (T1, T2, or T3) is recommended if there is evidence of curvature above the seventh or eighth thoracic vertebra (the usual upper limit of Dwyer correction).

 Postoperative Care. The great advantage of both anterior and posterior spinal fusion is that early mobilization of the patient is possible. A molded plastic jacket for 9 months to 1 year postoperatively suffices. The patient can begin sitting in his chair after the spinal orthosis has been fitted.

Hip

CONTRACTURES

Adduction contractures interfere with perineal hygiene and sitting balance due to pelvic obliquity. Usually only adductor myotomy and anterior branch obturator neurectomy are necessary for treatment (for operative technique see Chapter 6).

 If the lower limbs are crossed over the other (see Fig. 5–4) and the patient has spastic paralysis, intrapelvic obturator neurectomy is indicated.

 Before adductor myotomy and obturator neurectomy are performed, the presence of tension athetosis, which is often mistaken for spasticity, should be ascer-

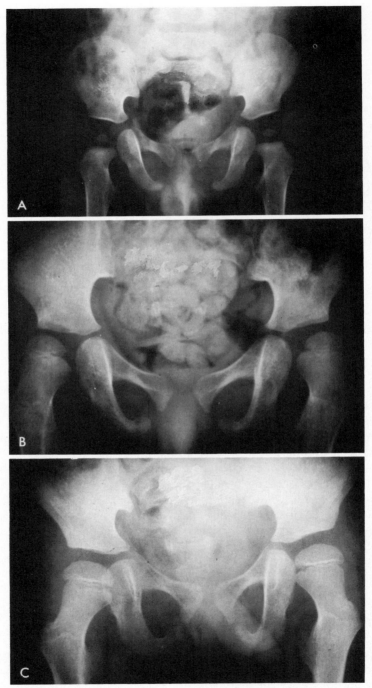

Figure 7–25 Anteroposterior radiographs of hips. A. Patient H.H.R., an 11-month-old spastic quadriplegic. Hips are in normal position. B. Now age 2 years, 9 months and non-ambulatory. Subluxation of both hips is present. Absence of acetabular dysplasia at this age distinguishes this acquired subluxation from the congenital type. C. Two years, ten months after iliopsoas tenotomy, adductor myotomy, and anterior branch obturator neurectomy. Hips are now perfectly located (courtesy of A. Holstein, M.D., Berkeley, California).

tained. Adductor weakening procedures in athetoid patients can result in excessive hip abduction postoperatively (Horning, 1977). Preoperative obturator nerve blocks with lidocaine or Marcaine are recommended in patients in whom athetosis is suspected.

Flexion contractures of the hip need not be relieved in non-ambulatory patients by reason of the contracture alone. If there is evidence of subluxation of the hip in the child, iliopsoas tenotomy is indicated. Cristofaro et al. (1977) reported conversion of flexed hip postures into extension postures in five of six non-ambulatory children an average of 3.2 years after iliopsoas "release" and stated that it should be avoided in non-ambulatory patients. I suspect that these patients, who had disabling extensor tone, also had tension athetosis rather than spastic paralysis.

DISLOCATION

Incidence.   Dislocation of the hip occurs almost exclusively in the total body involved patient who is non-ambulatory. Of 284 patients who had dislocated hips in Samilson's study (1972), 90 percent had quadriplegia. Only 11 percent had some limited ambulation. Baker et al. (1962) analyzed the incidence of subluxation and dislocation in 129 patients (258 hips), and found that 42 hips were subluxed and 31 were dislocated (28 percent). In 20 bed-ridden patients, Hoffer et al. (1972) reported dislocation of the hip in 15 (75 percent). With these percentages, we cannot deny the existence of a major and serious problem in the total body involved person.

Mechanism.   Dislocation of the hip is an acquired deformity that can be amply demonstrated by serial radiographic examinations from infancy to childhood. The hips at first are normal; then lateral subluxation *without* acetabular dysplasia occurs, and finally there is dislocation (Fig. 7–25). Acetabular dysplasia occurs later as a response to the lack of contact of the femoral head in the acetabulum (Fig. 7–26). The mean age at the time of dislocation is 7 years (Samilson, 1972).

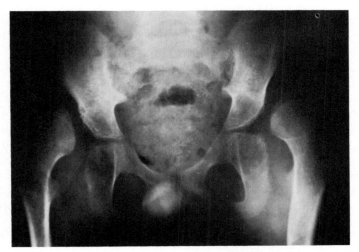

Figure 7–26   Anteroposterior radiograph of hips of an 8-year-old spastic quadriplegic. Note marked acetabular dysplasia resulting from the dislocation. Also illustrates failure to prevent dislocation with adductor myotomy and anterior branch obturator neurectomy performed four years previously.

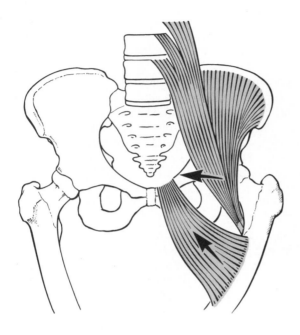

Figure 7–27   Spastic iliopsoas and adductor muscles are the initiating deforming force in hip dislocation.

The abnormal pull of spastic hip muscles is the initiating cause. The two muscles responsible are the iliopsoas and the adductors (Fig. 7–27), especially the iliopsoas. Adductory myotomy and obturator neurectomy alone have not prevented dislocation (Fig. 7–26) or subluxation (Fig. 7–28). In 75 dislocated hips, 69 failed to improve with adductor myotomy (Samilson, 1972).

Excessive femoral anteversion has been found consistently in subluxated and dislocated hips. Misleading radiographic diagnoses of coxa valga on anteroposterior projections have caused surgeons to believe that simple adduction contracture and increased femoral neck angles of inclination were the only mechanisms involved.

When overactivity and contracture of the iliopsoas occurs, its tendon first compresses the medial joint capsule and pushes the femoral head lateral (Fig. 7–29). This mechanism in congenital dislocation of the hip was established by Ferguson (1975). Excessive femoral anteversion in the non-ambulatory patient is an added deforming mechanism of dislocation. When such a patient sits or lies down, the hip flexes and rotates externally without bearing weight. The head and neck of the femur point forward. As lateral drift of the femoral head occurs, the iliopsoas insertion on the lesser trochanter becomes the center of rotation (Sharrard, 1975) (Fig. 7–30). Acetabular development ceases, and when the femoral head is completely displaced laterally, further hip flexion pushes the head posteriorly to complete the dislocation. Eventually, the femoral head comes to rest on the lateral superior and posterior aspect of the ilium.

Prevention.   O'Brien and Sirkin (1977) reported that in their patients with dislocated hips, pain, poor perineal care, and loss of "functional status" were not major problems, but in my experience and that of others (Hoffer et al., 1972; Sharrard, 1975; Root, 1977a; Cristofaro, 1977), these problems are of major importance in the adolescent and adult patient.

Prevention of hip dislocation by early surgical treatment appears to be a good policy based upon the experience of orthopaedic surgeons.

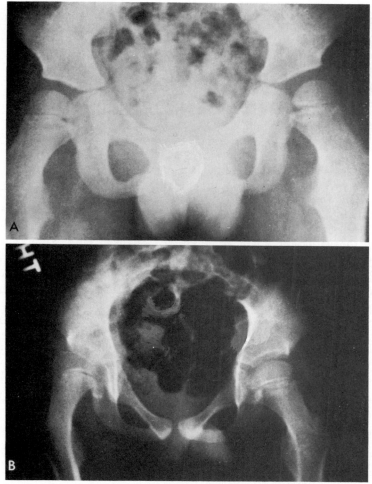

Figure 7–28 Anteroposterior radiographs of hips of patient P.C., a 4-year-old spastic quadriplegic. A. Hips are located with slight lateral subluxation of left hip. Adductor myotomy and anterior branch obturator neurectomy, bilateral, were performed. B. Four years postoperatively, subluxation of the right hip has occurred.

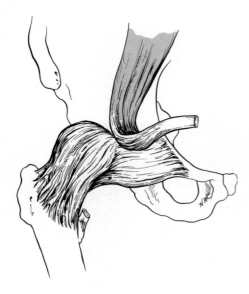

Figure 7–29 The spastic and contracted iliopso-
as compresses the joint capsule medial to the femoral
head and initiates lateral displacement of the hip.
(Redrawn from Ferguson, A. B. (1975) *Orthopaedic
Surgery in Infancy and Childhood,* 4th Ed., Baltimore,
Williams and Wilkins Company.)

Orthotics of any kind have failed to prevent subluxation or dislocation.

Physical therapeutic methods have not demonstrated efficacy in prevention no
matter how long or how continuously they are applied.

Surgery that is limited solely to adductor ''release'' with or without obturator
neurectomy has not proved to be uniformly successful when patients are followed
long enough postoperatively (Figs. 7–31 and 7–32). Iliopsoas tenotomy appears to be
the essential preventive surgery. Adductor myotomy with anterior branch obturator
neurectomy is also necessary if there is an adduction contracture.

Iliopsoas tenotomy has resulted in reduction of subluxated hips and has prevented dislocation when it is performed before the age of 7 or 8 years. After this age,
skeletal reconstruction is also required (see details in Chapter 6) (Figs. 7–33 through

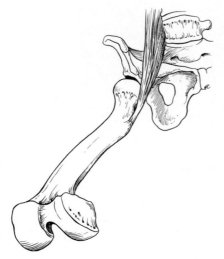

Figure 7–30 With excessive femoral anteversion
(non–weight-bearing) and spasticity and contracture of the
iliopsoas, the hip externally rotates during flexion with the
patient seated or lying down. The femoral head slips out
laterally and finally rests posteriorly. Acetabular dysplasia
results.

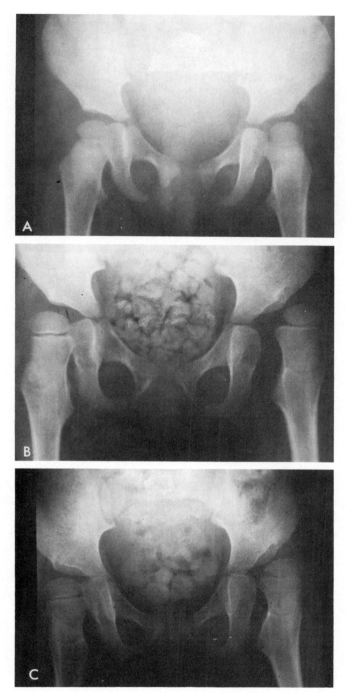

Figure 7–31 Anteroposterior radiographs of hips of patient J.L., a spastic quadriplegic with bilateral hip flexion and adduction contractures. A. Hips are located. B. Subluxation of left hip is more severe than on right. Only bilateral adductor myotomy and anterior branch obturator neurectomy were performed. C. Two years postoperatively, neither hip has reduced. (Courtesy of A. Holstein, M.D., Berkeley, California.)

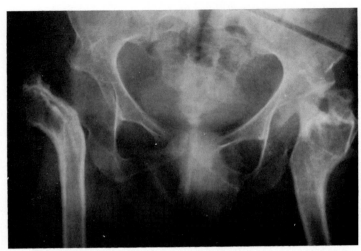

Figure 7–32   Anteroposterior radiograph of hips of a 17-year-old spastic quadriplegic, capable of wheelchair transfers. Patient had bilateral adductor myotomy and anterior branch obturator neurectomy for subluxation of both hips. Then, because reduction failed to occur, bilateral varus derotation femoral osteotomy was performed (iliopsoas tenotomy was not done). Finally, because painful subluxation of the hips was present, patient had bilateral head and neck resections combined with angulation subtrochanteric osteotomies.

7–35). Sharrard (1975) documented similar good results with iliopsoas elongation and adductor myotomy with anterior branch obturator neurectomy in 101 of 134 hips.

Acetabular reconstruction alone by iliac osteotomy or shelf procedures has not been consistently successful. Acetabular shelf procedures in particular are outdated, and, even if successful in preventing further subluxation, they result in limited motion due to arthrofibrosis of the joint and capsular ossification (Fig. 7–36).

OPERATIVE TECHNIQUE OF ILIOPSOAS TENOTOMY.   The concept of iliopsoas tenotomy in the surgical treatment of spastic paraplegia was introduced by Peterson (1950). The medial thigh incision and exposure of the proximal third of the femur was devised by Ludloff (Edmunson, 1963) and brought to my attention by Young (1954). Bleck and Holstein (1963) reported the same approach for iliopsoas tenotomy in cerebral palsy. Keats and Morgese (1967) clearly described the operation.

One major error of iliopsoas tenotomy and adductor myotomy is the failure to perform the procedure on both hips when both have spasticity and contracture even though only one has subluxation. In unilateral procedures, the opposite untreated hip is prone to dislocate postoperatively (Samilson, 1970).

Beginning 1 to 1.5 cm distal to the origin of the adductor longus, an incision is made directly over the adductor longus and extended distally for 5 cm. If necessary, adductor myotomy and anterior branch obturator neurectomy are then performed. By blunt dissection, one can retract the fibers of the adductor brevis and palpate the lesser trochanter of the femur with the hip in flexion and external rotation. A blunt retractor is placed medially and posterior to the iliopsoas tendon where it inserts on the lesser trochanter, and another retractor uncovers the fibers of the pectineus from the lesser trochanter.

Over the iliopsoas tendon there is a veil of fat that can be swept off the tendon with a peanut or stick sponge. A blunt retractor such as a Chandler or Cobra

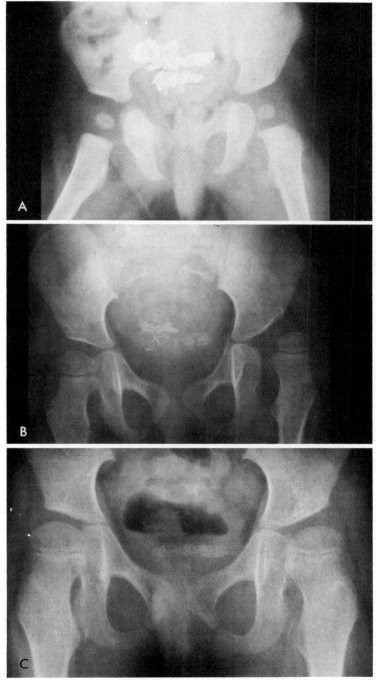

Figure 7–33 Anteroposterior radiographs of the hips of patient H.C.K., a 5-month-old spastic quadriplegic. A. Hips are in normal position. B. Age 3 years. Subluxation of left hip is present. C. Three and a half years after bilateral iliopsoas tenotomy, adductor myotomy with anterior branch obturator neurectomy. Although markedly improved and hips are reasonably located, patient remains non-ambulatory. (Courtesy of A. Holstein, M.D., Berkeley, California.)

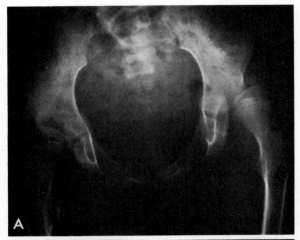

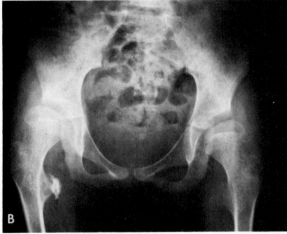

Figure 7–34 Anteroposterior radiographs of hips of patient C.D., a 9-year-old, non-ambulatory, spastic quadriplegic. A. Impending dislocation of left hip. Because of her general condition, osteotomies were not performed and only bilateral iliopsoas tenotomy, and adductor longus and gracilis myotomy with anterior branch obturator neurectomy were done. B. Age 11 years, two years after muscle surgery. Hips are not perfectly located but sufficiently so that bone surgery could be deferred.

retractor is placed on the lateral side of the iliopsoas tendon, which is sectioned with the scalpel or scissors (Figs. 7–37 through 7–39). Closed suction drainage of the wound is instituted. Wound closure is performed in the usual way, using subcutaneous and subcuticular synthetic absorbable sutures reinforced with sterile adhesive closures.

Postoperative care. Plaster immobilization after iliopsoas tenotomy in the very young child with an early subluxation of the hip is not routinely used. If there is hamstring spasm or if the hamstrings have been lengthened, plaster immobilization in long leg plasters is necessary, and a spreader bar is used to abduct each hip no more than 40 degrees and to hold the position for 3 weeks. Long-term night bracing has not been necessary. I allow these non-ambulatory patients to sit up as soon as the acute postoperative phase has passed. Special seats for the wheelchair can be constructed to hold the hips in moderate abduction (Figs. 7–14 and 7–15).

Surgical Treatment of Dislocation. There is a question whether dislocation of the hip should be treated at all. Often children aged 7 to 16 years have no pain with a dislocated hip. In later years, pain does become a problem often enough to merit

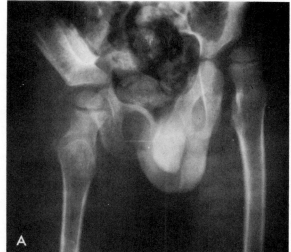

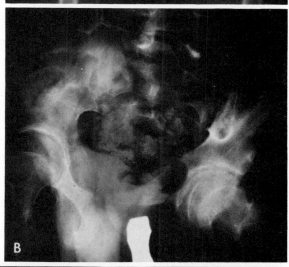

Figure 7–35 Anteroposterior radiographs of hips of patient D.K., a 4-year-old with total body involvement tension athetosis and spasticity. A. Impending dislocation of left hip. B. Age 16 years. Twelve years after bilateral ilipsoas tenotomy, adductor longus and gracilis myotomy with anterior branch obturator neurectomy. He is wheelchair dependent. Hips have remained located.

Figure 7–36 Anteroposterior radiograph of hip of crutch-walking spastic quadriplegic, ten years after bilateral acetabular shelf procedures for subluxation. The subluxation has not progressed, but motion is limited, the joint space is narrow, and there is partial ossification of the lateral joint capsule.

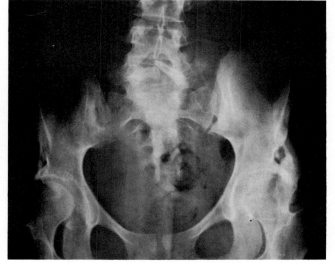

237

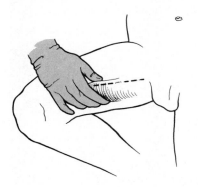

Figure 7–37 Medial thigh incision over adductor longus muscle for medial approach to iliopsoas tendon. (Redrawn from Keats, S., and Morgese, A. N. (1967) A simple anteromedial approach to the lesser trochanter of the femur for the release of the iliopsoas tendon. *Journal of Bone and Joint Surgery* 49A:632–636.)

Figure 7–38 Adductor longus and brevis (if not cut) retracted medially and pectineus laterally. Lesser trochanter and iliopsoas tendon are exposed. Hip is flexed, abducted, and externally rotated. (From Keats, S., and Morgese, A. N. (1967) A simple anteromedial approach to the lesser trochanter of the femur for the release of the iliopsoas tendon. *Journal of Bone and Joint Surgery* 49A:632–636.)

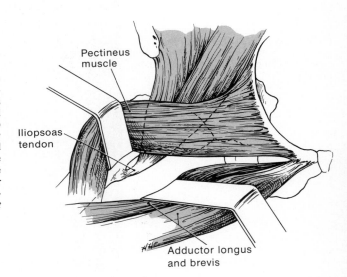

Pectineus
muscle

Iliopsoas
tendon

Adductor longus
and brevis

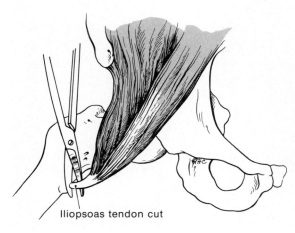

Iliopsoas tendon cut

Figure 7–39 A retractor (cobra or Chandler type) is placed posterior to the lesser trochanter and the iliopsoas tendon cut. (Redrawn from Keats, S., and Morgese, A. N. (1967) A simple anteromedial approach to the lesser trochanter of the femur for the release of the iliopsoas tendon. *Journal of Bone and Joint Surgery* 49A: 632–636.)

surgical relocation while the child is still growing. In the study by Hoffer et al. (1972), 7 of 15 unilateral dislocations were painful (47 percent). Root (1977a,b) has reported the results of hip arthrodesis and total hip replacements for pain relief in adults with cerebral palsy who had dislocated or subluxated hips. Others (Cristofaro et al., 1977) have used total hip replacement in an attempt to relieve pain in wheelchair-dependent patients. I have relocated painful dislocated hips in patients 14 to 18 years of age.

Although O'Brien and Sirkin (1977) reported that pain was not a major problem in the dislocated hips of their non-ambulatory patients, there is considerable evidence that the late onset of pain is a major problem. Because of the complexity and morbidity of adult reconstructive procedures (e.g., total hip replacement or arthrodesis), it is probably not a wise policy to "wait and see" if pain develops in children before performing surgical relocation. The problem with delay is that degeneration of the articular surfaces of the cartilage occurs when the cartilage out of contact with opposing articular cartilage. Once the degeneration of cartilage is advanced, the placement of the femoral head in the acetabulum is likely to result in a painful relocated hip.

Nor are "simple" solutions such as femoral head and neck resections satisfactory for pain relief (Fig. 7–40). Cristofaro et al. (1977) reported 100 percent failure to relieve pain by modified Girdlestone procedures. Root (1977a) also had had poor results.

Relocation of the dislocated hip in the child and adolescent is indicated (1) to prevent a painful hip in adult life that may compromise the patient's limited mobility; (2) to prevent and correct severe pelvic obliquity that interferes with sitting balance; (3) to prevent and correct severe adduction of the femur that makes perineal hygiene difficult; (4) to prevent painful bursal formation over the greater trochanter on the dislocated side and over the ischial tuberosity when pelvic obliquity becomes fixed.

OPERATIVE PLAN OF ONE-STAGE RELOCATION. I have had most success in children and adolescents whose femoral head articular cartilage is in reasonably good condition with techniques performed at *one stage* as follows:

1. Adductor longus, gracilis, and adductor brevis myotomy, anterior branch obturator neurectomy, and iliopsoas tenotomy.
2. Capsulotomy (to inspect the femoral head).
3. Femoral shortening with varus and derotation subtrochanteric femoral osteotomy and internal fixation (90-degree hip osteotomy compression nail plate).
4. Salter innominate osteotomy in patients under age 10 years.
5. Chiari (1974) iliac osteotomy in patients over 10 years (presumably Sutherland's [1977] modified iliac osteotomy or Steel's [1977] triple innominate osteotomy could be used).
6. Capsulorrhaphy.

Femoral shortening has been successfully used for reduction of congenital dislocation of the hip (Klisić and Jankovic, 1976). Larson (1971) introduced this method to us. The concept and technique of Sutherland's (1977) modification of the iliac osteotomy (Salter, 1961) is described in Chapter 6.

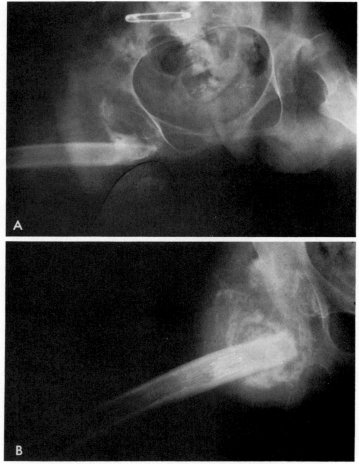

Figure 7–40 Anteroposterior radiographs of hips of patient with total body involvement at ages 22 (A) and 32 (B). After femoral head and neck resection for painful dislocated hip, hip was still painful and became hyperabducted with limited motion owing to heterotopic ossification. (Courtesy of Jacob Sharp, M.D., Porterville State Hospital, California.) Castle and Schneider (1978) appear to have a solution: proximal femoral resection interposition arthroplasty. (See *Journal of Bone and Joint Surgery* 60A: 1051–1054.)

OPERATIVE TECHNIQUE

1. Through a separate groin incision paralleling the adductor longus muscle an adductor myotomy and anterior branch obturator neurectomy are performed, and the iliopsoas tendon is divided as described in the preceding section on iliopsoas tenotomy.

The second incision is an anterior iliofemoral approach that starts at the mid-crest of the ilium and continues distally along the crest over the anterior superior iliac spine and then is curved gently laterally to the tip of the greater trochanter, where it is then again curved distally along the lateral aspect of the shaft of the femur. The sartorius and the rectus femoris are detached to expose the anterior capsule of the hip. The capsule is then incised along the labrum of the acetabulum and then parallel to the neck of the femur of the dislocated hip. The femoral head is then inspected; if the cartilage is in reasonably normal condition, reduction of the dislocation proceeds. The inner face of the ilium is exposed by subperiosteal stripping of the iliacus muscle and laterally by stripping the gluteus medius and minimus from the wing of the ilium and from the capsule of the dislocated hip.

2. The ligamentum teres is removed. The subtrochanteric region of the femur is stripped of the origin of the vastus lateralis muscle, and the shaft is exposed subperiosteally. Next, utilizing radiographic controls (we prefer the image intensifier), guide pins for the ASIF 90-degree hip compression nail are inserted through the greater trochanter and across the head and neck of the femur at an angle of 65 to 75 degrees to the shaft in order to provide a 35- to 25-degree varus osteotomy (Fig. 6–38 A and B). The channel is cut with the specially constructed ASIF chisel to match the blade portion of the nail, and the blade of the nail is then inserted in this track as far as it will go. The femoral shaft is then cut obliquely with a power saw at an angle of 70 degrees to the shaft of the femur and parallel to the nail inserted at the base of the greater trochanter. A second cut is made 1½ cm distal to the first cut in the femur, perpendicular to the femoral shaft. The segment of bone is removed, and the ASIF nail is driven all the way into the neck of the femur. With the nail holder attached, the hip can now be reduced easily into the acetabulum and then internally rotated to correct the femoral anteversion. The distal femur is then brought up so that the osteotomy sites are coapted, and it is rotated externally to leave approximately 30 degrees of internal rotation remaining when the osteotomy has been fixed. When this position has been attained, the Lowman or Richards bone-holding clamps fix the plate to the femoral shaft, and the compression device is applied so that the osteotomy site is compressed. The plate is fixed to the femoral shaft with the screws. The capsule can then be imbricated to take up any redundancy.

3. To perform the iliac osteotomy (Chiari), a guide pin is placed just at the edge of the capsular attachment on the ilium and angled 10 degrees cephalad with radiographic control. When the correct site of osteotomy has been ascertained, the ilium is cut along the line of the guide pin with either an osteotome or a reciprocating saw. The distal portion of the osteotomy, which consists of the iliac portion of the acetabulum, the ischium, and the pubis, is shifted medially to create a shelf of ilium that rests on the capsule of the hip joint. A 50 percent displacement is advisable. Abduction and internal rotation of the hip assist the medial displacement. The osteotomy of the ilium is fixed with two threaded Steinmann pins introduced through the crest of the ilium and continued across the osteotomy site but outside of the acetabulum. Again, radiographic control is invaluable (Fig. 7–41). The redundant capsule is excised and the remaining capsule snugly imbricated.

POSTOPERATIVE CARE. Immobilization in a plaster hip spica is required for 6 weeks. After 6 weeks mobilization of the hip and knee is begun, and a bed-chair regimen is possible. At 8 weeks, the healing of the femoral osteotomy is sufficiently advanced to permit weight-bearing in wheelchair transfers.

RESULTS. Our results appear to be satisfactory enough to merit this extensive procedure. We have follow-up data only for up to 5 years in a small number of cases. Only one hip out of 10 has shown recurrence of lateral subluxation. Hoffer (1972) reported good results of muscle "release" and varus derotation femoral osteotomy in 17 of 20 patients who before surgery could not sit longer than 1 hour, whereas after surgery sitting was possible for over 6 hours. In Samilson's (1972) experience of 48 hips on which subtrochanteric varus derotation osteotomy was performed, dislocation recurred in 12.

Even if degenerative arthritis of the relocated hip occurs and causes pain in later life, total hip replacement or arthrodesis can be done more easily and probably has

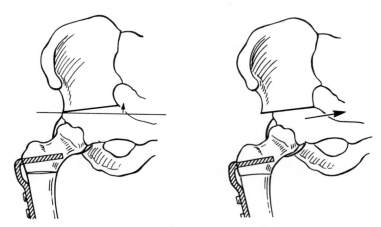

Figure 7–41 Operative technique for Chiari iliac osteotomy. Note that osteotomy begins laterally just at the attachment of the hip joint capsule and is directed 10 degrees cephalad from the horizontal plane. The dislocated hip is then reduced by femoral shortening and varus derotation osteotomy. Fixation is with the 90 degree compression nail-plate.

better results. Both procedures are more difficult in the dislocated hip (Figs. 7–42 and 7–43).

PITFALLS AND COMPLICATIONS

1.   Redislocation of the hip appears to be related to an insufficient varus angle of the femoral neck (Samilson, 1972). Probably a femoral neck angle of 100 to 115 degrees is best. Samilson did report the occurrence of fatigue fractures of the femoral neck after osteotomy; this late complication is probably related to an exaggerated varus inclination of the osteotomy.

My patient who had a lateral subluxation of the hip postoperatively did not have the capsulotomy, excision of the ligamentum teres, or capsulorrhaphy.

2.   Obvious degeneration of the femoral head articular cartilage is a contraindication for relocation. If this is discovered, hip arthrodesis to accommodate the sitting position may be a satisfactory solution.

3.   Aseptic necrosis of the femoral head is a possible complication of surgery. We have not seen it, but Samilson (1972) reported it in 6 of 48 hips. Preservation of the femoral head blood supply by avoidance of dissection of the posterior, lateral, and medial aspects of the femoral neck should minimize this complication.

4.   The main risk in the technique of the Chiari iliac osteotomy is placing the osteotomy too high to be effective or too low, so that the acetabulum is cut. This can be avoided by locating the intended site of the osteotomy with a guide pin under radiographic control during the procedure.

HIP ARTHRODESIS AND TOTAL HIP REPLACEMENT

Both arthrodesis and total hip replacement have been performed to relieve pain in adult total body involved patients who have dislocated or subluxated hips (Root, 1977a,b).

Arthrodesis is probably the best procedure in the non-ambulatory patient who cannot sit or rest because of hip pain. Root (1977a) had good results with an intra-articular fusion, an iliac crest muscle pedicle graft (Davis, 1954), and inter-

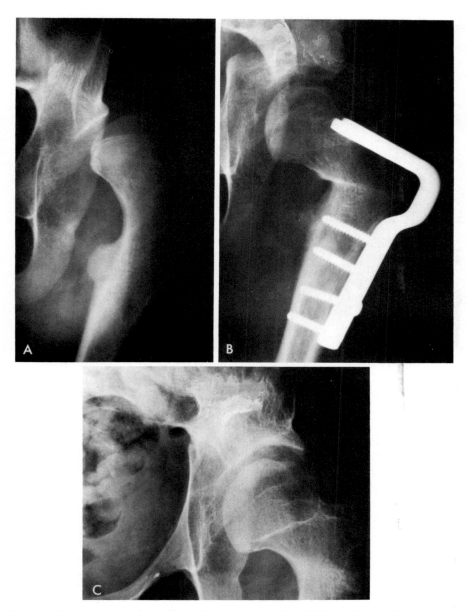

Figure 7–42 Anteroposterior radiographs of hip of patient F.C., a 16-year-old, crutch-walking spastic quadriplegic. A. Painful subluxated hip. B. Immediately after reduction with iliopsoas tenotomy, adductor longus myotomy, anterior branch obturator neurectomy, femoral shortening (1.5 cm), varus and derotation subtrochanteric osteotomy, and Chiari iliac osteotomy (operating time 4.5 hours). C. Three years postoperatively, hip was painless and stable.

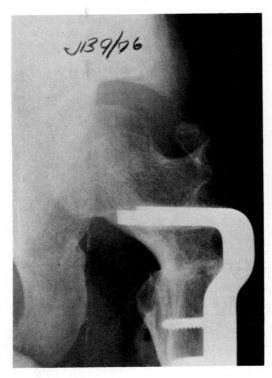

Figure 7–43 Anteroposterior radiograph of hip of patient J.B., a spastic quadriplegic capable of independent wheelchair transfers. At age 15 years, had a painful dislocated hip. Iliopsoas tenotomy, adductor longus myotomy, anterior branch obturator neurectomy, femoral shortening with derotation subtrochanteric osteotomy, and Chiari iliac osteotomy were performed. Note that little, if any, varus inclination was necessary in the osteotomy. Two years postoperatively, hip was painless and functional status was maintained.

trochanteric fixation. The hip should be fused in a comfortable sitting position with 45 to 50 degrees flexion, 15 to 20 degrees abduction, and neutral rotation.

Because the iliac crest muscle pedicle graft is so successful in obtaining rapid arthrodesis, the *femoral head should always be inspected* before stripping the ilium of its muscle attachments in preparation for an iliac osteotomy.

Total hip replacement is probably best reserved for ambulatory patients who have hip pain due to a subluxation. Root (1977*b*) used this procedure successfully in seven patients, five of whom were ambulatory. Cristofaro et al. (1977) did total hip replacements in four total body involved patients who were able to sit but had intractable hip pain. Their range of hip motion did not improve but sitting tolerance increased from zero to 10 hours per day. At follow-up (mean time followed, 16 months), hip pain was still present but did not prevent sitting.

In these procedures, presumably the deforming spastic muscles (abductor and iliopsoas) are released.

Knee

Knee deformities in totally involved patients consist mainly of knee flexion, which need be corrected only if such flexion deformities interfere with assistive transfers from the wheelchair or if positioning in bed becomes uncomfortable. It has not been determined how far a knee flexion deformity should be allowed to progress in a patient who is capable of sitting and cannot even do assistive transfers. The high incidence of postoperative supracondylar femoral fractures on the non-operated limb in those who had surgery to relocate the hip (Samilson, 1972) may have been due not only to osteoporosis but also to the knee flexion deformity.

Without doubt the knee flexion deformity should not be permitted to progress to more than to 15 to 20 degrees in patients who have wheelchair transfer ability, either assistive or independent.

Too much hamstring spasticity should not be relieved because quadriceps spasticity usually coexists in such patients, and it is possible to convert a comfortable wheelchair-sitting patient with his knees flexed to one whose knees are almost completely extended and are unable to flex because of the unopposed quadriceps spasticity that becomes evident postoperatively.

Before the knee flexion deformity becomes a knee flexion contracture, the hamstring tendons can be lengthened selectively. It does not seem to make much difference whether or not the semitendinosus is tenotomized, lengthened, or transferred.

If the knee flexion deformity becomes fixed due to joint capsular contracture, hamstring weakening surgery alone will not correct the deformity, and capsulotomy of the knee joint may be necessary. In these cases, sudden extension of the knee should be avoided, since postoperative sciatic stretch paralysis occurs frequently.

In the adult, correction of the knee flexion deformity by soft tissue surgery alone is a very difficult surgical problem because of the coexistent shortening of the neurovascular bundle. In such cases, which are rare indeed, supracondylar closed wedge osteotomy combined with hamstring lengthening may be the only safe solution.

Foot and Ankle

Foot and ankle deformities in the totally involved patient need correction only if they interfere with sitting posture or the mobility of the patient who is incapable of assistive transfers due to severe deformity.

The equinus deformity can interfere with either sitting or standing for transfers and should be corrected. It interferes with sitting because the foot cannot be rested firmly on the footrest of the wheelchair and the toe is apt to drag on the ground. Achilles, tendon lengthening by the Hoke or White method and a posterior capsulotomy of the ankle (if the contracture has progressed far enough to warrant it) are relatively simple solutions. Even in the total body involved patient who does not ambulate, overlengthening should be avoided because a spastic ankle dorsiflexor muscle can result in a disabling calcaneus deformity with all of the weight being borne on the heel.

Severe valgus or varus deformities can be corrected by triple arthrodesis and selective tendon lengthening. In a varus deformity, it is usual to lengthen the posterior tibial tendon above the medial malleolus, and in valgus deformity the peroneus brevis tendon is lengthened. Complicated tendon transfers are usually not required.

If overzealous Achilles tendon lengthening results in the unanticipated emergence of a spastic anterior tibial muscle leading to a calcaneus deformity, a satisfactory solution has been to transfer the anterior tibial tendon through the interosseous membrane to the os calcis posteriorly. In patients over the age of 12 years, this can be combined with a triple arthrodesis for maximum stability of the foot and security of correction.

REFERENCES

Bachman, W. H. (1972) Variables affecting post-school economic adaptation of orthopaedically handicapped and other health impaired students. *Rehabilitation Literature* 3:98–114.

Baker, L. D., Dodelin, N. D., and Bassett, F. H. (1962) Pathological changes in the hip in cerebral palsy: incidence, pathogenesis, and treatment. *Journal of Bone and Joint Surgery* 44A:1131–1342.

Balmer, G. A., and MacEwen, G. D. (1970) The incidence of scoliosis in cerebral palsy. *Journal of Bone and Joint Surgery* 52B:134–136.

Bleck, E. E. (1975) Deformities of the spine and pelvis in cerebral palsy. *Orthopaedic Aspects of Cerebral Palsy* (Ed. Samilson, R. L.), Philadelphia, J. B. Lippincott Co.

Bleck, E. E., and Holstein, A. (1963) Iliopsoas tenotomy for spastic hip flexion deformities in cerebral palsy. Paper presented at the annual meeting of the American Academy of Orthopaedic Surgeons, Chicago.

Bliss, C. K. (1965) *Semantography – Bliss Symbolics,* Sydney, Australia, Semantography Publications.

Bonnett, C. A. (1972) Anterior spinal fusion with Dwyer instrumentation for lumbar scoliosis in cerebral palsy. Paper presented at the annual meeting of the Western Orthopaedic Association, Houston.

Bonnett, C. A., Brown, J. C., and Sakai, D. N. (1976) Thoracolumbar scoliosis in cerebral palsy; results of surgical treatment. Paper presented at the annual meeting of the American Academy for Cerebral Palsy and Developmental Medicine, Los Angeles.

Bourgeois, O., Chaigne, M. O., Cherpin, J., Minaire, P., and Weber, D. (1977) Diminués physiques et transports collectifs. Institut de Récherche des Transports, Centre d'Evaluation et de Récherche des Nuisances, Bron, France.

Bunnell, W. P., and MacEwen, G. D. (1977) Non-operative treatment of scoliosis in cerebral palsy: preliminary report on the use of a plastic jacket. *Developmental Medicine and Child Neurology* 19:45–49.

Chiari, K. (1974) Medial displacement osteotomy of the pelvis. *Clinical Orthopedics and Related Research* 98:55–71.

Cotton, E. (1977) A bedroom routine for cerebral palsied children. Paper presented at the Study Group on Integrating the Care of Multiply Handicapped Children, St. Mary's College, Durham, England. London, The Spastics Society Medical Education and Information Unit.

Cristofaro, R., Koffman, M., Woodward, R., and Baxter, S. (1977) Treatment of the totally involved cerebral palsy problem sitter. Paper presented at the annual meeting of the American Academy for Cerebral Palsy and Developmental Medicine, Atlanta.

Davis, J. B. (1954) The muscle-pedicle bone graft in hip fusion. *Journal of Bone and Joint Surgery* 33A:513–616.

Edmundson, A. S. (1963) *Campbell's Operative Orthopaedics,* St. Louis, C.V. Mosby Co.

Ferguson, A. B. (1975) *Orthopaedic Surgery in Infancy and Childhood,* Baltimore, The Williams & Wilkins Co.

Grove, N. (1972) Personal communication.

Hagen, C., Porter, W., and Brink, J. D. (1973) Non-verbal communication: an alternative mode of communication for the child with severe cerebral palsy. *Journal of Speech and Hearing Disorders* 38:448–445.

Hoffer, M. M., Abraham, E., and Nickel, V. (1972) Salvage surgery at the hip to improve sitting posture of mentally retarded, severely disabled children with cerebral palsy. *Developmental Medicine and Child Neurology* 14:51–55.

Horning, M. R. (1977) A post-surgical hip deformity in cerebral palsy. Paper presented at the annual meeting of the American Academy for Cerebral Palsy and Developmental Medicine, Atlanta.

James, W. V. (1977) Spinal bracing for children with atonic cerebral palsy. *Prosthetics and Orthotics International* 1:105–106.

Keats, S., and Morgese, A. N. (1967) A simple anteromedial approach to the lesser trochanter of the femur for the release of the iliopsoas tendon. *Journal of Bone and Joint Surgery* 49A:632–636.

Klisić, P., and Jankovic, L. (1976) Combined procedure of open reduction and shortening of the femur in treatment of congenital dislocation of the hips in older children. *Clinical Orthopedics and Related Research* 119:60–69.

Larson, L. (1971) Lecture at Orthopaedic Grand Rounds, Stanford University School of Medicine, Palo Alto.

LeBlanc, M. (1977) Proposal for research and development of versatile, portable speech prosthesis. Department of Rehabilitation Engineering. Children's Hospital at Stanford, Palo Alto.

Letts, R. M., Fulford, R., and Hobson, D. A. (1976) Mobility aids for the paraplegic child. *Journal of Bone and Joint Surgery* 58A:38–41.

MacEwen, G. D. (1968) The incidence and treatment of scoliosis in cerebral palsy. Paper presented at the annual meeting of the American Academy for Cerebral Palsy, Miami Beach.

McNaughton, S. (1975) Visual symbols: a system of communication for the nonverbal physically handicapped child. Regional Course, American Academy for Cerebral Palsy, Palo Alto.

Motloch, W. M. (1973) Crutchless standing. *Canadian Orthotics-Prosthetics* 7:7.

Motloch, W. M. (1975) Personal communication.

Motloch, W. M. (1977) Seating and positioning for the physically impaired. *Orthotics and Prosthetics* 31:11–21.

O'Brien, J. J., and Sirkin, R. B. (1977) The natural history of the dislocated hip in cerebral palsy. Paper presented at the annual meeting of the American Academy for Cerebral Palsy and Developmental Medicine, Atlanta.

Peterson, L. T. (1950) Tenotomy in the treatment of spastic paraplegia with special reference to the iliopsoas. *Journal of Bone and Joint Surgery* 32A:875–885.

Robson, P. (1968) The prevalence of scoliosis in adolescents and young adults with cerebral palsy. *Developmental Medicine and Child Neurology* 10:447–452.

Root, L. (1977a) The totally involved cerebral palsy patient. Instructional Course Lectures, annual meeting of the American Academy of Orthopaedic Surgeons, Las Vegas.

Root, L. (1977b) Total hip replacement in cerebral palsy. Paper presented at the annual meeting of the American Academy for Cerebral Palsy and Dvelopmental Medicine, Atlanta.

Rosenthal, D. K., Levine, D. D., and McCarver, C. L. (1974) The occurrence of scolisois in cerebral palsy. *Developmental Medicine and Child Neurology* 16:664–667.

Russell, G., Sharp, E., and Iles, G. (1976) Clinical biofeedback applications in pediatric rehabilitation. *Inter-Clinics Information Bulletin* 15:1–6.

Salter, R. B. (1961) Innominate osteotomy in the treatment of congenital dislocation and subluxation of the legs. *Journal of Bone and Joint Surgery* 43B:518–539.

Samilson, R. L. (1970) Personal communication.

Samilson, R. L. (1972) Dislocation and subluxation of the hip in cerebral palsy. *Journal of Bone and Joint Surgery* 54A:863–873.

Samilson, R. L., and Bechard, R. (1973) Scoliosis in cerebral palsy. *Current Practice in Orthopaedic Surgery* (Ed. Adams, J. P.), St. Louis, C.V. Mosby Co.

Sharrard, W. J. W. (1975) The hip in cerebral palsy. *Orthopaedic Aspects of Cerebral Palsy* (Ed. Samilson, R. L.), Philadelphia, J.B. Lippincott Co.

Stagnara, P. (1971) Traction cranienne par le "halo" de Rancho Los Amigos. *Revue de Chirurgie Orthopaedique et Reparative de l'Appareil Moteur* (Paris) 57:287–300.

Sutherland, D. H., Miller, K. E., Cooper, L., and Matthews, J. V. (1977) Surgical treatment of hip subluxation and dislocation in the older child with spastic cerebral palsy. Scientific Exhibit at annual meeting of the American Academy of Orthopaedic Surgeons, Las Vegas.

United States, Bureau of Educational Handicaps, Department of Health, Education, and Welfare (1977) Estimated population of non-verbal individuals in the United States. Confence on Communication Aids for the Non-vocal Severely Physically Handicapped Person, Alexandria, Va.

Young, C. (1954) Personal communication.

Appendix A

MEASUREMENT OF PEDOGRAPH*

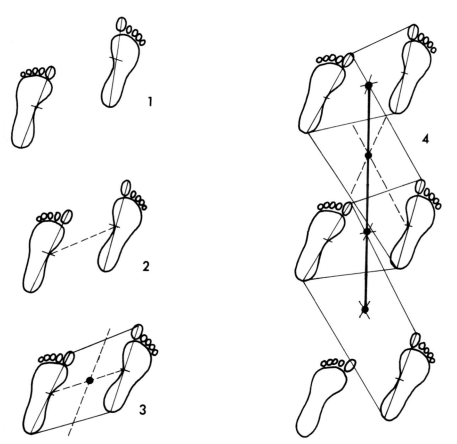

Figure 1 How to find the centroid in order to plot the changing line of progression of the gait.
1. Mark the footprint from the tip of the great toe to the posterior border of the heel and measure 1/2 the distance.
2. Connect the midfoot to the midfoot mark.
3. Mark toe to toe on opposite foot and heel to opposite heel; measure 1/2 this distance.
4. Connect centroids to find the line of progression.

---

*Adapted by Ford, F. from Chodera and Levell (1973).

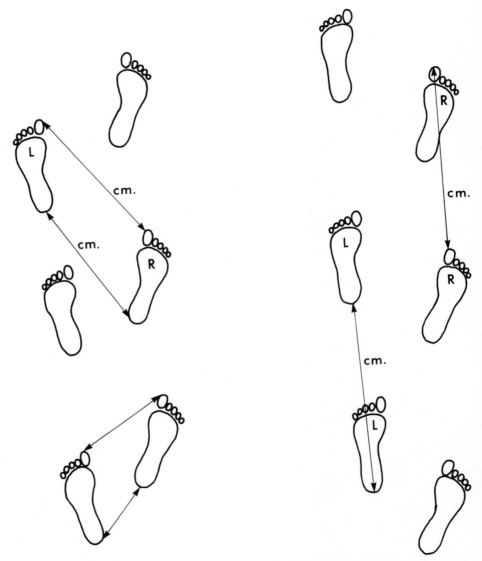

Figure 2 Step length is the distance between two successive footprints: either right to left (left step) or left to right (right step). Stride length is the distance between two successive footprints of the same foot: right to right, left to left.

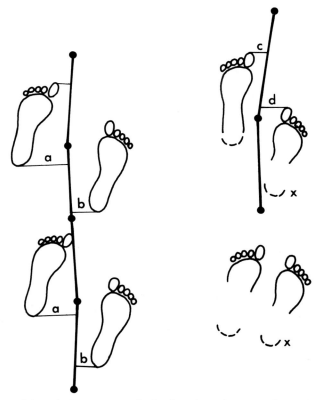

Figure 3 Base of the gait. Draw perpendicular lines from the center line to the tip of great toe and to posterior border of heel. Base of gait is the sum of $a+b$. If toe walker base of gait is the sum of $c+d$. To find heel on print of toe walker, measure actual length of foot from toe to heel of patient, transpose this measurement to footprint, and mark posterior border of heel (x).

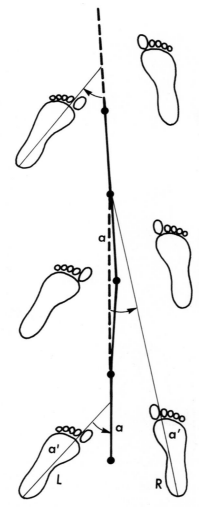

Figure 4 Angle of foot placement from line of progression. Angle of foot placement is measured by constructing line between the first and second metatarsals and through the posterior heel center, and extending this line to the line of progression for that foot. In this drawing left foot (L) *a'* should intersect with its line of progression, *a*; right foot (R) *a'* must intersect with projection of its line of progression *a* which has been extended with broken line in order to construct the angle of toe-in for the right foot.

Appendix B

REHABILITATION DEVICES

SPEECH OUTPUT — Communication

1. Speech Plus Talking Calculator
   James Bliss, Ph.D. (EE), President
   Telesensory Systems, Inc.
   1889 Page Mill Road
   Palo Alto, California 94304

2. Master Specialties Talking Calculator
   and Master Specialties Voice Read-Out
   System
   Master Specialties Company
   1640 Monrovia Avenue
   Costa Mesa, California 92627

3. Phonic Mirror/Handivoice
   H. C. Electronics
   Rick Pimentel
   250 Camino Alto
   Mill Valley, California 94941

4. Votrax Division
   Alfred Lubienski, General Manager
   Vocal Interface Division
   Federal Screw Works
   500 Stephenson Highway
   Troy, Michigan 48084

VISUAL OUTPUT — Communication

1. Bliss Symbolics Foundation
   Shirley McNaughton
   Bliss Symbol Foundation
   862 Eglinton Avenue E
   Toronto, Ontario
   Canada M4G 2L1

2. Matrix Communicator
   Armand F. DuFresne
   DUFCO
   901 Iva Court
   Cambria, California 93428

3. Zygo Communicator
   Laurence Weiss
   P.O. Box 1008
   Portland, Oregon 97207

4. Bliss Symbol Scanner
   Prentke-Romich Company
   R.D. 2, Box 191
   Shreve, Ohio 44676

PRINTED OUTPUT — Communication

1. Strip Printer
   Prentke-Romich Company
   R.D. 2, Box 191
   Shreve, Ohio 44676

2. Canon Communication Aid
   James Bliss, Ph.D. (EE)
   Telesensory Systems, Inc.
   1889 Page Mill Road
   Palo Alto, California 94304

3. IBM Selectric Typewriters
   Cathy Clemens
   IBM Corp.
   411 Borel Avenue, Suite 500
   San Mateo, California 94402

MOBILITY AIDS

1. ABEC Powered Wheelchair
   (United States)
   ABEC Electric Wheelchair, Inc.
   10889 Wilshire Blvd., Suite 2
   Los Angeles, California 90024

   (United Kingdom)
   Ray Biddel, Engineer
   103 Stourbridge Road
   Halesowen
   West Midland B63   3UB
   United Kingdom

2. MacLaren Buggy (now called Pogan Wagons)
   Genac, Inc.
   2220 Norwood Avenue
   Boulder, Colorado 80302

3. Stanford Slot Control
   Charles Chevillon, President
   Medical Equipment Distributors, Inc.
   1215 S. Harlem Avenue
   Forest Park, Illinois 60131

4. Stanford Weight-Relieving Walker
   Everest and Jennings Inc.
   1803 Pontius Avenue
   Los Angeles, California 90025

AID TO DAILY LIVING

1. Cerebral Palsy Feeders
   (United States)
   E. Alfred Burrill
   Orthopop
   P.O. Box 272
   Aptos, California 95003

   Canadian C.P. Feeders
   Physico-Medical Systems Corp.
   500 Buchanan St., Suite 505
   Montreal, Quebec
   Canada H4P 1T2

2. Environmental Control Systems
   Prentke-Romich Company
   R.D. 2, Box 191
   Shreve, Ohio 44676

3. Bath Chair Lift
   Abbey Rents, Inc.
   2841 S. El Camino Real
   San Mateo, California 94403

4. Standing "A" Frame
   Variety Village Electro Limb Center
   3701 Danforth Avenue
   Scarborough, Ontario
   Canada

Index